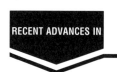

RECENT ADVANCES IN

Respiratory Medicine

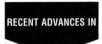

Respiratory Medicine

Edited by

David M. Mitchell MA MD FRCP

Consultant Physician, and Honorary Senior
Lecturer in Medicine, Respiratory Unit,
St Mary's Hospital,
London, UK

NUMBER FIVE

CHURCHILL LIVINGSTONE
EDINBURGH LONDON MELBOURNE NEW YORK AND TOKYO 1991

CHURCHILL LIVINGSTONE
Medical Division of Longman Group UK Limited

Distributed in the United States of America by Churchill
Livingstone Inc., 1560 Broadway, New York, N.Y. 10036,
and by associated companies, branches and representatives
throughout the world.

First published 1991

ISBN 0-443-04467-8
ISSN 0–308–6623

British Library Cataloguing in Publication Data
A catalogue record for this book is available from the British
Library

Library of Congress Cataloging in Publication Data is
available

Produced by Longman Singapore Publishers Pte Ltd
Printed in Singapore

Foreword

It is an honour for me to write the foreword for No. 5 of *Recent Advances in Respiratory Medicine*. It had been my great pleasure to contribute and co-edit the third and fourth issues in this series with my longterm friend, the late David C Flenley of Edinburgh. Together, we had produced reviews of the most important contemporary advances of relevance to the practising pulmonologist and primary care physician who was interested in diseases of the lungs and thorax. Progress in new understanding of mechanisms of disease and potential new therapeutic strategies, caused us to change the emphasis of each issue, but the unsolved problems of chronic obstructive pulmonary disease (COPD), lung cancer, adult respiratory distress syndrome (ARDS), and worldwide infections including tuberculosis were always featured.

I will always remember David Flenley for his huge contributions throughout the field of pulmonary medicine in general, but most particularly for his insight and understanding of the treatment of COPD. He was instrumental in helping me organize the First World Congress on Home Oxygen Therapy in Denver, Colorado, in 1986, and played a similar role in the First International Conference on Pulmonary Rehabilitation and Home Care also held in Denver in 1987. It was my privilege to be co-summarizer of both conferences, along with my friend, David.

The greatest single advance since *Recent Advances in Respiratory Medicine 4*, published in 1986, has been the growing success of lung and heart–lung transplantation for fibrotic lung disease states, emphysema, cystic fibrosis, and states of irreversible pulmonary hypertension. Thus these advances are appropriately featured in this new issue. Still greater advances await us in the important areas of smoking cessation, the prevention of AIDS pneumonias, and better approaches to the ever-challenging problem of worldwide tuberculosis. Thus, we can look forward to the dissemination of new knowledge in these areas in future volumes.

Now, I salute the present editor, David Mitchell, who kindly invited me to write this foreword as well as a chapter contained in this volume. He has organized an excellent compendium of timely chapters, all authored by experts in the field. Dr Mitchell has carried on the splendid tradition of excellence of David Flenley, who initiated this series.

Denver 1991   T. Petty MD

Preface

This volume aims to provide authoritative up to date reviews of the important areas in respiratory medicine both for the practising physician and for doctors in training. In the five years since the last issue of *Recent Advances in Respiratory Medicine*, there have been major clinical and scientific advances in many aspects of the subject. Although this expansion in knowledge has been partly paralleled by more journals and monographs, there is a need for a single volume of review chapters focusing on important contemporary developments in respiratory medicine, written by experts in the field. The editor is most grateful to all the authors who, despite their heavy clinical and research commitments, have found the time to write chapters on their areas of interest with great clarity and depth. The editor is also grateful to Yvonne O'Leary of Churchill Livingstone for her help and encouragement during the preparation of this book.

The following main topics are reviewed in this volume. The adult distress syndrome is still a difficult clinical problem despite improvements in understanding of its pathogenesis and developments in invasive monitoring. New support measures such as extracorporeal membrane oxygenators and new knowledge regarding the role of cytokines may mean that we are on the brink of seeing improvements in therapy for these patients. Over the last few years a major interest has developed in several new methods of ventilatory support for exacerbations of chronic obstructive disease and for longer term domiciliary ventilation for a variety of chronic conditions. This fruitful area will lead to improvements both in survival and quality of life for these patients. With the alarming increase in asthma morbidity and mortality a review of current knowledge of pathogenesis is timely in the hope that this will allow development of new effective agents or improved application of old ones. The paradox of increasing mortality from asthma in the face of increasingly effective drugs has stimulated interest in the problems of mis-diagnosis, under-treatment and problems of compliance. These crucial issues are also reviewed in this volume. Infection is clearly an increasing rather than a decreasing problem in respiratory medicine despite advances and changes in many aspects of both community acquired pneumonia and AIDS related pneumonia. It is also clear that the interaction between the human immunodeficiency virus and tuberculosis is potentially devastating and is going to result in a tragic increase in tuberculosis in areas of the world where the prevalence of both infections is high.

Since the last issue there have been major breakthroughs in cystic fibrosis including the identification of the cystic fibrosis gene. An extended chapter is devoted to these advances in view of their great importance and interest. Interstitial lung disease, sarcoidosis, chronic obstructive pulmonary disease and thrombo-embolic disease remain important and difficult areas, yet progress has been made in many aspects of these diseases over the last few years. Much new interest now focuses on the occupational lung diseases as a result of our heightened awareness of environmental pollution both generally and in the work place.

Without doubt the most exciting clinical development of the last 5 years has been the establishment of heart–lung and lung transplantation as successful treatments for a range of irreversible lung diseases. The good results now being obtained will inevitably lead to an enormous increase in demand for these procedures. This increase in demand may be easier to fulfil with the advent of the more economical single lung transplant. With this increase in mind the last section of the book is devoted to discussing the key aspects of lung transplantation. It is hoped that all these review chapters will be found to be of interest and of use to all those in the field of respiratory medicine.

London 1991   D.M. Mitchell

Contributors

D. J. Aravot MD
Transplant Senior Registrar, Transplant Unit, Papworth Hospital, Cambridge, UK

Peter J. Barnes MA DM DSc FRCP
Chairman, Department of Thoracic Medicine, and Honorary Consultant Physician, Royal Brompton Hospital, London, UK

S. R. Benatar MBChB FFA FRCP
Professor and Chairman, Department of Medicine, University of Cape Town and Groote Schuur Hospital, South Africa

Robert M. Bogin MD
Assistant Professor of Medicine, University of Colorado Health Sciences Center; Staff Physician, National Jewish Center for Immunology and Respiratory Medicine, Denver, Colorado, USA

Paul A. Corris MD FRCAP
Consultant Physician, Freeman Hospital, Newcastle Upon Tyne, UK

John H. Dark FRCS
Consultant Cardiothoracic Surgeon, Freeman Hospital, Newcastle Upon Tyne, UK

Christopher Dennis FRCAP
Research Fellow, Papworth Hospital, Cambridge, UK

M. W. Elliott MA MRCP
Senior Registrar, Royal Brompton and National Heart Hospital, London, UK

Donald A. Enarson BSc MD FRCP(C)
Professor, Department of Medicine, University of Alberta; Officer, International Union against Tuberculosis and Lung Disease, Paris, France

Timothy W. Evans BSc MD MRCP PhD
Senior Lecturer in Thoracic Medicine, and Consultant in Thoracic

Medicine and Intensive Care, Royal Brompton and National Heart
Hospital, London, UK

Duncan M. Geddes MD FRCP
Consultant Physician, Royal Brompton and National Heart Hospital,
London, UK

Annika Graham MRCP
Cystic Fibrosis Research Trust Clinical Research Fellow, Royal
Brompton and National Heart Hospital, London, UK

Timothy W. Higenbottam BSc MA MD FRCP
Director of Respiratory Physiology, and Consultant Physician, Papworth
and Addenbrookes Hospitals, Cambridge, UK

Talmadge E. King Jr MD FACP FCCP
Associate Professor of Medicine, University of Colorado Health Sciences
Center; Director of the Cohen Clinic, National Jewish Center for
Immunology and Respiratory Medicine, Denver, Colorado, USA

J. T. Macfarlane MA DM FRCP
Consultant Physician in General and Respiratory Medicine, City
Hospital, Nottingham, UK

Peter D. Macnaughton MBBS MRCP FCAnaes
MRC Training Fellow, Departments of Clinical Physiology and Intensive
Care, Royal Brompton and National Heart Hospital, London, UK

David M. Mitchell MA MD FRCP
Consultant Physician, and Honorary Senior Lecturer in Medicine,
Respiratory Unit, St Mary's Hospital, London, UK

Donald N. Mitchell MD FRCP
Consultant Physician, Royal Brompton and National Heart Hospital,
London, UK

Rebecca L. Mortenson MD
Assistant Professor of Medicine, University of Colorado Health Sciences
Center; Staff Physician, National Jewish Center for Immunology and
Respiratory Medicine, Denver, Colorado, USA

John Moxham MD FRCP
Professor of Thoracic Medicine, King's College Hospital; Senior
Lecturer, National Heart and Lung Institute, London, UK

Anthony Newman Taylor FRCP FFOM
Consultant Physician, Royal Brompton and National Heart Hospital;
Director, Department of Occupational and Environmental Medicine,
National Heart and Lung Institute, London, UK

Martyn R. Partridge MD FRCP
Consultant Physician, Whipps Cross Hospital, London, UK

T. L. Petty MD
Professor of Medicine, and President, Presbyterian/St Luke's Center for Health Sciences Education, Denver, Colorado, USA

Karel Styblo MD DSc
Director of Scientific Activities, International Union Against Tuberculosis and Lung Disease, Paris, France

John Wallwork BSc MB ChB FRCS(E) MA
Consultant in Cardiothoracic Surgery, Papworth Hospital, Cambridge, UK

Contents

Adult respiratory distress syndrome

P. D. Macnaughton   T. W. Evans

In 1967 the association of respiratory failure with non-cardiogenic pulmonary oedema was first described in a group of patients with a variety of serious pathologies not directly involving the lung (Ashbaugh et al 1967). Histological examination of pulmonary biopsies suggested superficial similarities with the infantile respiratory distress syndrome and the term adult respiratory distress syndrome (ARDS) was coined. In the last decade it has become apparent that ARDS is commonly associated with failure of other organ systems including the brain, kidneys, liver, heart and blood (the multiple organ failure syndrome or MOF). It is now thought that ARDS is the pulmonary manifestation of a generalized abnormality of cellular metabolic function, precipitated most commonly by sepsis or trauma and resulting in a defect of oxygen utilization.

DEFINITION

As ARDS represents one end of the spectrum of acute lung injury, the definition of the syndrome is somewhat arbitrary. Nevertheless, the current criteria for diagnosis are:

1. Antecedent history of precipitating condition
2. Refractory hypoxaemia (arterial oxygen tension (PaO_2) < 8.0 kPa (60 mmHg) on 40% inspired oxygen (FiO_2) and positive end-expiratory pressure (PEEP) of 5 cm or more)
3. Radiological evidence of newly evolving bilateral pulmonary infiltrates suggestive of oedema (Fig. 1.1)
4. A pulmonary artery occlusion pressure (PAOP) less than 15–18 mmHg in the presence of normal colloid oncotic pressure
5. Total thoracic compliance less than 30 ml/cmH$_2$O.

There is no uniform agreement regarding these criteria, in particular the need for the measurement of PAOP. As balloon-tipped pulmonary artery catheters tend to be inserted only in the most severely affected cases, it has been suggested that inclusion of PAOP as a diagnostic requirement may result in selection bias, contributing to the apparent association between ARDS and MOF (Rinaldo & Heyman 1990). Furthermore, a normal value

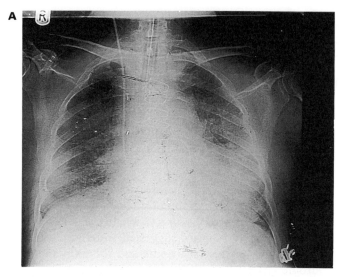

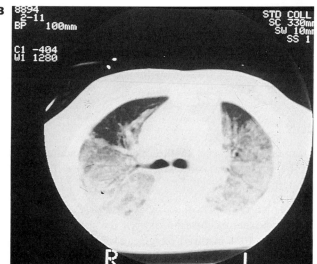

Fig. 1.1 A Chest X-ray (upper panel) and CT scan (lower panel) appearance of ARDS. Note pulmonary artery catheter in situ and extensive lower zone consolidation. **B** CT scan of the same patient reveals that this is a dependent phenomenon.

does not exclude cardiogenic pulmonary oedema secondary to transient myocardial dysfunction.

ARDS is clearly an umbrella term for a heterogeneous group of pulmonary insults that can result in the same clinical manifestations of acute severe lung injury. When considering such factors as therapeutic intervention and mortality data it would appear to be inappropriate to consider ARDS as a single disease entity. Most studies of ARDS have not categorized patients by underlying condition, thus making comparisons difficult. Murray et al (1988) have defined ARDS as the most severe form of lung damage, distinguishable from lesser degrees of lung injury by a score which takes into account chest X-ray appearance, degree of hypoxaemia, level of PEEP and thoracic compliance, as well as the underlying condition. ARDS can be divided into acute and chronic phases.

EPIDEMIOLOGY

There are estimated to be upwards of 150 000 cases of ARDS per annum in the USA and 10 000–15 000 per annum in the UK, although the incidence of established disease among patients in high-risk groups admitted to hospital may be as low as 5% (Bauman et al 1986). Recent evidence has suggested, however, that even patients only at risk of developing ARDS can display signs of a loss of endothelial integrity (Rocker et al 1989), which is the pathological hallmark of the condition. Estimates of mortality vary from 50% to 60%, but the eventual outcome seems to be unrelated to the severity of pulmonary pathology. Risk factor analysis indicates that the majority of early deaths are due to complications of the underlying illness, while later (i.e. greater than 72 hours after onset) mortality is a consequence of sepsis, which develops up to six times more frequently in patients with ARDS when compared to a critically ill control population (Montgomery et al 1985, Seidenfield et al 1986).

AETIOLOGY

Associated clinical conditions

The pathophysiology of ARDS, discussed in detail below, represents the outcome of a chain of events following insults to the pulmonary vascular endothelium or alveolar epithelium, which may be direct (e.g. aspiration of gastric contents or inhalation of toxic fumes) or indirect (e.g. septicaemia, massive haemorrhage or blood transfusion, major trauma, obstetrical crises). The incidence and fatality rates from ARDS for the population most at risk from developing the syndrome according to their predisposing illness are shown in Table 1.1 (Fowler et al 1983). The exact sequence of events that follows the initial pulmonary insult remains unknown, although a number of potential cellular and humoral components have been identified.

Underlying mechanisms

During respiratory failure inflammatory cells (principally neutrophils) sequester in the pulmonary vascular bed adjacent to areas of endothelial damage. Large numbers of neutrophils have also been isolated from bronchoalveolar lavage fluid obtained from patients with ARDS, and animals

Table 1.1 Incidence and fatality rates for ARDS by predisposed groups (Reproduced, in part, with permission from Fowler et al 1983)

Predisposing risk factor	Incidence rate (/100)	Fatality rate (/100)
Cardiopulmonary bypass	1.7	50.0
Burns	2.3	50.0
Bacteraemia	3.8	77.8
Hypertransfusion	4.6	44.4
Trauma	5.3	–
Pneumonia (ventilated)	11.9	60.0
Disseminated intravascular coagulation	22.2	50.0
Pulmonary aspiration	35.6	93.8

depleted of neutrophils display attenuated alveolar oedema formation when exposed to endotoxin. Nevertheless, despite the evidence suggesting a key role for the neutrophil in the generation of ARDS, the precise mechanism underlying neutrophil activation is unknown (Tate & Repine 1983) (Fig. 1.2). The complement system is stimulated in many disorders associated with ARDS, and can itself increase vascular permeability when administered intravenously to animals, but has few other direct effects on lung pathology. Other potential mediators of neutrophil activation include fibrin, bradykinin, histamine, tumour necrosis factor (TNF) and platelet-activating factor (PAF); several of these are inflammatory mediators with intrinsic vasoactive properties (Evans et al 1987). Neutrophil activation leads to the generation of toxic oxygen radicals and to the breakdown of arachidonic acid with production of cyclooxygenase (e.g. prostaglandins, thromboxane) and lipoxygenase (e.g. leukotrienes) products. PAF is also generated in these circumstances, is chemotactic for neutrophils and eosinophils, and leads to platelet activation and aggregation and may modulate changes in pulmonary vascular control (McCormack et al 1990). Factors released by human platelets include proteases, kallikrein and fibronectin, which are themselves cytotoxic and have potent effects on vasomotor control (Heffner et al 1987). Platelets also release a growth factor which stimulates fibroblast replication and collagen production. A dense fibrotic reaction is a feature of ARDS and may lead to death in a minority of patients some weeks after the initial illness.

Recent evidence suggests that ARDS is a multisystem disease and that the changes that occur in the pulmonary endothelium are a reflection of a more generalized endothelial disorder. Fleck et al (1985) demonstrated increased transcapillary escape of albumin after septic shock and surgery which they attributed to generalized changes in capillary permeability. In a study of patients after major trauma a positive correlation was found between extravascular lung water and the appearance of β_2-macroglobulin

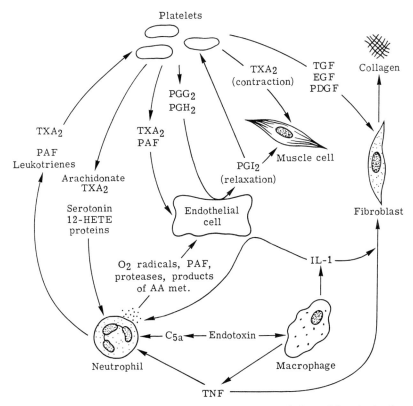

Fig. 1.2 Schematic representation of possible consequences of neutrophil activation by the cytokines tumour necrosis factor (TNF) and interleukin-1 (IL-1). Note the redundancy built into the system, such that if one pathway to endothelial damage is blocked another may produce the same end result. AA, arachidonic acid; 12-HETE, 12-hydroxyeicosatetraenoate; EGF, epidermal growth factor; PAF, platelet-activating factor; PG, prostaglandins; TGF, transforming growth factor; TXA_2, thromboxane A_2; PDGF, platelet-derived growth factor. (Reproduced with permission from Keogh et al 1990.)

in the urine, the latter being a marker of increased renal capillary permeability (Kreuzfelder et al 1988).

What mechanisms account for the activation of the inflammatory cascades described above which result in generalized endothelial injury? It has been proposed that persistent stimulation of these inflammatory processes is required in order for the panendothelial injury which leads to MOF to occur (Rinaldo & Heyman 1990). Chronic pulmonary sepsis or the absorption of gastrointestinal bacterial products may be the causes of ongoing inflammatory stimulation which can precipitate MOF. Nosocomial Gram-negative bacterial infection is common in patients with ARDS (Montgomery et al 1985). This may result in the release of endotoxin, which will stimulate lung macrophages to release cytokines such as TNF and interleukin-1. The gut is a large reservoir of potential bacterial pathogens, and the development of a panendothelial injury may damage the integrity of the gut mucosa, resulting in the absorption of bacterial products into the portal circulation (Cheung 1984). This may result in the stimulation of hepatic macrophages (Kupffer cells) to release inflammatory mediators, further fuelling the inflammatory processes. A positive feedback mechanism may then occur, resulting in increasing mucosal damage and bacterial product absorption, leading to the progressive downward spiral of MOF, eventually terminating in death (Rinaldo & Heyman 1990).

PATHOPHYSIOLOGY

Pathology

Despite the diverse causes of ARDS, the associated pulmonary pathology is uniform and characterized by increased permeability of the alveolar–capillary membrane. This may be measured at the simplest level through the detection of intravenously injected radiolabelled albumin in bronchoalveolar lavage fluid (Anderson et al 1979). More sophisticated techniques involve assessing the rate of clearance of an inhaled marker (e.g. radiolabelled diethylenetriaminepentaacetic acid, DTPA) into the blood and the measurement of the movement of intravenously injected radiolabelled transferrin from blood to the alveolar space (Hunter et al 1990). Loss of endothelial integrity leads to pulmonary oedema and extravasation of inflammatory cells, with the formation of fibrin and platelet thrombi in microvessels and lymphatics. As the condition develops, hyaline (eosinophilic) membrane formation occurs, with capillary congestion and interstitial oedema. These changes are most apparent in specimens obtained within the first 5 days of the insult. In those patients who survive the acute phase, interstitial fibrosis (primarily in the alveolar ducts) ensues and a measurable increase in total lung collagen content occurs after the first 10 days (Zapol et al 1979b). The healing process in ARDS has been little studied, but involves proliferation of type I pneumocytes, and the resultant surfactant deficiency has important implications in both acute and chronic forms of the illness. Microscopic examination of the lungs at necropsy reveals hyperaemia, dilated engorged capillaries and areas of alveolar atelectasis, although diffuse interstitial inflammatory changes with fibrosis may also be observed.

Pulmonary physiology

Changes in net fluid flux from the intra- to extravascular compartments occur according to the Starling equation, which is defined by the product of the net driving pressure across the alveolar–capillary membrane and the membrane conductance (Sibbald et al 1985). Experimental and clinical studies have shown that the protein content of the pulmonary oedema fluid in ARDS approaches that of plasma, indicating a loss of integrity of the alveolar–capillary membrane. Physiological studies also suggest that the normal protective increase in the lymphatic clearance of fluid does not occur in ARDS, causing a further accumulation of interstitial and alveolar oedema. The presence of circulating proteins in the alveolar compartment greatly reduces surfactant surface activity (Lachmann 1989). The physiological consequences are a fall in total lung capacity (TLC) and in functional residual capacity (FRC) of up to 50%. Profound ventilation–perfusion mismatch results in a marked increase in shunt fraction and alveolar dead space, leading to refractory hypoxaemia (Dantzker et al 1979). Reduced lung compliance results in an increase in the work of breathing. The high lung recoil pressure at FRC leads to early airway closure and alveolar collapse. Once this has occurred, very high inflation pressures are needed to reinflate the lung. The application of PEEP prevents airway pressure falling to atmospheric and moves functioning alveoli higher up their individual pressure–volume curves, leading to a considerable increase in FRC. However, studies using computerized axial tomography have revealed that the lungs are not homogeneously affected in these circumstances and a three-zone model of healthy, diseased and recruitable alveoli has been demonstrated. Thus the maximal consolidation tends to concentrate in the dependent regions of the lung when the patient is supine (Fig. 1.1). The application of PEEP has been shown to cause a variable clearing of these densities, reflecting an opening of previously non-aerated lung (Gattinoni et al 1988).

Cardiac performance and oxygen delivery

Most of the diseases with which ARDS is associated are characterized by increased peripheral oxygen requirements. Oxygen delivery (DO_2) is a function of cardiac output and arterial oxygenation (Table 1.2). ARDS has adverse effects on both parameters. As a result of hypoxia and the mechanisms outlined above, pulmonary hypertension of varying severity occurs and its effects on cardiac output can be severe, depending in part upon the presence of pre-existing cardiac and/or pulmonary vascular disease (Zapol & Snider 1977). The consequent increase in right ventricular afterload moves the intraventricular septum, thereby reducing left ventricular stroke volume. In the absence of right ventricular hypertrophy (as occurs, for example, in chronic obstructive pulmonary disease) it is unlikely that cardiac performance can be maintained beyond a mean pulmonary artery pressure of 35–40 mmHg. Moreover, there is evidence to suggest that ventricular contractility is depressed further in patients with sepsis by the presence of a circulating myocardial depressant factor (Reilly et al 1989).

An abnormal relationship between DO_2 and oxygen consumption (VO_2) has been demonstrated in patients with ARDS and sepsis (Danek et al 1980). At rest VO_2 is normally delivery independent if DO_2 is maintained above a critical level (DO_2 crit) (Shibutani et al 1983). As DO_2 increases

Table 1.2 Indices to be calculated in the haemodynamic management of patients with ARDS. Note that a balloon-tipped, flow-directed pulmonary artery catheter of the haemodilution type is necessary for the collection of the relevant data[a]

Systemic vascular resistance (SVR)	(MAP–CVP)/cardiac output
Pulmonary vascular resistance (PVR)	(MPAP–PAOP)/cardiac output
Oxygen delivery (DO_2)	$CI \times SaO_2 \times Hb \times 13.9$
Oxygen consumption (VO_2)	$CI \times (SaO_2 - SvO_2) \times Hb \times 13.9$

[a] MAP, mean arterial pressure; CVP, central venous pressure; MPAP, mean pulmonary artery pressure; PAOP, pulmonary artery occlusion pressure; SaO_2, arterial saturation; SvO_2, mixed venous saturation (both expressed as fraction); Hb, haemoglobin concentration (g/dl); CI, cardiac index (l min^{-1} m^{-2}). The contribution of oxygen dissolved in the blood has been ignored as it contributes little to oxygen carriage under normobaric conditions.

VO_2 remains constant and therefore oxygen extraction ratio falls. Below DO_2 crit there is a linear relationship between VO_2 and DO_2 (Fig. 1.3). In some patients with ARDS and sepsis, delivery dependence of oxygen consumption has been demonstrated even when DO_2 is above DO_2 crit, suggesting a covert oxygen debt (Bihari et al 1987). In these patients the oxygen extraction ratio remains constant. The mechanisms underling this abnormal oxygen utilization are not understood. A primary defect in mitochondrial oxygen utilization could partially explain the phenomenon, but a more likely explanation is an abnormality in the diffusion of oxygen from the blood to the tissues due to interstitial oedema, abnormal distribution of blood flow, the formation of microemboli or the release of various vasoactive mediators (Schumacker & Cain 1987).

Whatever the explanation, this abnormality is associated with a high mortality and DO_2 may need to be increased to supranormal levels by pharmacological means in order that tissue oxygen requirements are met (Bihari et al 1987). Oxygen uptake supply dependency can be demonstrated by measuring the change in oxygen consumption after an acute increase in oxygen transport either by fluid loading or pharmacological means (Haupt et al 1985, Bihari et al 1987, Vincent et al 1990). An increased plasma lactate level, reflecting an imbalance between metabolic requirements and DO_2 also appears to predict those patients with oxygen uptake supply dependency (Rashkin et al 1984, Haupt et al 1985, Vincent et al 1990).

CLINICAL FEATURES AND DIAGNOSIS

The diagnosis of ARDS depends upon the recognition of predisposing pathology in the presence of non-cardiogenic pulmonary oedema. Patients usually present with dyspnoea, either acute in onset or developing over a number of hours. Cyanosis may not be apparent despite marked hypoxaemia. Accompanying tachypnoea leads to hypocapnia in unventilated patients,

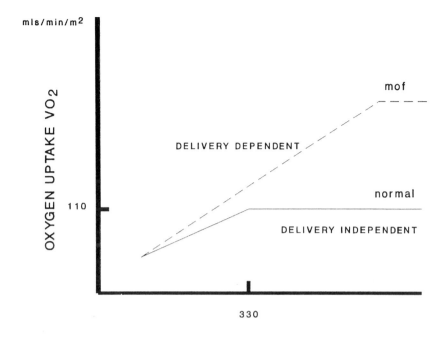

Fig. 1.3   Relationship between oxygen supply and consumption in normal and critically ill patients. MOF, multiple organ failure syndrome. DO_2 crit, 330 ml min^{-1} m^{-2} (see text).

causing superficial vasoconstriction and a pale, waxy complexion. Alternatively, patients with established ARDS due to sepsis may have a hyperdynamic circulation due to increased basal metabolism, with warm, vasodilated peripheries (in contrast to the peripheral vasoconstriction of cardiac failure). Auscultation of the chest reveals signs of pulmonary oedema.

Investigations

Arterial blood gas analysis

Arterial blood gas analysis demonstrates hypoxaemia. In established ARDS the FiO_2 and PEEP required to maintain a PaO_2 of 8 kPa (60 mmHg) are in excess of 0.4 and 5 cmH_2O, respectively. Extreme dyspnoea usually results in a low arterial carbon dioxide tension ($PaCO_2$), producing a respiratory alkalosis and a leftward shift of the haemoglobin–oxygen dissociation curve, such that patients may not appear to be cyanosed.

The chest radiograph

The chest radiograph shows diffuse alveolar shadowing suggestive of pulmonary oedema, often with air bronchograms (Fig. 1.1). An absence of cardiac enlargement or lobar consolidation helps to differentiate ARDS from left ventricular failure or infection.

Haemodynamic measurements

The insertion of a balloon-tipped, flow-directed pulmonary artery catheter of the thermodilution type can help exclude hydrostatic causes of pulmonary oedema if the PAOP is less than 18 mmHg and there is normal plasma oncotic pressure. If the latter is reduced, pulmonary oedema develops at a lower PAOP. Estimations of PAOP may be affected by the position of the catheter tip (which should be below the level of the left atrium, in 'zone 3' lung) and the presence or absence of PEEP. In the severely hypoxaemic, mechanically ventilated patient, it may be impossible to complete the necessary measurements without PEEP, in which circumstances some authors have advocated subtracting 50% of this value from the measured PAOP. However, in a recent study PEEP did not affect the correlation between PAOP and left ventricular end-diastolic pressure measurements in patients with severe ARDS (Teboul et al 1989). If cardiac output is measured then pulmonary and systemic vascular resistances (PVR, SVR) can be calculated (Table 1.2). The SVR is normally low in ARDS, reflecting decreased peripheral vascular resistance in the face of an increased metabolic rate. PVR can be markedly elevated and reflects the severity of the lung injury. VO_2 and DO_2 can be calculated if samples of arterial and mixed venous blood are obtained and cardiac output is measured (Table 1.2). A VO_2 below 8 ml min^{-1} kg^{-1} has been associated with an increased mortality (Rashkin et al 1984).

Pulmonary compliance

Pulmonary compliance is decreased, usually to less than 30 ml/cmH$_2$O. Static lung compliance measurements made with the patient anaesthetized and paralysed have been used as an indicator of the severity of the lung injury.

Vascular permeability

The measurement of an increase in pulmonary microvascular permeability confirms the presence of the definitive characteristic of ARDS, but requires technology not readily available to the average intensive care unit (Hunter et al 1990).

Underlying condition

The underlying condition should be fully investigated and steps taken to correct any factors precipitating ARDS. Evidence of multiple organ dysfunction is common in the form of abnormal haematological indices (reduced platelet count, increased fibrinogen degradation products or frank disseminated intravascular coagulopathy), cerebral dysfunction (confusion, coma), or renal and hepatic impairment. A full bacteriological screen should be undertaken.

MANAGEMENT

Therapy in ARDS is essentially supportive and aimed at maintaining DO_2 at adequate levels by appropriate respiratory and cardiovascular support. The underlying cause should be treated if possible. Any suspected sites of sepsis should be managed aggressively with broad-spectrum antibiotics and surgical drainage if indicated. Early fixation of unstable fractures may be important in the trauma patient (Svenningsen et al 1987). Patients with ARDS do not usually die from respiratory failure, but from the associated MOF (Montgomery et al 1985).

Respiratory support

The spontaneously breathing patient

Satisfactory oxygenation can be achieved in patients with mild ARDS using continuous positive airways pressure (CPAP). The patient breathes an oxygen–air mixture spontaneously, either through an endotracheal tube or a tightly fitting face mask. In order to maintain the intrathoracic pressure at the required level of CPAP throughout the respiratory cycle, high gas flows (in excess of 70 l/min) or a large pressurized reservoir bag are required. If there are significant falls in pressure during inspiration the work of breathing may be increased. The level of CPAP used varies between 5 and 10 cmH_2O and is most easily obtained by placing the expiratory limb of the breathing circuit under water. CPAP recruits collapsed alveoli, increasing FRC and reducing compliance such that the work of breathing is reduced and gas exchange improved. If, despite these measures, PaO_2 cannot be maintained above 8 kPa (60 mmHg) or respiratory fatigue develops, then full mechanical respiratory support must be initiated.

Conventional mechanical ventilation

Ventilatory support in ARDS should provide adequate oxygenation in the face of reductions in pulmonary compliance and lung volumes and increased alveolar dead space. Controlled mandatory ventilation (CMV) or synchronized intermittent mandatory ventilation (SIMV) may be utilized. SIMV allows the patient to initiate preset ventilator breaths and enables spontaneous ventilation in between. Proposed advantages of SIMV include improved cardiocirculatory function and a reduced requirement for sedation. However, ARDS often produces a high respiratory drive, resulting in increased respiratory muscle oxygen consumption. This is clearly undesirable in the face of critical oxygen transport and in these circumstances CMV with sedation is indicated. Neuromuscular blockade should also be considered to reduce oxygen consumption further, and has the additional advantage of increasing thoracic compliance.

The increase in alveolar dead space means that high minute and tidal volumes (10–15 ml/kg) are required to achieve satisfactory CO_2 removal. A large tidal volume also recruits collapsed alveoli, thus improving shunt, but may result in high peak airway pressures due to the reduced compliance. Pressures above 50 cmH_2O have been associated with an increased risk of barotrauma (Peterson & Baier 1983) and may exacerbate lung injury. However, barotrauma is possibly influenced more by the severity of the underlying pathology rather than by absolute airway pressures. Nevertheless, most clinicians attempt to keep peak airway pressure below 40 cmH_2O, although this is frequently difficult using conventional means of respiratory support. The pressure–volume relationship of the lung is not linear (Fig. 1.4) and a tidal volume should be selected that maintains the lung on the steepest, most compliant portion of the curve. In practice this is achieved by increasing the tidal volume by small (100 ml) increments, the optimal

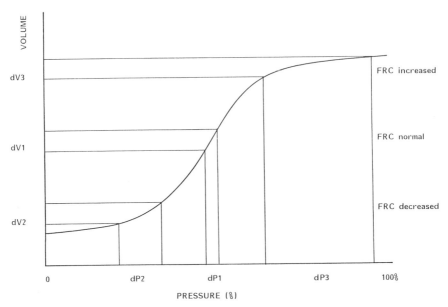

Fig. 1.4 Pressure–volume relationship of the lungs. Note that when FRC is decreased, as in ARDS, applying a volume dV2 results in a large increase in airway pressure (dP2). Applying the identical volume dV1 on a favourable portion of the curve (attained through the use of PEEP) causes a much smaller rise in pressure (dP1). Overdistension of the lung through the application of an overlarge tidal volume or excessive PEEP will again result in large increase in airway pressure (dP3).

volume being exceeded when there is a disproportionate increase in the peak airway pressure, which may be further reduced by prolonging the inspiratory time.

The hypoxaemia of ARDS is due to a large increase in intrapulmonary shunt and is therefore difficult to correct even with a high FiO_2. Although there is no good evidence that an FiO_2 above 0.6 further exacerbates the lung injury most authorities suggest it is kept below this value.

PEEP prevents alveolar collapse at the end of expiration, thereby increasing FRC, improving lung compliance and reducing intrapulmonary shunt. However, PEEP increases mean intrathoracic pressure, reduces venous return and therefore cardiac output. Even though PaO_2 may increase with PEEP, oxygen transport may fall overall due to the decrease in cardiac output, and the optimal use of PEEP requires that DO_2 is monitored (Suter et al 1975). Fluid loading can overcome the effects of PEEP on venous return, but may be undesirable in the face of increasing lung water. PEEP is usually applied in the range of 5–15 cmH_2O, but its prophylactic use in patients at risk of ARDS has not been shown to be beneficial (Pepe et al 1984).

There is a wide variation in the ventilation time constants of individual alveoli in ARDS. The use of an inspiratory pause improves ventilation–perfusion matching by increasing the ventilation of alveoli with large time constants (slow alveoli). This may cause significant improvements in gas exchange although the associated increase in mean intrathoracic pressure may reduce cardiac output and therefore DO_2.

New approaches to ventilatory management

The rationale behind a number of new approaches to ventilation is to maintain a mean airway pressure high enough to recruit unstable alveoli and therefore improve gas exchange, whilst avoiding the high peak airway pressures associated with barotrauma.

Inverse ratio ventilation

Inverse ratio ventilation (IRV) utilizes a prolonged inspiratory phase, such that the inspiratory to expiratory (I : E) ratio is between 1 : 1 and 4 : 1. Volume-controlled IRV (VC-IRV) delivers a preset tidal volume regardless of inspiratory pressure and therefore allows a predictable clearance of CO_2. Increased mean airway pressure may improve oxygenation when conventional ventilation has failed, although significant air trapping may result in excessive lung volumes, high peak airway pressures and a profound reduction in cardiac output. Pressure-controlled IRV (PC-IRV) delivers a constant preset inspiratory pressure for the desired inspiratory time and therefore avoids the risks of air trapping associated with VC-IRV. The results of PC-IRV have been encouraging in improving gas exchange and reducing peak airway pressure without impairing cardiac performance (Tharratt et al 1988, Lain et al 1989), but a reduction in mortality has not been demonstrated. Airway pressure release ventilation allows the patient to breathe spontaneously while mean airway pressure and therefore oxygenation is maintained with CPAP. Carbon dioxide clearance is increased by the transient release of the airway pressure, allowing lung volume to fall (Downs & Stock 1987). This technique has been used successfully in ARDS, although its influence on outcome is as yet unknown.

High-frequency jet ventilation

High-frequency jet ventilation (HFJV) delivers a high-pressure pulse (driving pressure) of oxygen–air mixture at a rate between 60 and 600 times per minute for a preset percentage of each respiratory cycle (inspiratory or I time). Tidal volumes are smaller than the dead space volume and the mechanisms of gas exchange in HFJV are not fully understood (Rouby et al 1983). Carbon dioxide clearance tends to increase as rate falls. Airway pressures are less than with conventional ventilation and the risk of barotrauma may be reduced. A controlled trial of HFJV demonstrated that this mode of ventilation can be used safely in ARDS, although it failed to show any improvement in outcome (Carlon et al 1981). Research is in progress to assess if aggressive alveolar recruitment and maintenance of lung volume with high mean airway pressures and frequencies close to the natural resonant frequency of the lung (5–7 Hz) can improve outcome in ARDS (Keogh et al 1990).

Extracorporeal membrane oxygenation

Extracorporeal membrane oxygenation (ECMO) involves the removal of blood from the inferior vena cava via a femoral vein catheter, which then passes through a gas-exchanging membrane, the oxygenated blood being returned to the aorta via a femoral artery catheter. A National Institutes of Health (NIH) trial in the USA failed to demonstrate any overall improvement in mortality compared with conventional ventilation when ECMO was used in ARDS (Zapol et al 1979a), but the 5-day mortality was reduced, suggesting that the technique was successful in treating acute respiratory failure. In order to achieve adequate oxygenation ECMO requires high blood flows of up to 80% of cardiac output. This increases the incidence of blood trauma, a major complication of the procedure, and may also result in inadequate pulmonary perfusion compromising lung repair (Gattinoni et al 1986).

Extracorporeal carbon dioxide removal

Recently there have been encouraging results using extracorporeal carbon dioxide removal ($ECCO_2R$). This is a veno-venous technique whereby blood is removed from the femoral vein and returned to the inferior vena cava via relatively small cannulae. Adequate carbon dioxide clearance can be achieved due to its high diffusibility, using a combination of low blood flow (1–2 l/min) and high gas flow (40 l/min) through the membrane oxygenator. Such flow rates reduce blood trauma and provide approximately 50% of the total oxygen requirement. The technique is combined with positive pressure ventilation in order to achieve adequate oxygenation, although as carbon dioxide is being cleared through the membrane low frequencies (six breaths/min) maintain satisfactory overall gas exchange and limit pulmonary barotrauma. It has been suggested that the resultant combination of normal pulmonary perfusion and minimum ventilation provides optimal conditions for lung repair in ARDS. In an uncontrolled trial of $ECCO_2R$, patients with the same entry criteria as the NIH trial had a mortality of less than 50%, when the predicted mortality was more than 90% (Gattinoni et al 1986). A controlled trial comparing $ECCO_2R$ combined with PC-IRV and conventional ventilation is currently in progress at the University of Utah.

A device placed in the inferior vena cava which allows gas exchange to occur through microbore tubes has recently been developed (intravascular oxygenation device (IVOX), Cardiopulmonics, USA). Animal work suggests that it can supply up to 90% of basal oxygen requirements, and clinical trials in ARDS are planned.

Fluid balance and renal support

The increase in pulmonary vascular permeability that characterizes ARDS means that the rate of fluid transudation into the pulmonary interstitium is directly related to the mean pulmonary capillary pressure. A reduction in circulating volume may therefore improve oxygenation. Achieving optimal fluid balance is assisted greatly by the insertion of a balloon-tipped pulmonary artery catheter. The goal of fluid therapy is to maintain the lowest PAOP compatible with an adequate cardiac output and therefore DO_2, which usually means a value of 8–12 mmHg. Judicious use of diuretics and fluid restriction are possible in patients with normal renal function, but this approach may be inappropriate if reduced circulating volume improves PaO_2 at the expense of cardiac output, therefore reducing DO_2. Patients with ARDS may have reduced ventricular compliance such that a small increase in circulating volume may produce a large increase in PAOP and therefore extravascular lung water (Sibbald et al 1985).

Due to the increase in endothelial permeability, artificial attempts to increase colloid osmotic pressure are unlikely to reduce pulmonary oedema. Plasma albumin concentration is not an accurate estimate of colloid osmotic pressure in the critically ill, and attempts to maintain albumin concentration above certain arbitrarily defined limits are not justified (Grootendorst et al

1988). Renal failure is a common complication of the underlying conditions associated with ARDS and haemofiltration has proved useful both in correcting the serum chemistry and achieving the desired negative fluid balance.

Circulatory support

As ARDS is associated with a defect of peripheral oxygen utilization the primary objective must be to maximize DO_2. Cardiac output may be compromised due to a number of mechanisms, including low filling pressures secondary to fluid therapy, the effect of high levels of CPAP or PEEP, elevated pulmonary vascular resistance (PVR) and the presence of a circulating myocardial depressant factor (Reilly et al 1989). Inotropes are often required to maintain DO_2. Dobutamine may be the drug of choice, increasing DO_2 both through positive inotropic effects and due to peripheral vasodilation from a β_2 effect (Shoemaker et al 1988). In septic shock, when vital organ perfusion is compromised due to the drop in SVR, the use of vasoconstrictors such as noradrenaline can be beneficial (Meadows et al 1988), but excessive vasoconstriction will reduce DO_2.

Due to the poor specificity of currently available drugs, attempts to selectively reduce PVR do not necessarily improve DO_2 (Melot et al 1989). Prostacyclin has been shown to reduce PVR and improve right ventricular function in patients with increased pulmonary artery pressures secondary to ARDS (Rademacker et al 1990). Prostacyclin infusion increases DO_2 and VO_2 in critically ill patients with ARDS, but has not been shown to improve mortality (Bihari et al 1987). Adenosine appears to be a highly selective pulmonary vasodilator when infused into the pulmonary artery of patients with primary pulmonary hypertension (Morgan et al 1990) and may therefore be useful in ARDS.

As previously described, delivery dependence of VO_2 in ARDS and sepsis is associated with a high mortality. Recently, therapy in septic shock has been guided by defining specific goals for DO_2 and VO_2 (Edwards et al 1989, Shoemaker et al 1990), which are those haemodynamic values identified as predicting survivors in previous studies. This approach to the therapy of shock has been developed whereby the goals are defined 'operationally' (Shoemaker et al 1990). DO_2 is increased by fluid loading, inotropes and/or vasodilators as long as VO_2 continues to rise. Using the combination of dobutamine and noradrenaline Edwards et al (1989) were able to increase DO_2 and VO_2 from mean values of 605 and 130 ml min^{-1} m^{-2}, respectively, to 843 and 170 ml min^{-1} m^{-2} in a group of patients with severe septic shock. Mortality in this uncontrolled trial was 48%, which was considerably less than predicted. Further trials are required to confirm if this type of haemodynamic goal-directed therapy is associated with improved survival.

Nutrition and gastrointestinal tract

Nutritional support may be sacrified in the short term to reduce fluid input. Once hypoxaemia has been alleviated, parenteral or enteral feeding should be commenced. There is some evidence that the use of enteral feeds, even in low volumes, by supplying essential nutrients to the gut mucosa, may have a protective effect in maintaining the integrity of the mucosa and prevent the absorption of bacterial products into the portal circulation (Cheung 1984). The enteral route should be used whenever possible, with parental supplementation as necessary. Intravenous lipids have been shown to exacerbate the lung injury seen in neonates, and infusion of lipid has been demonstrated to result in a transient deterioration in respiratory function in patients with ARDS (Hwang et al 1990). Proposed mechanisms include the accumulation of fats in the pulmonary lymphatics exacerbating pulmonary oedema and the increase in free fatty acids acting as substrate for the production of vasoactive mediators such as thromboxane. However, the respiratory quotient of lipids is greater than 1 and lipid metabolism therefore produces less carbon dioxide than an equivalent amount of dextrose. The use of lipids in enteral feeds may thus be appropriate in severe ARDS, when carbon dioxide elimination is critical and has been shown to reduce the time taken to wean patients from mechanical ventilation (Al-Saady et al 1989). The widespread use of histamine$_2$ receptor blockers as prophylaxis against stress ulceration may increase the risk of nosocomial pulmonary infection secondary to bacterial colonization of the upper gastrointestinal tract (Driks et al 1987). A number of studies have shown that selective gut decontamination with non-absorbable antibiotics reduces the incidence of nosocomial infection in ventilated patients (Unertl et al 1990), but a significant reduction in mortality has not been demonstrated.

Pharmacotherapy in acute lung injury

The loss of integrity of the pulmonary endothelial barrier with increased microvascular permeability is probably a late, and possibly irreversible, manifestation of the processes underlying ARDS. To date, the rationale for pharmacotherapy has been based on our understanding of the mechanisms leading to endothelial damage and has therefore been aimed at the inflammatory process. Indeed, a wide variety of anti-inflammatory agents have been tried in experimental and human ARDS, with variable results. The initial report of Ashbaugh et al (1967) suggested that steroid therapy might have had a favourable effect in patients with underlying fat embolism and viral pneumonia. Corticosteroids ameliorate the increase in lung permeability seen in endotoxin-treated sheep, and may, in massive doses, reduce vascular leakage in humans. Nevertheless, there is no evidence that steroid therapy improves survival in patients with ARDS (Bernard et al

1987) and may even worsen prognosis in patients with impaired renal function (Bone et al 1987).

Most research into other potential treatments for ARDS has involved animal models, but the results have been similarly disappointing. Thromboxanes, which with prostaglandins are the principal products of the cyclooxygenase pathway of arachidonic acid metabolism, may partially mediate the vascular effects of endotoxin, and the experimental use of established inhibitors of cyclooxygenase metabolism has been found to reduce permeability changes. The possible involvement of oxygen radicals in certain forms of acute lung injury has led to the assessment of free radical scavengers and anti-oxidants in the treatment of experimentally induced ARDS, with some encouraging early results, particularly in protecting rats against the effects of hyperoxia.

Pharmacological manipulation of the immuno-inflammatory cascades thought to precipitate the endothelial injury associated with sepsis is an area of great interest. Antibodies to endotoxin, complement fragments and TNF have been developed and are undergoing evaluation. A methylxanthine, pentoxifylline, inhibits neutrophil adherance to the endothelium, and pretreatment of a pig model of sepsis resulted in an improvement in haemodynamic and histological changes (Tighe et al 1990).

There have been encouraging reports from the use of endogenous surfactant in ARDS (Lachmann 1989), and the development of synthetic surfactants for use in neonates (Ten Centre Study Group 1987) will allow this therapy to be assessed both in the prophylaxis and treatment of ARDS.

CONCLUSIONS

The average mortality amongst patients with ARDS is 50–60% and has remained unchanged since 1967. Although our understanding of the condition has grown rapidly, specific therapeutic advances have been few and treatment is almost entirely supportive in nature. As the understanding of the mechanisms precipitating ARDS increase, therapies directed at preventing the progression of lung injury and MOF may be developed in the near future.

REFERENCES

Al-Saady N M, Blackmore C M, Bennett E D 1989 High fat low carbohydrate enteral feeding lowers PaCO$_2$ and reduces period of ventilation in artificially ventilated patients. Intensive Care Medicine 15: 290–295
Anderson R R, Holiday R L, Driedger A A et al 1979 Documentation of pulmonary capillary permeability in the adult respiratory distress syndrome accompanying human sepsis. American Review of Respiratory Disease 119: 869–875
Ashbaugh D G, Bigelow D B, Petty T L, Levine B E 1967 Acute respiratory distress in adults. Lancet ii: 319–323
Bauman W R, Jung R C, Koss M, Boylen T, Navarro L, Sharma O P 1986 Incidence and mortality of adult respiratory distress syndrome: A prospective analysis from a large metropolitan hospital. Critical Care Medicine 14: 1–4

Bernard G R, Luce J M, Sprung C L et al 1987 High-dose corticosteroids in patients with the adult respiratory distress syndrome. New England Journal of Medicine 317: 1565–1570

Bihari D, Smithies M, Grimson A et al 1987 The effects of vasodilation with prostacyclin on oxygen delivery and uptake in critically ill patients. New England Journal of Medicine 317: 397–403

Bone R C, Fisher C J, Clemmer T P et al 1987 A controlled trial of high dose methylprednisolone in the treatment of severe sepsis and septic shock. New England Journal of Medicine 317: 653–658

Carlon G C, Khan R C, Howlard W S et al 1981 Clinical experience with high frequency jet ventilation. Critical Care Medicine 9: 1–6

Cheung L Y 1984 Gastric mucosal blood flow: its measurement and importance in mucosal defence. Journal of Surgical Research 36: 282–288

Danek S T, Lynch J P, Weg J G et al 1980 The dependence of oxygen uptake on oxygen delivery in the adult respiratory distress syndrome. American Review of Respiratory Disease 122: 387–395

Dantzker D R, Brook C J, Dehart P et al 1979 Ventilation perfusion distributions in the adult respiratory distress syndrome. American Review of Respiratory Disease 120: 1039–1052

Downs J B, Stock M G 1987 Airway pressure release ventilation: A new concept in ventilatory support. Critical Care Medicine 15: 459–461

Driks M R, Craven D E, Celli B R et al 1987 Nosocomial pneumonia in intubated patients given sucralfate as compared with antacids or histamine type 2 blockers. New England Journal of Medicine 317: 1376–1382

Edwards J D, Ceri S, Brown G, Nightingale P 1989 Use of survivors' cardiorespiratory values as therapeutic goals in septic shock. Critical Care Medicine 17: 1098–1103

Evans T W, Chung K F, Rogers D F, Barnes P J 1987 Effect of platelet activating factor on airway microvascular permeability: Possible mechanisms. Journal of Applied Physiology 63: 479–484

Fleck A, Howker F, Wallace P F et al 1985 Increased vascular removal: A major cause of hypoalbuminaemia in disease and injury. Lancet i: 781–784

Fowler A A, Hamman R F, Good J T et al 1983 Adult respiratory distress syndrome: Risk with common predispositions. Annals of Internal Medicine 98: 593–597

Gattinoni L, Pesenti A, Mascheroni D et al 1986 Low frequency positive pressure ventilation with extracorporeal CO_2 removal in severe respiratory failure. Journal of the American Medical Association 256: 881

Gattinoni L, Pesenti A, Bagliari S 1988 Inflammatory pulmonary oedema and positive end expiratory pressure: Correlation between imaging and physiological studies. Journal of Thoracic Imaging 3: 59–64

Grootendorst A F, Van Wilgenberg M G M, Last P H J M et al 1988 Albumin abuse in intensive care. Intensive Care Medicine 14: 554–557

Haupt M T, Gilbert E M, Carlson R W 1985 Fluid loading increases oxygen consumption in septic patients with lactic acidosis. American Review of Respiratory Disease 131: 912–916

Heffner J, Sahn S, Repine J E 1987 The role of platelets in the adult respiratory distress syndrome. American Review of Respiratory Disease 135: 482–492

Hunter D N, Morgan C J, Evans T W 1990 The use of radionucleotide techniques in the assessment of alveolar capillary membrane permeability on the ICU. Intensive Care Medicine 16: 363–371

Hwang T L, Huong S L, Chen M F 1990 Effects of intravenous fat emulsions on respiratory failure. Chest 97: 934–938

Keogh B F, Evans T W, Morgan C J 1990 Improved oxygenation with ultra high frequency jet ventilation in adult respiratory distress syndrome. Eur Respir J 3 (supp 10): 62s

Kreuzfelder E, Joka T Keinecke H et al 1988 Adult respiratory distress syndrome as a specific manifestation of a general permeability defect in trauma patients. Am Rev Respir Dis 137: 95–99

Lachmann B 1989 Animal models and clinical pilot studies of surfactant replacement in adult respiratory distress syndrome. European Respiration Journal (suppl 3): 98s–103s

Lain D C, Di Benedetto R, Morris S C et al 1989 Pressure controlled inverse ratio ventilation as a method to reduce peak inspiratory pressure and provide adequate ventilation and oxygenation. Chest 95: 1081–1088

McCormack D G, Barnes P J, Evans T W 1990 Platelet activating factor and hypoxic pulmonary vasoconstriction in the pig. Critical Care Medicine (in press)

Meadows D, Edwards J D, Wilkins R G et al 1988 Reversal of intractable shock with nor-epinephrine therapy. Critical Care Medicine 16: 663–666

Melot C, Lejune P, Leeman M et al 1989 Prostacyclin El in the adult respiratory distress syndrome. American Review of Respiratory Disease 132: 495–489

Montgomery A B, Stager M A, Carrico C J et al 1985 Causes of mortality in patients with the adult respiratory distress syndrome. American Review of Respiratory Disease 132: 485–489

Morgan J M, McCormack D J, Griffiths M J D et al 1990 Adenosine as a selective pulmonary vasodilator. Circulation 18: 1398–1401

Murray V F, Mathay M A, Luce J M et al 1988 Pulmonary perspectives: An expanded definition of the adult respiratory distress syndrome. American Review of Respiratory Disease 138: 720–723

Pepe P E, Hudson L D, Carrico C J 1984 Early application of positive end expiratory pressure in patients at risk for the adult respiratory distress syndrome. New England Journal of Medicine 311: 281–286

Peterson C W, Baier H 1983 Incidence of pulmonary barotrauma in a medical ICU. Critical Care Medicine 13: 786–791

Radermacher P, Santak B, Wust H J 1990 Prostacyclin and right ventricular function in patients with pulmonary hypertension associated with ARDS. Intensive Care Medicine 16: 227–232

Rashkin M C, Bosken C, Baughman R P 1984 Oxygen delivery in critically ill patients: relationship to lactate and survival. International Critical Care Digest 4: 37–39

Reilly J M, Cunnion R E, Burch-Whitman C et al 1989 A circulating myocardial depressant substance is associated with cardiac dysfunction and peripheral hypoperfusion (lacticacidaemia) in patients with septic shock. Chest 95: 1072–1080

Rinaldo J E, Heyman S J 1990 ARDS: A multisystem disease with pulmonary manifestations. Critical Care Report 1: 174–188

Rocker G M, Pearson D, Wiseman M S et al 1989 Diagnostic criteria for ARDS: A time for change. Lancet i: 120–123

Rouby J J, Fusciardi J, Bourgain J L 1983 High frequency jet ventilation in post operative respiratory failure: Determinants of oxygenation. Anaesthesiology 59: 281–287

Schumacker P T, Cain S M 1987 The concept of critical oxygen delivery. Intensive Care Medicine 13: 223–229

Seidenfield J J, Pohl D F, Bell R C et al 1986 Incidence, site and outcome of infection in patients with the adult respiratory distress syndrome. American Review of Respiratory Disease 134: 12–16

Shibutani K, Komatsu T, Kubal K et al 1983 Critical level of oxygen delivery in anaesthetised man. Critical Care Medicine 11: 640–643

Shoemaker W C, Appel P L, Kran H B 1988 Haemodynamic and oxygen transport effects of dobutamine in critically ill general surgical patients. Critical Care Medicine 14: 1032–1037

Shoemaker W C, Kram H B, Appel P L 1990 Therapy of shock based on pathophysiology, monitoring and outcome prediction. Critical Care Medicine 18: S19–S25

Sibbald W J, Short A I K, Warshawski F J et al 1985 Thermal dye measurements of Starling forces and extravascular lung water in adult respiratory distress syndrome. Chest 87: 585–592

Suter P M, Fairly H B, Isenberg M D 1975 Optimum end-expiratory pressure in patients with acute respiratory failure. New England Journal of Medicine 292: 284–289

Svenningsen S, Nesse O, Finsen V et al 1987 Prevention of the fat embolism syndrome in patients with femoral fractures: Immediate or delayed operative fixation. Annales Chirurgiae et Gynaecologiae 76: 163–166

Tate R M, Repine J E 1983 Neutrophils and the adult respiratory distress syndrome. American Review of Respiratory Disease 128: 552–559

Teboul J L, Zapol W M, Brun-Buisson C et al 1989 A comparison of pulmonary artery occlusion pressure and left ventricular end diastolic pressure during mechanical ventilation with PEEP in patients with severe ARDS. Anaesthesiology 70: 261–266

Ten Centre Study Group 1987 Ten centre trial of artificial surfactant (artificial lung expanding compound) in very premature babies. British Medical Journal 294: 991–996

Tharratt R S, Allen R P, Albertson T E 1988 Pressure controlled inverse ratio ventilation in severe adult respiratory failure. Chest 94: 755–762

Tighe D, Moss R, Hynd J et al 1990 Pretreatment with pentoxifylline improves the hemodynamic and histologic changes and decreases neutrophil adhesiveness in a pig fecal peritonitis model. Critical Care Medicine 18: 184–189

Unertl K E, Lenhart F-P, Ruckdeschel G 1990 Selective gut decontamination in ventilated patients. In: Update in intensive care and emergency medicine, vol 10. Springer, Berlin, pp 32–39

Vincent J L, Roman A, De Bacher D et al 1990 Oxygen uptake/supply dependency: Effects of short term dobutamine infusion. American Review of Respiratory Disease 142: 2–7

Zapol W, Snider M T 1977 Pulmonary hypertension in severe acute respiratory failure. New England Journal of Medicine 296: 476–480

Zapol W M, Snider M T, Hill J T et al 1979a Extracorporeal membrane oxygenation in severe acute respiratory failure: A randomized prospective study. Journal of the American Medical Association 242: 2193–2196

Zapol W M, Trelstad R L, Coffey J W et al 1979b Pulmonary fibrosis in severe acute respiratory failure. American Review of Respiratory Disease 119: 547–554

2

Non-invasive ventilation

M. W. Elliott   J. Moxham

The clinical use of a machine to maintain ventilation artificially was first described in 1928 when Drinker and McKhann successfully ventilated an 8-year-old girl with polio, using an iron lung (Drinker & Shaw 1929, Drinker 1931). Over the next few decades large numbers of patients with respiratory failure due to polio were successfully treated during the acute phase of the illness. Approximately 10% of these patients needed long-term ventilatory support and this was often continued in the patient's home. During a particularly severe epidemic in Copenhagen from 1951 to 1953 there were insufficient negative pressure devices available for those requiring artificial ventilation. Of necessity endotracheal intubation and positive pressure ventilation were tried and found to be effective and safe for prolonged treatment of patients in respiratory failure. Following the advent of an effective vaccine and the almost complete disappearance of polio from the developed world, the focus of attention for artificial ventilation shifted from patients with neuromuscular disease to those with primary disease of the lungs, requiring relatively short periods of ventilatory assistance. Control of the upper airway and more effective ventilation have made endotracheal intubation and positive pressure ventilation the modality of choice in these conditions. Increasingly sophisticated ventilators and monitoring equipment allow patients with major multisystem disease to be successfully treated on intensive care units. However, intubation and positive pressure ventilation are not without hazard, particularly for patients with chronic respiratory disease, and once initiated it may be difficult for the patient to resume spontaneous ventilation. In addition considerable medical and nursing care are required and ventilation, even following tracheostomy, is not easily continued at home. Therefore there has been a resurgence of interest in non-invasive methods of artificially maintaining ventilation, suitable for use in hospital and at home.

TECHNIQUES

EXTERNAL NEGATIVE PRESSURE DEVICES

With these devices a negative pressure is applied externally and results in a a fall in pressure within the thorax and gas flow into the lungs. The most effective device is the tank ventilator, which encloses the whole body with no restriction to the expansion of chest and abdomen. There may be problems in achieving an adequate seal around the neck and, although ports allow access to the patient, routine nursing care is difficult. All patients require help closing the tank and adjusting the neck seals. Patients with severe deformity may be uncomfortable lying in the supine position for long periods. The size and expense of tank ventilators make them unsuitable for wide-scale home use and in-hospital use is limited to specialist units.

Simpler, less expensive devices, such as cuirass and jacket ventilators, enclosing only the thorax and abdomen, have been developed but at the cost of some loss in efficiency (Kinnear & Shneerson 1985). Modern cuirasses comprise a single shell with padded edges which fits over the patient's chest and abdomen anteriorly. Optimal sealing of the cuirass, with adequate room for expansion, is best achieved by making a custom-built shell for each patient, but leakage and friction at pressure points may still be a problem (Brown et al 1985). Jacket respirators, e.g. the pneumosuit or Tunnicliffe jacket, overcome some of the problems of leakage by enclosing the patient's trunk in an airtight garment tied around the arms, neck and waist. An anterior shell and a back plate prevent collapse of the jacket during the negative pressure phase.

Both cuirasses and jackets are relatively inefficient, particularly when the impedance to inflation is high, and may not be able to maintain adequate ventilation. When effective ventilation can be achieved in the patient with stable chronic respiratory failure the extra load imposed by an acute exacerbation may necessitate tank ventilation or intermittent positive pressure ventilation (IPPV). Compared to the tank these devices are portable but the equipment is cumbersome and uncomfortable when compared with other methods of non-invasive ventilation. Most patients can fit the equipment themselves and are therefore less dependent on others than with the tank.

Accentuation or development of upper airway collapse, preventing effective ventilation, may occur with all negative pressure devices (Splaingard et al 1982, Simonds & Branthwaite 1985). The problem may be lessened by the use of protryptiline (Simonds et al 1986), a tracheostomy (Splaingard et al 1982), patient-triggered pumps or nasal continuous positive airway pressure (CPAP) (Goldstein et al 1987) (see below).

CONTINUOUS POSITIVE AIRWAY PRESSURE

A continuous positive pressure is delivered either by a portable compressor or from a flow generator, in conjunction with a high-pressure gas source. Confusion between CPAP and nasal intermittent positive pressure ventilation (NIPPV) has arisen because both can be used with a nasal mask and both are used at home for sleep-related disturbances of breathing. However, CPAP is only effective if the patient is breathing spontaneously, and it cannot provide ventilation if the patient becomes apnoeic. It reduces the work of breathing either by increasing functional residual capacity (FRC), so moving the patient onto a more beneficial part of the pressure–volume curve, or by acting as an inspiratory agonist (Katz 1984, Branson et al 1985). When used with a nasal mask low pressures, 5–10 cmH$_2$O, are effective in splinting the upper airway and prevent upper airway obstruction in patients with obstructive sleep apnoea (OSA) (Sullivan et al 1983).

POSITIVE PRESSURE VENTILATION

Intermittent or continuous positive pressure can be applied to the lungs via the mouth, nose or through a tracheostomy.

Ventilation via the mouth using a mouth-piece is only suitable for short periods, and weak patients may not be able to hold the device in position or maintain an effective seal. A tracheostomy allows continuous or nocturnal assisted ventilation and permits efficient suctioning of secretions. If aspiration of pharyngeal secretions is a problem a cuffed tube is necessary; however, the system is closed and spontaneous breaths are not possible in the event of ventilator failure or incoordination between the patient's respiratory efforts and machine-imposed breaths. The cuff must be deflated or a speaking tube inserted by day, to permit speech. Uncuffed tubes allow spontaneous breathing in the event of incoordination between the ventilator and the patient or ventilator failure, and permit speech. However, the major disadvantage is the morbidity and occasional mortality associated with a tracheostomy (Stauffer et al 1981). Potential complications include tracheal stenosis and dilatation, haemorrhage, tracheo-oesophageal fistula and obstruction of the tracheostomy tube by granulation tissue. In addition the upper airway is an important barrier to the ingress of pathogens and warms and humidifies inspired air. If it is bypassed humidification of the inspired gas is necessary and respiratory infections become more likely.

More recently the use of a well-fitting nasal mask has been described (Braun 1987, Kerby et al 1987, Ellis et al 1987) (Fig. 2.1). The nasal route obviates the need for cumbersome external equipment, is effective and well tolerated and maintains the patency of the upper airway. The mask is held in position over the nose by a series of straps and can easily be applied and removed by the patient, though those with weak upper limbs may require some assistance. The mask may need to be applied quite tightly to the face to maintain a good seal, leading to some soreness, particularly over the bridge of the nose. Most patients quickly get used to this and it does not usually cause difficulties during long-term domiciliary use. Pressure damage may be a problem in the acute situation, when patients are ventilated for much of the day, but excessive soreness and tissue breakdown can be prevented by the use of sticking plaster or other cushioning material over pressure areas. The barrier material used to protect the skin around abdominal stomata, e.g. granuflex, can be particularly effective. A wide range of commercially manufactured masks are now available and an

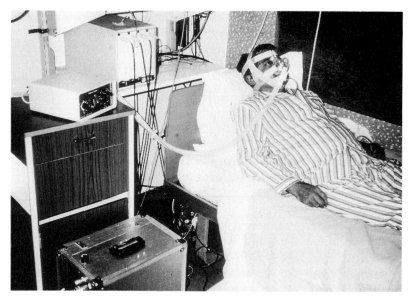

Fig. 2.1   A patient receiving intermittent positive pressure ventilation by nasal mask. The ventilator control unit is situated on the bedside table and the compressor on the floor. The nasal mask is held in position by commercially available straps and fastenings.

adequate seal can usually be achieved, but occasionally custom-built masks may be necessary. The Adams circuit, utilizing nasal plugs, is a recent innovation and may be more effective or be better tolerated in some patients. Leaks from the mouth, particularly during sleep, can be reduced by a chin strap. If control of hypoxia is inadequate, low-flow oxygen can easily be added through a port in the mask.

During nasal ventilation the oesophagus is not protected and this technique is not suitable for patients with bulbar weakness, at risk from aspiration. In all patients uncomfortable gastric distension may be a problem, particularly when high inflation pressures are used, but this is lessened by good coordination between spontaneous efforts by the patient and machine-imposed breaths.

Positive pressure can be delivered to the nose and the mouth using a full face mask, but many patients find this claustrophobic. It is difficult to achieve a satisfactory seal and, as with a tracheostomy, if ventilation is inadequate the patient cannot take spontaneous breaths.

Ventilators

Volume preset ventilators

A fixed tidal volume is delivered, and to achieve this the inflation pressure may vary from breath to breath. The technical specification of the machine used is important. It should be able to coordinate with the patient's spontaneous breaths and provide full ventilation in the event of apnoea. This requires a sensitive trigger with a short response time if the work of breathing is not to be increased during triggered ventilation. A more subtle difficulty exists if the patient breathes with the machine and continues to inspire after gas flow from the machine has ceased or a further inspiratory effort is detected before significant expiratory flow has occurred. If the machine is triggered into another inspiratory phase before the lungs have been allowed to empty, successive breaths summate and cause hyperinflation. This can be prevented if there is a closed window in the respiratory cycle, during which the trigger is refractory.

Ventilators used in the UK include the Lifecare PLV 100 (UK supplier: Medicaid Ltd, Hook Lane, Pagham, Sussex), the Monnal D (UK supplier: Deva Medical Electronics Ltd, 8 Jensen Court, Runcorn, Cheshire) and the Bromptonpac (Pneupac Ltd, Crescent Road, Luton, Beds). There are differences between the machines but all are volume-limited flow generators designed for home use. They are capable of delivering large minute volumes, which is important if the nasal route is used, since tidal volumes up to twice those used in intubated patients are necessary to compensate for leaks around the mask and through the mouth and to ventilate the increased dead space of the nasopharynx. All are portable and the Lifecare PLV 100 can be powered by batteries for short periods.

Pressure-limited ventilators

Inspiration is terminated when a preset pressure is reached and tidal volume may vary from breath to breath. These ventilators are therefore not suitable for use when the impedance to inflation is high, since adequate tidal volumes cannot be achieved. The principal models available in the UK are the Bird (M and IE Dentsply, Sowton Industrial Estate, Exeter) and the Bennett (UK supplier: Puritan Bennett, 152–176 Great South West Road, Hounslow, Middlesex). Both have sensitive triggers which ensure coordination of the patient's inspiratory efforts with the inspiratory phase of the ventilator.

A more recent innovation is the BIPAP (bi-level positive airway pressure), a development of CPAP. The level of pressure is set independently for inspiration and expiration, with the inspiratory pressure always greater than the expiratory. Different machines are available, the most sophisticated of which can be used in four different modes. The spontaneous (S) mode requires the patient to initiate every breath whereas using the timed (T) mode the machine cycles between inspiration and expiration based upon preset timing intervals independent of patient effort. In the S/T mode the machine cycles between inspiration and expiration in response to patient triggering but will automatically cycle into inspiration if the patient fails to initiate a breath. Alternatively it can be used to provide CPAP. An important advantage is that the machine automatically compensates for leaks through the mouth or around the mask and automatically adjusts the trigger threshold. Preliminary experience has shown that it provides effective ventilation and control of nocturnal hypoventilation in some patients (Simonds 1990). Limitations are that current machines are only capable of generating pressures up to 20 cmH_2O and may not be effective when the impedance to inflation is high.

OTHER TECHNIQUES

Gravity and/or passive descent of the diaphragm have been utilized to promote ventilation using positive pressure applied to the chest or abdomen or a rocking bed (Kinnear & Shneerson 1985). Compression of the chest during expiration, so that the end-expiratory volume is below FRC, utilizes the passive elastic recoil of the chest as an inspiratory agonist. Alternatively, compression of the abdomen when the patient is upright forces the diaphragm upwards, which then descends passively with gravity as the pressure is released. The pneumobelt is the most familiar of such devices and has the advantage that it is easily applied by the patient and is relatively compact. It is very inefficient when used alone, but can be used to augment ventilation using other devices, though this may be uncomfortable. With a rocking bed the patient is tilted between the horizontal position and approximately 60° head up. The equipment is cumbersome and some patients find it hard to adjust to the rocking motion. It has the advantage that the patient is free to change position but it is inefficient and has only been used successfully in selected patients with central hypoventilation and neuromuscular disorders.

Electrical stimulation of the phrenic nerves by implanted electrodes has been used in patients with high cervical cord lesions and in those with central hypoventilation (Glenn & Sairenji 1985, Lozewicz et al 1981). Normal phrenic nerve function, good diaphragm contractility and an intact rib cage are prerequisites (Moxham & Potter 1988). Successful pacing may be difficult to achieve and it may need to be combined with some other form of ventilatory assistance, but a major advantage is the possibility of independence from the ventilator in dependent patients. If used for long periods without a break the diaphragm may become fatigued, and over time the phrenic nerve may be damaged and become fibrosed.

CONDITIONS EFFECTIVELY MANAGED USING NON-INVASIVE VENTILATION

RESPIRATORY FAILURE IN PATIENTS WITH A PRIMARY ABNORMALITY OF THE VENTILATORY APPARATUS
(Table 2.1)

Idiopathic and congenital kyphoscoliosis (Bergofsky et al 1959)

Patients at the greatest risk of developing cardiorespiratory failure are those

Table 2.1 Diseases causing respiratory failure

1. Abnormalities of the spine
   Kyphoscoliosis
     Idiopathic
     Congenital
     Paralytic
       Previous polio
       Spinal muscular atrophy
       Syringomyelia
       Motor neurone disease

2. Abnormalities of the ribs and costotransverse joints
     Thoracoplasty
     Ankylosing spondylitis
     Congenital abnormalities

3. Neuromuscular disease affecting respiratory muscles
   — Anterior horn cell
       Poliomyelitis
       Syringomyelia
       Motor neurone disease
       Spinal muscular atrophy
   — Nerve roots (C3–C5) Guillain–Barré syndrome
   — Phrenic nerve
       Tumour
       Trauma (cardiac surgery)
       Peripheral neuropathy
       — Congenital, e.g. Charcot–Marie–Tooth
       — Acquired, e.g. neuralgic amyotrophy, carcinomatous, hypothyroidism
   — Neuromuscular junction
       Myasthenia gravis
       Lambert–Eaton syndrome
   — Muscle
       Muscular dystrophies
       Myopathies — acid maltase deficiency and nemaline myopathy
       Polymyositis

4. Abnormalities of central ventilatory control
   — Congenital
   — Acquired — associated with other neurological disease
   Obesity hypoventilation syndrome

who have an early onset of their scoliosis, usually before the age of 7 (Branthwaite 1986). An early onset probably impairs lung maturation and development. Other risk factors are vital capacity less than 50% predicted, patients with a high dorsal curve and marked twisting of the spine (Branthwaite 1986). Spinal surgery, performed to stabilize the spine, may occasionally improve respiratory function but often leads to fusion of the costotransverse joints, with resulting deterioration in lung volumes and earlier onset of respiratory failure. When assessing lung function in patients with marked skeletal deformity, predicted values should be based on the span rather than height since the latter may be misleading. Respiratory failure usually occurs in the 4th and 5th decades, and its occurrence earlier, or in patients without known risk factors, should prompt a search for co-existent cardiac and neuromuscular conditions.

Paralytic kyphoscoliosis

The commonest cause is previous poliomyelitis (Howard et al 1988, Lane et al 1974) but other conditions (Table 2.1) may also be responsible. The age at onset of respiratory failure is variable and depends upon the relative contribution of chest wall deformity and muscle weakness. The identification of a paralytic element to the kyphoscoliosis is important since treatment of an underlying neurological disorder, e.g. decompression of a syrinx, may occasionally obviate the need for respiratory support, and an understanding of the natural history of a particular neurological condition may affect the decision to institute ventilation.

Neuromuscular disorders

Respiratory muscle involvement may be a presenting feature, e.g. in acid maltase deficiency or nemaline myopathy, or may be part of a more obviously generalized process (Braun et al 1983, Mier et al 1990). Ventilatory failure as a consequence of respiratory muscle weakness is unlikely if the maximal inspiratory mouth pressure (PI_{max}) is greater than 30 cmH$_2$O. However, if there is coexisting lung, cardiac or chest wall disease lesser degrees of weakness may be critical. In cases of doubt specialist assessment including measurement of oesophageal and transdiaphragmatic pressures are important. Patients with 'pure' diaphragm paralysis, e.g. following phrenic nerve trauma at cardiac surgery or as a sequel to neuralgic amyotrophy, are unlikely to develop chronic respiratory failure or nocturnal hypoventilation (Laroche et al 1988). The finding of abnormal ventilation in such patients should prompt a search for coexistent lung or cardiac disease or suggests that additional respiratory muscles are involved.

Myasthenia gravis may present a particular difficulty. Ventilatory failure may be the presenting feature (Mier et al 1990) but more commonly occurs relatively late in the disease. Respiratory muscle involvement is best diagnosed by measuring the change in mouth pressures or sniff oesophageal pressure following intravenous edrophonium (Tensilon) (Mier-Jedrzejowicz et al 1988). Measurement of the change in vital capacity, though simpler, is less sensitive for respiratory muscle involvement.

Other causes of chest wall deformity (Bergofsky 1979, Sawicka et al 1983)

Patients with a past history of tuberculosis and either a thoracoplasty or severe pleural thickening may develop respiratory failure. Pleural thickening due to asbestos exposure is rarely sufficient to cause respiratory failure. Thoracic kyphosis, unless very severe, and pectus excavatum do not cause respiratory failure but abnormalities of the ribs, particularly fusion of the costotransverse joints, may cause severe lung restriction and ventilatory failure.

Treatment

Unlike respiratory failure in patients with abnormal lungs where hypoxia can usually be corrected simply by increasing the inspired oxygen tension, increasing the fraction of inspired oxygen (FiO_2) in patients with severe chest wall deformity and neuromuscular disease almost always leads to symptomatic hypercapnia (Spencer 1977). The primary indication for assisted ventilation is to correct abnormal arterial blood gas tensions, and this can be done effectively using positive or negative pressure devices (see below). However, the onset of overt respiratory failure is often preceded by many months of gradual symptomatic decline with increasing breathlessness, lethargy, daytime sleepiness, early morning headaches and disturbed sleep (Spencer 1977, Branthwaite 1990). Recurrent episodes of 'bronchitis' are common which are seldom due to infection but are a consequence of mucosal engorgement because of right heart failure and pulmonary venous congestion (Branthwaite 1990).

Nocturnal hypoventilation is important in the pathogenesis of these symptoms (Mezon et al 1980). Daytime symptoms and signs reflect the abnormalities occurring during sleep. Wakefulness is an important stimulus to breathe and mild hypoventilation during sleep (Stradling et al 1985, Douglas et al 1982), with an increment in CO_2 tension of up to 6 mmHg, is normal; however, in patients with little respiratory reserve marked oxygen desaturation and hypercapnia can occur. Respiratory reserve is reduced in scoliosis because the work of breathing is increased by deformity and rigidity of the chest wall and reduced lung compliance (Bergofsky 1979). Rapid eye movement (REM) sleep may be associated with severe hypoxaemia and worsening hypercapnia (Sawicka & Branthwaite 1987), since during this phase of sleep there is a profound loss of postural muscle activity and ventilation is largely dependent upon diaphragm function (Remmers 1981). Diaphragm contractility may be impaired as part of a primary neuromuscular disease or by poor perfusion, hypoxia and hypercapnia caused by inadequate ventilation, or its action compromised because of working at a mechanical disadvantage as a consequence of an abnormal chest configuration (Jardim et al 1981, Juan et al 1984, Smith et al 1987). In these patients, mainly dependent upon accessory muscles, the diaphragm alone is unable to maintain ventilation during REM sleep and marked oxygen desaturation and hypercapnia occur. Repeated episodes of hypoxaemia and hypercapnia during sleep lead, in time, to the development of daytime respiratory failure, pulmonary hypertension, right heart failure and death (Guilleminault et al 1981).

Correction of nocturnal hypoventilation improves daytime symptoms and respiratory failure (Goldstein et al 1987, Ellis et al 1987, Hoeppner et al 1984, Carroll & Branthwaite 1988, Heckmatt et al 1990). Its early detection and treatment is the cornerstone of the management of the respiratory consequences of these disorders. Since the onset of nocturnal hypoventilation is often insidious, patients at high risk should be seen frequently, with regular monitoring of lung function and daytime arterial blood gas tensions. Residual volume and total lung capacity may fall before there is a significant reduction in vital capacity, reflecting the tendency to atelectasis in these patients (Branthwaite 1990). Nocturnal hypoventilation becomes increasingly likely when the FVC falls below 1 litre, and although arterial blood gas tensions during the day may be normal an unexplained rise in the base excess suggests the presence of significant nocturnal hypoventilation (Branthwaite 1990). If nocturnal ventilatory failure is suspected oxygen saturation and carbon dioxide tensions should be monitored overnight. There are no clear-cut guidelines of when nocturnal hypoventilation should be treated, but the presence of symptoms, pulmonary hypertension or cardiorespiratory failure are indications for therapy.

Not all patients require mechanical ventilatory support. For those in whom nocturnal hypoventilation is mild and associated with minimal derangement of daytime blood gas tensions all that may be required is a reduction of the time spent in REM sleep. This can be achieved with small doses (e.g. 10 mg at night) of the non-sedative tricyclic drug protriptyline (Simonds et al 1986) (Fig. 2.2). Daytime arterial blood gas tensions frequently improve and many patients remain in good health for long periods, though anticholinergic side effects may be troublesome. Some patients, with more severe respiratory failure, require an initial period of in-hospital assisted ventilation to restore arterial blood gas tensions and bicarbonate concentration, and the improvement can then be maintained

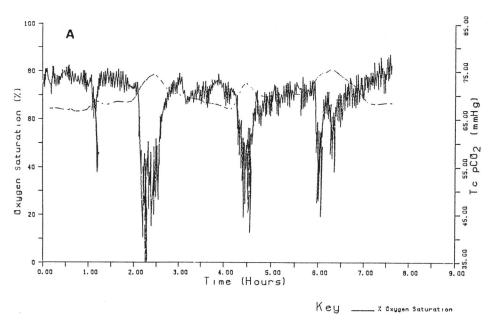

Fig. 2.2 See p. 34 for caption.

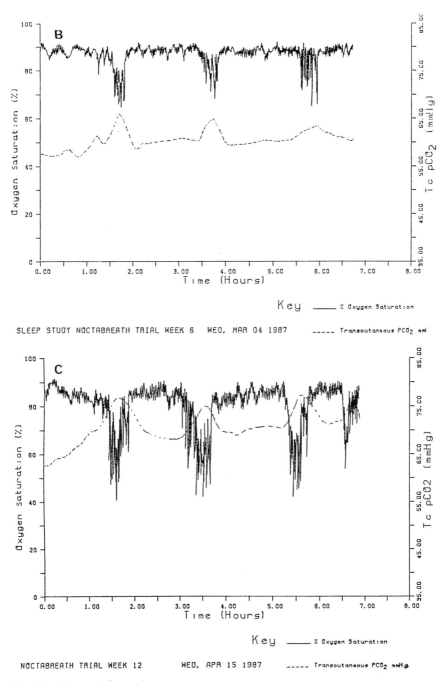

SLEEP STUDY NOCTABREATH TRIAL WEEK 6   WED, MAR 04 1987

NOCTABREATH TRIAL WEEK 12   WED, APR 15 1987

Fig. 2.2 See p. 34 for caption.

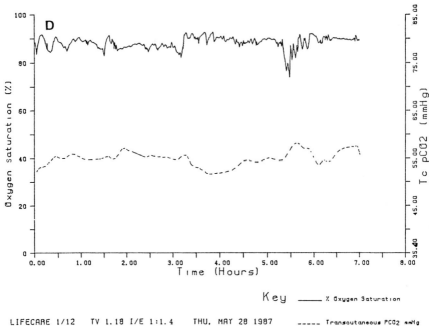

LIFECARE 1/12   TV 1.18 I/E 1:1.4   THU. MAY 28 1987   ----- Transcutaneous PCO2 mmHg

Fig. 2.2 A series of overnight studies of oxygen saturation (SaO_2, left axis) and transcutaneous carbon dioxide ($TcCO_2$, right axis) in a patient with kyphoscoliosis and mild COPD. **A** Breathing air spontaneously. Note the low baseline saturation at the start of the night and the episodes of profound desaturation associated with a rise in the $TcCO_2$. **B** After 6 weeks' treatment with protriptyline 10 mg nocte. Improved baseline SaO_2 and $TcCO_2$ and with less marked desaturation during the night. **C** After 12 weeks daytime blood gas tensions and the sleep study were deteriorating and NIPPV was started. **D** After 4 weeks home NIPPV. Note the improved overnight SaO_2 and the markedly lower $TcCO_2$. Benefit in this patient from protriptyline was short lived, but some patients maintain the improvement indefinitely. (Sleep studies courtesy of Dr A. K. Simonds.)

by protriptyline. If these measures are not successful domiciliary nocturnal ventilation should be considered. When possible a gradual escalation of treatment is helpful since domiciliary ventilation is a large undertaking for the patient, requiring considerable motivation, and the perception that it is beneficial is an important ingredient in determining a successful outcome. A number of centres have reported the efficacy of domiciliary nocturnal ventilation in improving quality of life, daytime blood gas tensions and reducing the requirement for hospitalization, with some series reporting experience over two decades (Leger et al 1989, Robert et al 1982, Sawicka et al 1988, Splaingard et al 1983, Robert et al 1983).

Possible explanations for the improved arterial blood gas tensions by day include a restoration of central drive, resting of fatigued respiratory muscles and improvements in chest wall or pulmonary compliance, improved sleep and the resolution of cardiac failure. Both negative pressure and positive pressure devices have been used effectively at home in these patients but NIPPV is now the preferred option in most centres.

In patients with respiratory impairment because of slowly progressive neuromuscular disease, nocturnal ventilation is easy to apply and highly effective. Indeed, because the impedance to inflation is low, marked hypocapnia may occur overnight. When the patient resumes spontaneous ventilation his own ventilatory apparatus is unable to match that of the machine, and as carbon dioxide rises the patient experiences severe respiratory discomfort. This can easily be documented by overnight monitoring of oxygen and carbon dioxide and corrected by reducing the ventilator settings. The place of ventilatory assistance in patients with rapidly progressive neuromuscular disease, e.g. motor neurone disease, is less clear but at least some patients, in whom respiratory symptoms predominate, may benefit, albeit for a limited time (Sivak & Streib 1980). A summary of the investigation and treatment of patients with neuromuscular disease and scoliosis is shown in Fig. 2.3.

A small number of patients who are unable to breathe adequately at any time, e.g. following high cervical cord injury, require continuous ventilatory assistance. This is best provided by positive pressure ventilation via tracheostomy. A battery power source allows some mobility, though the

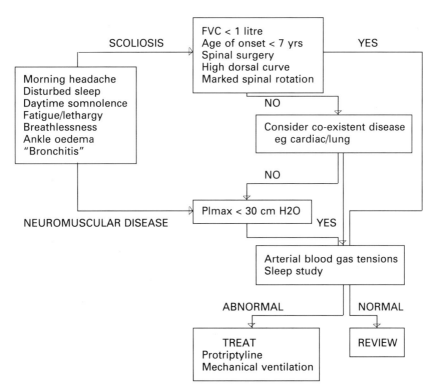

Fig. 2.3   An algorithm for the management of patients with chest wall deformity or neuromuscular disease at risk of developing respiratory failure.

constraints of size limit this to a few hours. Ventilator malfunction or power failure can be catastrophic and suitable arrangements must be made to cater for this possibility.

CHRONIC RESPIRATORY FAILURE IN PATIENTS WITH A PRIMARY ABNORMALITY OF THE LUNGS

The effectiveness of assisted ventilation in patients unable to maintain adequate ventilation because of an inadequate respiratory muscle pump is not surprising. A logical case can also be made for the extension of this technique to patients with lung disease characterized by alveolar hypoventilation. Most work has been done in patients with chronic obstructive pulmonary disease (COPD). These patients, particularly those hypercapnic by day, hypoventilate during sleep and this is particularly marked during REM sleep (Hudgel et al 1983, Douglas & Flenley 1990, Wynne et al 1979) (Figs 2.4 and 2.5). A consequence of nocturnal hypoventilation is renal retention of bicarbonate ions to buffer the acidosis consequent upon transient increases in arterial carbon dioxide tension ($PaCO_2$) leading to a reduction in central ventilatory drive. Finally the respiratory muscles are at a mechanical disadvantage because of hyperinflation (Sharp et al 1974) and this has led to the proposal that ventilatory failure occurs, in part, because of chronic fatigue of the respiratory muscles (Macklem 1986).

Various trials of 'in hospital' assisted ventilation in patients with COPD have been reported (Guttierez et al 1988, Cropp & Dimarco 1987, Ambrosino et al 1990, Celli et al 1989, Sczno et al 1990). These have usually used negative pressure devices and the period of ventilation has ranged from 3–6 hours for 3 days to 8 hours once weekly for several months. Improvements have been seen in arterial blood gas tensions during spontaneous breathing, maximal inspiratory and expiratory mouth pressures, transdiaphragmatic pressures, quality of life and exercise capacity. The focus of treatment has been rest of purportedly chronically fatigued muscles, and the improvements, particularly in mouth pressures, have been cited as evidence for the effectiveness of respiratory muscle rest therapy and the existence of chronic fatigue. In many studies respiratory muscle rest has not been documented and patients have often been recruited during recovery from an acute exacerbation. Individual patients have shown large improvements in arterial blood gas tensions despite decreases in mouth pressures, and the contributions of changes in load and central drive have not been evaluated. Further data are needed before the large-scale application of respiratory muscle rest therapy is justified.

The use of negative pressure devices at home in patients with COPD has been largely unsuccessful (Zibrak et al 1988, Celli et al 1989). The main reasons have been an inability to sleep with the equipment because of discomfort and upper airway collapse. The large-scale intermittent positive pressure breathing (IPPB) trial, using pressure-limited ventilators and mouth-pieces during the day, showed no advantage over conventional therapy (IPPB trial group 1983). Patients were asked to use IPPB for 10 minutes three times a day, during which time they inhaled a β-agonist generated by the machine's nebulizer. Despite this relatively undemanding treatment

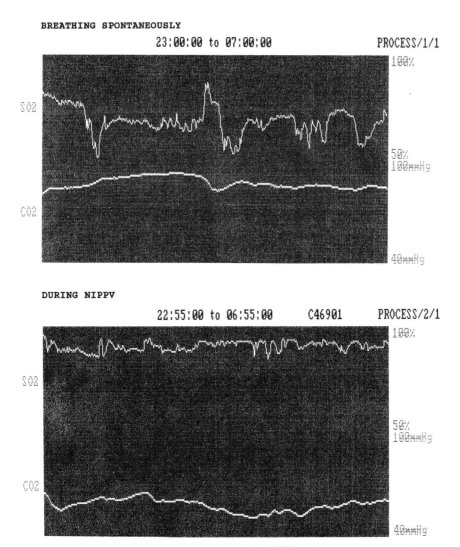

Fig. 2.4 Overnight monitoring of oxygen saturation (SaO$_2$) and transcutaneous carbon dioxide (TcCO$_2$) in a patient with COPD. The top panel is with the patient breathing air spontaneously. SaO$_2$ is very low throughout most of the night, with dips down to 50% and with a high TcCO$_2$, which rises further through the night. The improvement in SaO$_2$ and TcCO$_2$ occurring in the middle of the night is due to the patient waking for nebulized bronchodilators. The bottom panel shows much improved oxygenation and a much lower TcCO$_2$ during NIPPV with air.

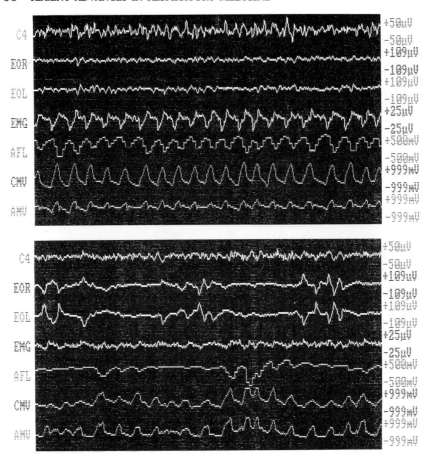

Fig. 2.5   One-minute epochs from the study in Fig. 2.4. The top panel shows regular chest (CMV) and abdominal (AMV) wall motion and oronasal airflow (AFL) during stage 2 sleep. The lower panel shows REM sleep with marked hypoventilation associated with bursts of eye movement.

schedule only 50% of the patients complied with the protocol. Nocturnal positive pressure ventilation via a tracheostomy has shown no additional benefit to domiciliary oxygen therapy (Robert et al 1983) and the necessity for a tracheostomy is a significant disincentive to this approach. The study of Carroll and Branthwaite using NIPPV included four patients with COPD and the outcome in these patients was less successful than in those with extrapulmonary restrictive disease. Possible reasons included technical deficiencies of the ventilators used, particularly the ability to trigger in response to spontaneous respiratory efforts. A further study is in progress using a purpose-built ventilator specifically in COPD, and initial results are encouraging. Nocturnal hypoventilation was successfully controlled and 7 out of 12 patients recruited were still using the equipment after 12 months. Important ingredients for success included adequate patient education,

motivation and pre-existing symptomatic sleep disturbance unrelieved by oxygen therapy (Elliott et al 1990a, b). The further place of NIPPV in the management of COPD needs to be clarified by formal comparison with long-term domiciliary oxygen therapy. However, it would seem reasonable to offer this therapy to selected motivated hypercapnic patients deteriorating despite domiciliary oxygen.

PATIENTS FAILING TO WEAN FROM MECHANICAL VENTILATION

Negative pressure devices have been used successfully in encouraging a return to spontaneous ventilation, but the necessary equipment is not widely available. The patient can be extubated in the tank and receive immediate ventilatory support. NIPPV has the advantage that it can be used on any intensive care unit. Most modern ventilators are suitable and the only additional equipment necessary are the nasal mask and head straps. A proportion of patients may require long-term domiciliary assistance, particularly those with pre-existing chronic respiratory failure or those who have sustained a lasting insult to the ventilatory apparatus, e.g. damage to the phrenic nerves during cardiac surgery.

NON-INVASIVE VENTILATION IN ACUTE RESPIRATORY FAILURE

The specialized knowledge and technical back-up needed to institute negative pressure ventilation mean that this can only be performed in specialized centres (Corrado et al 1990). By contrast the technique of NIPPV is easily learnt by anyone with some knowledge of ventilators and can be performed in any hospital. It is the treatment of choice in most patients with acute or chronic respiratory failure due to chest wall deformity and neuromuscular disease and can be applied to selected patients with lung disease (Elliott et al 1990c). It is usually possible to improve oxygenation without worsening hypercapnia. Advantages are that intensive care unit admission and intubation can be avoided. Haemodynamic instability is unusual because anaesthetic drugs are not necessary and changes, particularly in $PaCO_2$, occur more slowly than with intubation and IPPV. The patient is able to participate with physiotherapy and to take part in discussions about future management, and nutrition can be maintained. The place of NIPPV in patients presenting to hospital with acute respiratory failure due to COPD, but not necessarily severe enough to warrant intubation and ventilation, is currently the subject of a multicentre trial.

COST AND LOGISTICS OF NON-INVASIVE VENTILATION

The financial implications of non-invasive ventilation need to be addressed as larger numbers of patients are recruited. The average cost of a suitable machine for non-invasive positive pressure ventilation is approximately £3000 and the ongoing maintenance costs about £500 a year. At first sight this is high, but compared to the costs of in-patient or intensive care admission or to that of other established treatments capable of restoring and maintaining well-being, e.g. haemodialysis, it is relatively inexpensive. With provision of domiciliary ventilation many patients return to gainful employment and can participate in normal family life (Robert et al 1983, Goldstein et al 1987, Carroll & Branthwaite 1988). Most patients can be acclimatized to the technique in less than a week in hospital. After-care is important, with a programme of regular machine servicing, provision of an effective emergency breakdown service and replacement of masks and head gear, which need renewing approximately 6-monthly.

The number of patients in the UK requiring some form of domiciliary ventilatory support is unknown and an important priority is the establishment of a national register. If the concept of home ventilation is to be developed further the UK needs to follow the lead of other nations, which have developed a comprehensive system of home respiratory care (Goldberg 1986, Branthwaite 1989). Most respiratory physicians are unlikely to see many patients requiring domiciliary ventilation, and the setting up of regional centres, along the lines of haemodialysis units, seems a logical step. The regional centre can provide the necessary medical, nursing and physiotherapy expertise and facilities for monitoring gas exchange during sleep. Mutual support between patients can be facilitated and centralized administration and bulk buying help to keep costs down.

CONCLUSIONS

The history of ventilatory assistance started with non-invasive ventilation and the wheel has now come full circle. The ability to ventilate patients using positive pressure and the nasal route is an important development in respiratory medicine. The simple nature of the equipment, its portability and efficiency make it, for most patients, the preferred method for providing ventilation in the home. NIPPV, which is feasible in any hospital, is a useful addition to the armamentarium of thoracic and intensive care physicians. The challenges for the future are the development of a comprehensive programme of home care and research into the mechanisms of benefit. Further improvements of mask design and ventilator specification will widen the potential applications of this exciting technique.

KEY POINTS FOR CLINICAL PRACTICE

1. A high index of suspicion for nocturnal hypoventilation is important in 'at risk' patients.

2. Non-specific symptoms suggestive of nocturnal hypoventilation or abnormal arterial blood gas tensions are indications for overnight monitoring of oxygen and carbon dioxide tensions.

3. Non-invasive ventilation should be considered in patients presenting with acute respiratory failure, in whom the morbidity and mortality associated with intubation is known to be high.

4. Patients requiring domiciliary ventilation should be managed in specialized centres.

REFERENCES

Ambrosino N, Montagna T, Nava S et al 1990 Short term effect of intermittent negative pressure ventilation in COPD patients with respiratory failure. European Respiratory Journal 3: 502–508
Bergofsky E H 1979 Respiratory failure in disorders of the thoracic cage. American Review of Respiratory Disease 119: 643–669
Bergofsky E H, Turino G M, Fishman A P 1959 Cardiorespiratory failure in kyphoscoliosis. Medicine (Baltimore) 38: 263–317
Branson R D, Hurst J M, DeHaven C B 1985 Mask CPAP: State of the art. Respiratory Care 30: 846–857
Branthwaite M A 1986 Cardiorespiratory consequences of unfused idiopathic scoloiosis. British Journal of Diseases of the Chest 80: 360–369
Branthwaite M A 1989 Mechanical ventilation at home. British Medical Journal 298: 1409
Branthwaite M A 1990 Ventilatory support in the home. Proceedings of the Royal Society of Physicians of Edinburgh 20: 262–265
Braun N M T 1987 Nocturnal ventilation: A new method. American Review of Respiratory Disease 135: 523–524
Braun N M T, Arora N S, Rochester D F 1983 Respiratory muscle and pulmonary function in polymyositis and other proximal myopathies. Thorax 38: 616–623
Brown L, Kinnear W J M, Sergeant K A et al 1985 Artificial ventilation by external negative pressure: A method for making cuirass shells. Physiotheraphy 71: 181–183
Carroll N, Branthwaite M A 1988 Control of nocturnal hypoventilation by nasal intermittent positive pressure ventilation. Thorax 43: 349–353
Celli B, Lee H, Criner G et al 1989 Controlled trial of external negative pressure ventilation in patients with severe chronic airflow limitation. American Review of Respiratory Disease 140: 1251–1256
Corrado A, Bruscoli G, De Paola E et al 1990 Respiratory muscle insufficiency in acute respiratory failure of subjects with severe COPD: Treatment with intermittent negative pressure ventilation. European Respiration Journal 3: 644–648
Cropp A, Dimarco A F 1987 Effects of intermittent negative pressure ventilation on respiratory muscle function in patients with severe chronic obstructive pulmonary disease. American Review of Respiratory Disease 135: 1056–1061
Douglas N J, Flenley D C 1990 Breathing during sleep in patients with obstructive lung disease. American Review of Respiratory Disease 141: 1055–1070
Douglas N J, White D P, Pickett C K et al 1982 Respiration during sleep in normal man. Thorax 37: 840–844
Drinker P 1931 Prolonged administration of artificial respiration. Lancet ii: 1186–1188
Drinker P, Shaw L A 1929 An apparatus for the prolonged administration of artificial ventilation. Journal of Clinical Investigation 7: 229
Elliott M W, Carroll M A, Wedzicha J A, Branthwaite M A 1990a Nasal positive pressure ventilation can be used successfully at home to control nocturnal hypoventilation in COPD. American Review of Respiratory Disease 141: A322 (abstract)
Elliott M W, Carroll M, Wedzicha J A, Branthwaite M A 1990b Domiciliary nasal positive pressure ventilation in chronic obstructive pulmonary disease (COPD). Thorax 45: 793
Elliott M W, Steven M H, Phillips G D, Branthwaite M A 1990c Non-invasive mechanical ventilation for acute respiratory failure. British Medical Journal 300: 358–360

Ellis E R, Bye P T B, Bruderer J W, Sullivan C E 1987 Treatment of respiratory failure during sleep in patients with neuromuscular disease. American Review of Respiratory Disease 135: 148–152

Glenn W W L, Sairenji H 1985 Diaphragm pacing in the treatment of chronic ventilatory insufficiency. In: Roussos C, Macklem P T (eds) The thorax: Lung biology in health and disease. Marcel Dekker, New York, pp 1407–1440

Goldberg A L 1986 Home care for life-supported persons: Is a national approach the answer? Chest 90: 744–748

Goldstein R S, Moloyiu N, Skrastins R et al 1987 Reversal of sleep-induced hypoventilation and chronic respiratory failure by nocturnal negative pressure ventilation in patients with restrictive ventilatory impairment. American Review of Respiratory Disease 135: 1049–1055

Guilleminault C, Kurlan G, Winkle R et al 1981 Severe kyphoscoliosis, breathing and sleep: The Quasimodo syndrome during sleep. Chest 79: 626–630

Guttierez M, Beroiza T, Contreras G et al 1988 Weekly cuirass ventilation improves blood gases and inspiratory muscle strength in patients with chronic airflow limitation and hypercarbia. American Review of Respiratory Disease 138: 617–623

Heckmatt J Z, Loh L, Dubowitz V 1990 Night-time ventilation in neuromuscular disease. Lancet 335: 579–582

Hoeppner V H, Cockcroft D W, Dosman J A, Cotton D J 1984 Nighttime ventilation improves respiratory failure in secondary kyphoscoliosis. American Review of Respiratory Disease 129: 240–243

Howard R S, Wiles C M, Spencer G T 1988 The late sequelae of poliomyelitis. Quarterly Journal of Medicine 66: 219–232

Hudgel D W, Martin R J, Capeheart M et al 1983 Contribution of hypoventilation to sleep oxygen desaturation in chronic obstructive pulmonary disease. Journal of Applied Physiology 55: 669–677

Intermittent positive pressure breathing trial group 1983 Intermittent positive pressure breathing therapy of chronic obstructive pulmonary disease. Annals of Internal Medicine 99: 612–620

Jardim J, Farkas G, Prefant C et al 1981 The failing inspiratory muscles under normoxic and hypoxic conditions. American Review of Respiratory Disease 124: 274–279

Juan G, Calverley P, Talamo C et al 1984 Effect of carbon dioxide on diaphragmatic function in human beings. New England Journal of Medicine 310: 874–879

Katz J A 1984 PEEP and CPAP in perioperative respiratory care. Respiratory Care 29: 614–624

Kerby G R, Mayer L S, Pingleton S K 1987 Nocturnal positive pressure ventilation via nasal mask. American Review of Respiratory Disease 135: 738–740

Kinnear W J M, Shneerson J M 1985 Assisted ventilation at home: Is it worth considering? British Journal of Diseases of the Chest 79: 313–351

Lane D J, Hazelman B, Nichols P J R 1974 Late onset respiratory failure in patients with poliomyelitis. Quarterly Journal of Medicine 172: 551–568

Laroche C M, Carroll N, Moxham J, Green M 1988 The clinical significance of severe isolated diaphragmatic weakness. American Review of Respiratory Disease 138: 862–865

Leger P, Jennequin J, Gerard M et al 1989 Home positive pressure ventilation via nasal mask for patients with neuromusculoskeletal disorders. European Respiratory Journal 2 (suppl 7): 640s–645s

Lozewicz S, Potter D, Costello J et al 1981 Diaphragm pacing in ventilatory failure. British Medical Journal 283: 1015–1016

Macklem P T 1986 The clinical relevance of respiratory muscle research: J Burns Amberson Lecture. American Review of Respiratory Disease 134: 812–815

Mezon B L, West P, Israels J, Kryger M 1980 Sleep breathing abnormalities in kyphoscoliosis. American Review of Respiratory Disease 122: 617–621

Mier A, Laroche C, Green M 1990 Unsuspected myasthenia gravis presenting as respiratory failure. Thorax 45: 422–423

Mier-Jedrzejowicz A K, Brophy C, Green M 1988 Respiratory muscle function in myasthenia gravis. American Review of Respiratory Disease 138: 876–873

Moxham J, Potter D 1988 Diaphragm pacing. Thorax 43: 161–162

Remmers J E 1981 Effects of sleep on control of breathing. International Review of Physiology 23: 111–147

Robert D, Gerard M, Leger P et al 1982 Long term intermittent positive pressure ventilation at home of patients with end stage chronic respiratory insufficiency. Chest 82: 249–250

Robert D, Gerard M, Leger P et al 1983 Domiciliary ventilation by tracheostomy for chronic respiratory failure. Revue Française des Maladies Respiratoires 11: 923–936

Sawicka E H, Branthwaite M A 1987 Respiration during sleep in kyphoscoliosis. Thorax 42: 801–808

Sawicka E H, Branthwaite M A, Spencer G T 1983 Respiratory failure after thoracoplasty: Treatment by intermittent negative pressure ventilation. Thorax 38: 433–435

Sawicka E H, Loh L, Branthwaite M A 1988 Domiciliary ventilatory support: An analysis of outcome. Thorax 43: 31–35

Scano G, Gigliotti F, Duranti R M et al 1990 Changes in ventilatory muscle function with negative pressure ventilation in COPD. Chest 97: 322–327

Sharp J T, Danon J, Druz W S et al 1974 Respiratory muscle function in patients with chronic obstructive lung disease: Its relationship to disability and to respiratory failure. American Review of Respiratory Disease 110: 154–167

Simonds A K 1990 Personal communication.

Simonds A K, Branthwaite M A 1985 Efficiency of negative pressure ventilatory equipment. Thorax 40: 213 (abstract)

Simonds A K, Parker R A, Sawicka E H, Branthwaite M A 1986 Protriptyline for nocturnal hypoventilation in restrictive chest wall disease. Thorax 41: 586–590

Sivak E D, Streib E W 1980 Management of hypoventilation in motor neurone disease presenting with respiratory insufficiency. Annals of Neurology 7: 188–191

Smith P E M, Calverley P M A, Edwards R H T et al 1987 Practical problems in the respiratory care of patients with muscular dystrophy. New England Journal of Medicine 316: 1197–1205

Spencer G 1977 Respiratory insufficiency in scoliosis: Clinical management and home care. In: Zorab P (ed) Scoliosis. Academic Press, London, pp 315–338

Splaingard M L, Jefferson L S, Harrison G M 1982 Survival of patients with respiratory insufficiency secondary to neuromuscular disease treated at home with negative pressure ventilation. American Review of Respiratory Disease 125: 139 (abstract)

Splaingard M L, Frates F C, Harrison G M et al 1983 Home positive pressure ventilation: Twenty years experience. Chest 84: 376–382

Stauffer J L, Olson D E, Retty T L 1981 Complications and consequences of endotracheal intubation and tracheostomy. American Journal of Medicine 70: 65–75

Stradling J R, Chadwick G A, Frew A J 1985 Changes in ventilation and its components in normal subjects during sleep. Thorax 40: 364–370

Sullivan C E, Berthon Jones M, Issa F G 1983 Reversal of obstructive sleep apnoea by continuous positive airway pressure applied through the nares. Lancet i: 862–865

Wynne J W, Block J, Hemenway J et al 1979 Disordered breathing and oxygen desaturation during sleep in patients with chronic obstructive lung disease (COPD). American Journal of Medicine 66: 573–579

Zibrak J D, Hill N S, Federman E C et al 1988 Evaluation of intermittent long term negative-pressure ventilation in patients with severe COPD. American Review of Respiratory Disease 138: 1515–1518

3

New concepts in asthma and the implications for therapy

P. J. Barnes

In recent years our views about asthma have changed rather strikingly. In the past asthma was viewed simply as allergen-induced mast cell degranulation, resulting in the release of mediators such as histamine and leukotrienes which contracted airway smooth muscle (Fig. 3.1). It is now becoming clear that asthma is a chronic inflammatory disease involving many interacting cells which release a whole variety of inflammatory mediators that activate several target cells in the airway, resulting in bronchoconstriction, microvascular leakage and oedema, mucus hypersecretion and stimulation of neural reflexes (Barnes 1989a). Although there may be several ways of initiating this inflammatory response, the type of inflammation which is characteristic of asthma is typified by infiltration with eosinophils and T-lymphocytes and by shedding of airway epithelial cells. These inflammatory changes may be seen even in the mildest of asthmatic patients (Laitinen et al 1985, Beasley et al 1989, Jeffery et al

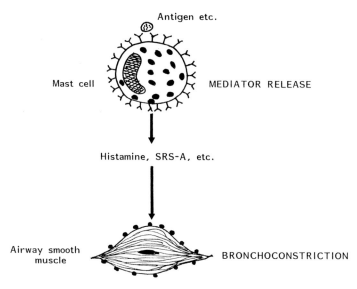

Fig. 3.1 The old view of asthma emphasized mast cells and airway smooth muscle contraction.

1989) and there is compelling evidence that inflammation underlies the phenomenon of airway hyperresponsiveness, which is the hallmark of asthma (Chung 1986, O'Byrne et al 1987). The precise relationship between airway inflammation, bronchial hyperresponsiveness and symptoms is still not certain, and the commonly used tests of bronchial responsiveness, such as histamine or methacholine challenge, may not relate as closely to clinical symptoms in individual patients as had been suspected (Fig. 3.2). This may be because inflammation may *directly* lead to symptoms, perhaps by activating sensitized sensory nerve endings.

There are no satisfactory animal models of asthma and previous 'models' have proved to be very misleading, since the information provided was not applicable to either normal or asthmatic humans, although animals may be useful in modelling certain aspects of the asthmatic process (Smith 1989).

INFLAMMATORY CELLS

Mast cells

For many years mast cells were assumed to play a pivotal role in the pathogenesis of asthma, but recent evidence argues strongly against a critical role for mast cells in either the late response which follows allergen challenge, or in airway hyperresponsiveness. Sodium cromoglycate was shown to stabilize rat peritoneal mast cells, and this seemed a reasonable explanation for its ability to prevent early and late bronchoconstrictor responses to allergen. More potent mast cell stabilizers which were later developed (more than thirty such compounds have now gone into clinical trial) failed to show any useful effect in clinical asthma and, although some of these drugs protected against early responses to allergen, they failed to prevent late responses and did not reduce subsequent airway hyper-responsiveness. In addition, β_2-agonists, such as salbutamol and terbutaline, which are potent stabilizers of human mast cells (Church & Hiroi 1987), fail to inhibit late responses or to reduce bronchial hyperresponsiveness (Cockroft & Murdock 1987, Kraan et al 1988, Kerrebijn et al 1987).

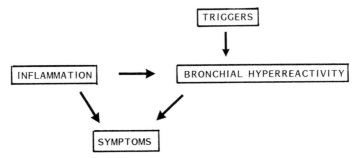

Fig. 3.2 Interrelationship between airway inflammation, bronchial hyperresponsiveness and symptoms in asthma. (From Barnes et al 1989a.)

Furthermore, corticosteroids, which have no effect on the early response when given in a single dose, are highly effective in preventing the late response and in preventing the subsequent increase in bronchial responsiveness, have no apparent direct action on human lung mast cells (Schleimer et al 1983). Thus, although mast cells are involved in immediate responses to allergens (and probably other acute challenges, such as exercise and fog), they are less likely to play a critical role in airway hyperresponsiveness and chronic asthma. Attention has now focused on other inflammatory cells which may play a role in the chronic inflammation of asthmatic airways. Indeed, asthma is likely to involve several inflammatory cells which interact in a complex manner, not yet fully understood (Fig. 3.3).

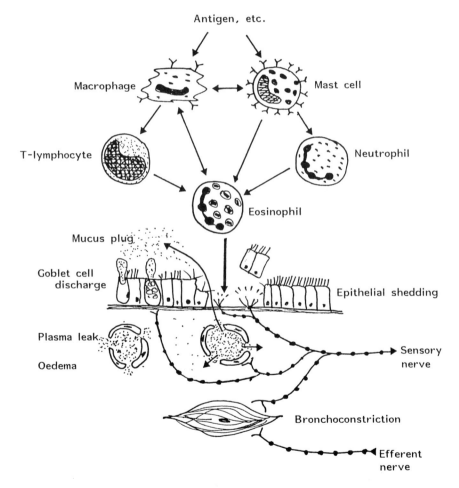

Fig. 3.3 The new view of asthma includes several inflammatory cells which interact in a complex manner and release multiple inflammatory mediators which act on various target cells of the airways to produce the characteristic pathophysiology of asthma.

Macrophages

The recent demonstration that macrophages may be activated by immunoglobulin E (IgE)-dependent mechanisms has suggested that these cells, which are present in the airway lumen and submucosa, may be involved in asthmatic inflammation (Joseph et al 1983). Indeed, macrophages from asthmatics release increased amounts of mediators, such as thromboxane, prostaglandins and platelet-activating factor (PAF). Allergen challenge results in a marked increase in the numbers of macrophages obtained by bronchoalveolar lavage (Metzger et al 1987). In contrast to mast cells, release of mediators from alveolar macrophages is inhibited by corticosteroids (Fuller et al 1986b), but not by β-agonists (Fuller et al 1988).

Eosinophils

Eosinophil infiltration is a characteristic feature of asthmatic airways and differentiates asthma from other inflammatory conditions of the airway. Indeed, asthma might more accurately be termed 'chronic eosinophilic bronchitis'. Allergen inhalation results in a marked increase in eosinophils in bronchoalveolar lavage fluid at the time of the late reaction (de Monchy et al 1985, Metzger et al 1987), and there is a close relationship between eosinophil counts in peripheral blood or bronchial lavage and airway hyperresponsiveness (Taylor & Luksza 1987, Wardlaw et al 1988). Eosinophils release a variety of mediators, including leukotriene C4, PAF, and also basic proteins such as major basic protein and eosinophil cationic protein, which are toxic to airway epithelium (Gleich et al 1988). Eosinophils cause marked epithelial shedding when stimulated to degranulate (Yukawa et al 1990a). Activated eosinophils in the airway lumen may thus lead to the epithelial shedding, which is so characteristic of asthma (Laitinen et al 1985, Beasley et al 1989). Eosinophils are sensitive to corticosteroids, with a reduction in tissue and peripheral eosinophils, although they are not very effectively inhibited by β-agonists or theophylline (Yukawa et al 1989, 1990b, Barnes et al 1990). Presumably inhaled steroids, by clearing airway eosinophils, allow epithelial cells to recover and regenerate.

The mechanisms by which circulating eosinophils are selectively recruited into the airways of asthmatic patients are of critical importance in understanding asthma pathophysiology. Such mechanisms involve adhesion of eosinophils to vascular endothelial cells in the airway circulation, their migration into the submucosa and their subsequent activation (Fig. 3.4). The role of individual cytokines and mediators in orchestrating these responses has yet to be clarified.

Adhesion of eosinophils involves the expression of specific glycoprotein molecules on the surface of eosinophils (integrins) and the expression of molecules such as intercellular adhesion molecule-1 (ICAM-1) on vascular

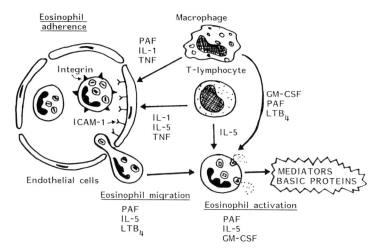

Fig. 3.4 Mechanisms of eosinophilic inflammation.

endothelial cells. A recent study has demonstrated that, in sensitized monkeys, an antibody directed at ICAM-1 markedly inhibits eosinophil accumulation in the airways after allergen exposure and also blocks the accompanying hyperresponsiveness (Wegner et al 1990).

Neutrophils

While neutrophil infiltration is found in some animal models of asthma (O'Byrne et al 1987), the role of neutrophils in human asthma is less certain. In some experimental studies neutrophil infiltration apparently *follows* the development of increased responsiveness, and neutrophil depletion with cyclophosphamide does not affect its development. Neutrophils are found in the airways of chronic bronchitics and patients with bronchiectasis who do not have the degree of airway hyperresponsiveness found in asthma. The neutrophil may, however, be involved in certain types of asthma (such as certain occupational asthmas) and may interact with other inflammatory cells.

T-lymphocytes

Although the role of B-lymphocytes in the synthesis of IgE is well established, it is only recently that a role for T-lymphocytes in asthma has been recognized. CD4+ (helper) lymphocytes are prominent in asthmatic biopsies (Jeffery et al 1989), and it seems likely that these lymphocytes may be involved in orchestrating the chronic inflammatory response in asthma through the secretion of a specific pattern of lymphokines, such as interleukin-5 (IL-5), which may be important in recruitment and maintenance of eosinophils in airway tissues (Yamaguchi et al 1988).

Airway epithelial cells

Airway epithelial damage may be a critical feature of airway hyper-responsiveness and may explain how several different mechanisms, such as ozone exposure, virus infection and allergen exposure, can lead to its development, since all these stimuli may lead to epithelial disruption. Epithelial damage may contribute to airway hyperresponsiveness in a number of ways:

1. Epithelial shedding may remove a protective barrier, thus allowing allergens and inhaled chemicals to reach cells in the submucosa which would normally be protected.
2. Recent studies have demonstrated that mechanical removal of epithelial cells in vitro results in increased responsiveness of airway smooth muscle to several spasmogens (Cuss & Barnes 1987), and suggests that epithelial cells may release a relaxant factor analogous to endothelial-derived relaxant factor in blood vessels. Damage of epithelium would thus remove the protective effect of this relaxant factor, leading to exaggerated bronchoconstrictor responses.
3. Epithelial damage will also expose sensory nerve endings, which may be activated by inflammatory mediators, leading to inflammation via an axon reflex mechanism (Barnes 1986b).
4. Epithelial cells themselves may release inflammatory mediators, such as lipoxygenase products, which are chemotactic for inflammatory cells (Hunter et al 1985).
5. Epithelial cells may produce enzymes which degrade inflammatory mediators. Thus, airway epithelial cells strongly express the ectoenzyme neutral endopeptidase which degrades bioactive peptides such as bradykinin and substance P.

Platelets

Various abnormalities of platelet function have been described in asthma, and animal studies suggest that platelets may be implicated in certain types of bronchial hyperresponsiveness (Barnes et al 1988a). Platelets may release a variety of mediators, such as serotonin, thromboxane and lipoxygenase products, and may also be activated by IgE-dependent mechanisms, although their role in asthma has not yet been determined.

INFLAMMATORY MEDIATORS

Many different mediators have been implicated in asthma and they may have a variety of effects on the airways which could account for the pathological features of asthma (Barnes et al 1988a). Mediators such as histamine, prostaglandins and leukotrienes contract airway smooth muscle, increase microvascular leakage, increase airway mucus secretion and attract other inflammatory cells (Table 3.1). It is therefore possible that interaction between inflammatory mediators might account for airway hyper-responsiveness.

Eicosanoids

Prostaglandin D_2 (PGD_2), via activation of thromboxane receptors, potentiates the bronchoconstrictor response to both histamine and methacholine in asthmatic subjects (Fuller et al 1986a). This sensitizing effect is transient and therefore unlikely to account for the sustained airway hyperresponsiveness of asthma. The sulphidopeptide leukotrienes LTC_4, LTD_4 and LTE_4 are potent constrictors of human airways, and both LTD_4 and LTE_4 increase airway responsiveness (Arm et al 1988, Kaye & Smith 1990) and may play an important role in asthma (Drazen & Austen 1987). The recent development of potent specific antagonists such as ICI 204,219 (Smith et al 1990) may soon reveal the contribution of these mediators to asthma. LTB_4 is chemotactic for neutrophils but, since neutrophil infiltration is less characteristic than eosinophil infiltration in asthmatic airways, it is not a primary candidate, although it may be synergistic with other mediators. Inhalation of LTB_4 does not appear to have any effect on airway responsiveness in normal subjects (Black et al 1989).

Platelet-activating factor

A mediator which has attracted considerable attention recently is PAF, since it mimics many of the features of asthma (Barnes et al 1988b). PAF,

Table 3.1 Effects of inflammatory mediators implicated in asthma

Mediator	Broncho-constriction	Airway secretion	Microvas-cular leakage	Chemotaxis	Bronchial hyperres-ponsive-ness
Histamine	+	+	+	+	−
Prostaglandins D_2, $F_{2\alpha}$	++	+	?	?	+
Prostaglandin E_2	−	+	−	+	−
Thromboxane	++	?	−	±	+
Leukotriene B_4	−	−	±	++	±
Leukotriene C_4, D_4, E_4	++	++	++	?	±
Platelet-activating factor	++	+	++	++	++
Bradykinin	+	+	++	−	−
Adenosine	+	?	?	?	−
Substance P	+	++	++	±	−
Neurokinin A	++	?	+	−	−
Complement fragments	+	+	+	++	−
Serotonin	±	?	+	−	−
Oxygen radicals	+	?	+	?	−

++, pronounced effect; +, moderate effect; ±; uncertain effect; ?, information not available; −, no effect.

like prostaglandins and leukotrienes, is formed by the action of phospholipase A_2 on membrane phospholipids and may be produced by several of the inflammatory cells implicated in asthma, such as macrophages, eosinophils and neutrophils. Inhaled PAF causes not only bronchoconstriction, but also a small increase in bronchial responsiveness in normal subjects, whereas lyso-PAF is without effect (Cuss et al 1986, Kaye & Smith 1990). The maximal effect is observed 3 days after inhalation and may persist for up to 4 weeks. Similar changes have also been observed in asthmatic subjects, although they do not achieve statistical significance because of the greater variability in airway reactivity (Chung & Barnes 1989). Because PAF is rapidly inactivated in vivo, this suggests that it must trigger a chain of inflammatory events which lead to the very prolonged increase in bronchial responsiveness. Perhaps this is related to its interaction with eosinophils. PAF, like antigen, stimulates selective accumulation of eosinophils in lung (Denjean et al 1988) and in the skin of atopic subjects (Henocq & Vargaftig 1988). PAF increases the adhesion of eosinophils to endothelial surfaces (Kimani et al 1988), which may be the initial step in eosinophil recruitment into tissues. Since eosinophils themselves are a rich source of PAF they can attract further eosinophils and there is the potential for a continued inflammatory reaction. PAF is very effective in stimulating human eosinophils to release basic proteins (Kroegel et al 1989), which may result in epithelial damage. PAF also causes an increased expression of IgE receptors on eosinophils (Moqbel et al 1990) and increased expression of low-affinity IgE receptors on monocytes (Paul-Eugene et al 1990).

PAF has other properties which may be relevant in asthma. In animals, PAF is a potent inducer of airway microvascular leak, being the most potent mediator so far described (Evans et al 1987). Several specific antagonists of PAF are available and their use in models of disease should now make it possible to evaluate the role of endogenous PAF. One such antagonist, ginkgolide B, is derived from the leaves of *Ginkgo biloba*, an ancient Chinese herbal remedy for chest disease. Ginkgolides, given orally, inhibit PAF-induced platelet aggregation and wheal and flare responses in the skin (Chung et al 1987), and may therefore be useful in determining the role of PAF in allergic disease. These PAF antagonists also inhibit the late response to allergen in human skin, which is characterized by eosinophil infiltration (Roberts et al 1988). Whether PAF antagonists have a role in human asthma is not yet known, but the development of several potent drugs in this class should soon answer this question. Clinical trials of the most potent antagonist, WEB 2086, which is effective in inhibiting ex vivo platelet aggregation in response to PAF after oral administration (Adamus et al 1988), are currently underway.

It is clear that no single mediator can be responsible for all the features of asthma, and it is likely that multiple mediators constitute an 'inflammatory soup' which may vary from patient to patient, depending on the relative state of activation of the different inflammatory cells (Fig. 3.5).

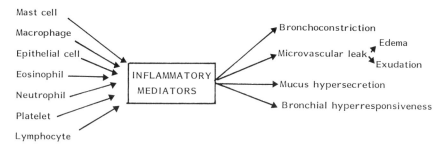

Fig. 3.5 Mediators may be released from a variety of inflammatory cells in asthma and make up a 'soup' of variable composition which then leads to the characteristic pathology of asthma.

Cytokines

Cytokines are peptide mediators released from inflammatory cells which are important in signalling between cells and may determine the type and duration of an inflammatory response. The role of the many cytokines implicated in asthma is uncertain but it seems likely that IL-3 may be important in persistence of mast cells in tissues, IL-4 may be important in programming certain B-lymphocytes to produce IgE, and IL-5 from T-lymphocytes may be involved in eosinophil recruitment, survival in tissues and priming (Yamaguchi et al 1988) (Fig. 3.6). Macrophages may also

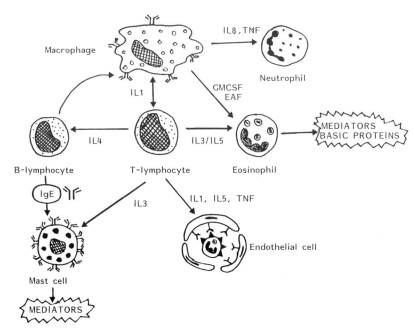

Fig. 3.6 The role of cytokines in asthma is increasingly recognized.

release a variety of cytokines, including granulocyte–macrophage colony-stimulating factor (GM-CSF) which may also contribute to eosinophil survival and priming. Mast cells may also synthesize cytokines (GM-CSF, IL-3 and IL-5) under certain conditions (Burd et al 1989).

Although there are no effective blockers of cytokine receptors, studies with monoclonal antibodies directed at specific cytokines are beginning to reveal the roles of individual cytokines in inflammation. Thus, an antibody against IL-5 inhibits eosinophilia in mice infested with worms (Coffman et al 1989).

MICROVASCULAR LEAKAGE

Microvascular leakage is an essential component of the inflammatory response, and many of the inflammatory mediators implicated in asthma produce this leakage. There is good evidence for microvascular leakage in asthma (Persson 1988, Chung et al 1990); this may result in plasma extravasation (which may inhibit mucociliary clearance and lead to the formation of plasma-derived mediators such as bradykinin) and mucosal oedema (which may contribute to airway hyperresponsiveness for geometric reasons). Therapeutic measures to reduce microvascular leakage may therefore be beneficial in asthma. In experimental animals neither i.v. β-agonists nor theophylline are very effective, whereas adrenaline (acting via α_1-receptors) and corticosteroids inhibit mediator-induced leak (Boschetto et al 1989, Boschetto et al 1990). Since both adrenaline and corticosteroids reduce airway microvascular leak it is possible that the circadian fall in these hormones at night may lead to increased mediator release and increased leakage, thus contributing to nocturnal exacerbations of asthma (Barnes 1988a).

NEURAL MECHANISMS

There has recently been a renewal of interest in neural mechanisms in asthma. In the nineteenth century, asthma was explained by neural mechanisms. Autonomic nervous control of the airways is complex, for in addition to classical cholinergic and adrenergic mechanisms non-adrenergic non-cholinergic nerves and several neuropeptides have been identified in the respiratory tract (Barnes 1986a). Several studies have investigated the possibility that defects in autonomic control may contribute to bronchial hyperresponsiveness and asthma, and abnormalities of autonomic function, such as enhanced cholinergic and α-adrenergic responses or reduced β-adrenergic responses, have been proposed (Barnes 1986c). Current thinking suggests that these abnormalities are likely to be secondary to the disease, rather than primary defects. It is possible that airway inflammation may interact with autonomic control by several mechanisms (Barnes 1986a).

Cholinergic mechanisms

Inflammatory mediators may stimulate cholinergic reflex bronchoconstriction by activation of afferent nerve endings, and may also facilitate release of acetylcholine from motor nerve endings in the airway. Anticholinergic drugs have not proved to be very effective in asthma, which has suggested that cholinergic mechanisms are not important. The recent demonstration of cholinergic autoreceptors in cholinergic nerves in human airways, which inhibit acetylcholine release (Barnes 1990c), means that this must be re-evaluated, since such currently available anticholinergic drugs may not be effective against reflex cholinergic bronchoconstriction since they will enhance acetylcholine release.

Neuropeptides

Many different neuropeptides have now been identified in human airways which have potent effects on airway function (Barnes 1987), and it is possible that these peptides might be implicated in asthma. Vasoactive intestinal peptide is a potent relaxant of human airways in vitro and is a cotransmitter of acetylcholine in cholinergic nerves. If this peptide is degraded more rapidly in asthma by enzymes released from inflammatory cells, this could reduce its 'braking' effect on cholinergic nerves, leading to exaggerated bronchoconstrictor responses (Barnes 1987). Sensory neuropeptides such as substance P, neurokinin A and calcitonin gene-related peptide may also be involved in asthma, since these peptides could be released by a local axon reflex (Barnes 1986b). Damage to airway epithelium may expose unmyelinated C-fibre afferent nerves, which may be sensitized by the action of mediators such as prostaglandins and cytokines, then triggered by mediators such as bradykinin (Fuller et al 1987). This might release sensory neuropeptides from collaterals of these nerves, resulting in broncho-constriction, microvascular leakage and mucus secretion. Axon reflexes, as in the skin and gut, may thus spread the inflammatory changes from areas of localized epithelial damage and so neurogenic inflammation may therefore contribute to bronchial hyperresponsiveness (Barnes 1990b). Airway epithelial cells contain an enzyme, neutral endopeptidase (enkephalinase), which rapidly breaks down substance P and neurokinin A, so epithelial shedding in asthma would greatly potentiate sensory neuropeptide effects in the airway (Frossard et al 1989, Sekizawa et al 1987).

IMPLICATIONS FOR THERAPY

Because airway obstruction in asthma involves more than spasm of airway smooth muscle, it follows that treatment must involve more than bronchodilators. β-Agonist bronchodilators not only fail to reduce bronchial hyperresponsiveness, but may even exacerbate it (Kraan et al 1985, Kerrebijn et al 1987, Vathenen et al 1988). By giving acute relief of symptoms, these drugs may therefore mask the underlying inflammatory process, and over-reliance on β-agonists may be a contributory factor to the recent increase in asthma mortality. It is important that some sort of prophylactic or anti-inflammatory therapy which reduces bronchial responsiveness is also used in the chronic treatment of asthma (Barnes 1989b).

Corticosteroids

Corticosteroids, which inhibit virtually every step in the inflammatory process, are very effective in reducing airway hyperresponsiveness in asthma (Barnes 1990a), but other drugs such as sodium cromoglycate and nedocromil sodium may also be useful. These drugs should probably be started at an earlier stage of treatment and there is a case to be made for introducing inhaled steroids, sodium cromoglycate or nedocromil sodium as the initial therapy, together with an inhaled β-agonist for symptom relief. Yet even high-dose steroid therapy is frequently unable to reduce the bronchial responsiveness and airway narrowing of asthma back to normal, suggesting that there is an irreversible component. This is most likely to be due to structural changes, such as hypertrophy of airway smooth muscle and subepithelial fibrosis (Roche et al 1989), which could result from the release of various growth factors (such as macrophage- and platelet-derived growth factors) from inflammatory cells. Although these changes cannot be reversed by therapy, it seems likely that they may be *prevented* by effective and continued suppression of the airway inflammation. Prolonged therapy with prophylactic drugs may thus prevent the later development of irreversible airflow obstruction, which may be seen in chronic asthma.

New approaches

It seems probable that there are several different types of asthma involving different mechanisms which may respond to different forms of therapy, but far more research is needed, particularly in human subjects, since animal models have proved to be so misleading in the past. There are several promising new drugs, such as leukotriene and PAF antagonists, and selective phosphodiesterase inhibitors, which may prove valuable in treating asthma in the future (Barnes 1988b), but improved understanding of how currently effective drugs work, such as steroids, sodium cromoglycate and nedocromil sodium, is also needed.

Drugs which modulate the abnormal immune response in asthma are also needed. While cyclosporin A, which inhibits certain functions of T-lymphocytes, may be useful for severe asthma, less toxic and more specific therapy that may block specific cytokines such as IL-4 and IL-5 may be the way forward in the future. It is hoped that a major research effort will lead to further understanding and reduced morbidity and mortality from asthma.

ACKNOWLEDGEMENT

I thank Madeleine Wray for kindly preparing the manuscript.

REFERENCES

Adamus W S, Heuer H, Meade C J, Frey G, Brecht H M 1988 Inhibitory effect of oral
  WEB-2086, a novel selective paf-acether antagonist on ex vivo platelet aggregation.
  European Journal of Clinical Pharmacology 35: 237–240
Arm J P, Spur B W, Lee T H 1988 The effects of inhaled leukotriene E4 on the airway
  responsiveness to histamine in subjects with asthma and normal subjects. Journal of
  Allergy and Clinical Immunology 82: 654–660
Barnes P J 1986a Neural control of human airways in health and disease. American Review
  of Respiratory Disease 134: 1289–1314
Barnes P J 1986b Asthma as an axon reflex. Lancet i: 242–245
Barnes P J 1986c Airway inflammation and automatic control. European Journal of
  Respiratory Disease 69 (suppl 147): 80–87
Barnes P J 1987 Neuropeptides in human airways: Function and clinical implications.
  American Review of Respiratory Disease 136: S77–83
Barnes P J 1988a Inflammatory mechanisms and nocturnal asthma. American Journal of
  Medicine 85: 64–70
Barnes P J 1988b The drug therapy of asthma: Directions for the 21st century. Agents and
  Actions (suppl) 23: 293–313
Barnes P J 1989a New concepts in the pathogenesis of bronchial hyperresponsiveness and
  asthma. Journal of Allergy and Clinical Immunology 83: 1013–1026
Barnes P J 1989b A new approach to asthma therapy. New England Journal of Medicine
  321: 1517–1527
Barnes P J 1990a Effect of corticosteroids on airway hyperresponsiveness. American Review
  of Respiratory Disease 140: S70–76
Barnes P J 1990b Neurogenic inflammation in airways and its modulation. Archives
  Internationales de Pharmacodynamie 303: 67-82
Barnes P J 1990c Muscarinic receptors in airways: Recent developments. Journal of
  Applied Physiology 68: 1777–1785
Barnes P J, Chung K F, Page C P 1988a Inflammatory mediators in asthma.
  Pharmacological Reviews 40: 49–84
Barnes P J, Chung K F, Page C P 1988b Platelet-activating factor as a mediator of allergic
  disease. Journal of Allergy and Clinical Immunology 81: 919–934
Barnes P J, Kroegel C, Yukawa T, Dent G, Chung K F 1990 Pharmacology of
  eosinophils. In: Kay AB (ed) Eosinophils in allergic disease. Blackwell, Oxford,
  pp 144–157
Beasley R, Roche W R, Roberts J A, Holgate S T 1989 Cellular events in the bronchi in
  mild asthma and after bronchial provocation. American Review of Respiratory Disease
  139: 806–817
Black P N, Fuller R W, Taylor G W, Barnes P J, Dollery C T 1989 Effect of inhaled
  leukotriene B4 alone and in combination with prostaglandin D2 on bronchial
  responsiveness to histamine in normal subjects. Thorax 44: 491–495
Boschetto P, Roberts N M, Rogers D F, Barnes P J 1989a Effect of anti-asthma drugs on
  microvascular leakage in guinea-pig airways. American Review of Respiratory Disease
  139: 416–421
Boschetto P, Rogers D F, Fabbri L M, Barnes P J 1991 Corticosteroid inhibition of airway
  microvascular leakage. American Review of Respiratory Disease 143: 605–609
Burd P R, Rogers H W, Gordon J R et al 1989 Interleukin 3-dependent and -independent
  mast cells stimulated with IgE and antigen express multiple cytokines. Journal of
  Experimental Medicine 170: 245–257
Chung K F 1986 Role of inflammation in the hyperreactivity of the airways in asthma.
  Thorax 41: 657–662
Chung K F, Barnes P J 1989 Effects of platelet activating factor on airway calibre, airway
  responsiveness and circulating cells in asthmatic subjects. Thorax 44: 108–115
Chung K F, Dent G, McCusker M, Guinot Ph, Page C P, Barnes P J 1987 Effect of a

ginkgolide mixture (BN 52063) in antagonising skin and platelet responses to platelet activating factor in man. Lancet i: 248–251

Chung K F, Rogers D F, Barnes P J, Evans T E 1990 The role of increased airway microvascular permeability and plasma exudation in asthma. European Respiration Journal 3: 329–337

Church M K, Hiroi J 1987 Inhibition of IgE-dependent histamine release from human dispersed lung mast cells by anti-allergic drugs and salbutamol. British Journal of Pharmacology 90: 421–429

Cockroft D W, Murdock K Y 1987 Comparative effects of inhaled salbutamol, sodium cromoglycate and beclomethasone diproprionate on allergen-induced early asthmatic responses, late asthmatic responses and increased bronchial responsiveness to histamine. Journal of Allergy and Clinical Immunology 79: 734–740

Coffman R L, Seymour B W P, Hudak S, Jackson J, Rennick D 1989 Antibody to interleukin-5 inhibits helminth-induced eosinophilia in mice. Science 245: 308–310

Cuss F M, Barnes P J 1987 Epithelial mediators. American Review of Respiratory Disease 136: S32–35

Cuss F M, Dixon C M S, Barnes P J 1986 Effects of inhaled platelet activating factor on pulmonary function and bronchial responsiveness in man. Lancet ii: 189–192

De Monchy J G R, Kauffman H F, Venge P et al 1985 Bronchoalveolar eosinophils during allergen-induced late asthmatic reactions. American Review of Respiratory Disease 131: 373–376

Denjean A, Arnoux B, Benveniste J 1988 Long-lasting effect of intratracheal administration of PAF-acether in baboons. American Review of Respiratory Disease 137: A283

Drazen J M, Austen K F 1987 Leukotrienes and airway responses. American Review of Respiratory Disease 136: 985–998

Evans T W, Chung K, Rogers D F, Barnes P J 1987 Effect of platelet-activating factor on airway vascular permeability: possible mechanisms. Journal of Applied Physiology 63: 479–484

Frossard N, Rhoden K J, Barnes P J 1989 Influence of epithelium on guinea pig airway responses to tachykinins: Role of endopeptidase and cyclooxygenase. Journal of Pharmacology and Experimental Therapeutics 248: 292–299

Fuller R W, Dixon C M S, Dollery C T, Barnes P J 1986a Prostaglandin D2 potentiates airway responses to histamine and methacholine. American Review of Respiratory Disease 133: 252–254

Fuller R W, Morris P K, Richmond R et al 1986b Immunoglobulin E-dependent stimulation of human alveolar macrophages: Significance of type I hypersensitivity. Clinical and Experimental Immunology 65: 416–426

Fuller R W, Dixon C M S, Cuss F M C, Barnes P J 1987 Bradykinin-induced bronchoconstriction in man: Mode of action. American Review of Respiratory Disease 135: 176–180

Fuller R W, O'Malley G, Baker A J, MacDermot J 1988 Human alveolvar macrophage activation: Inhibition by forskolin but not beta-adrenoceptor stimulation or phosphodiesterase inhibition. Pulmonary Pharmacology 1: 101–106

Gleich G J, Flavahan N A, Fujisawa T, Vanhoutte P M 1988 The eosinophil as a mediator of damage to respiratory epithelium: A model for bronchial hyperreactivity. Journal of Allergy and Clinical Immunology 81: 776–781

Henocq E, Vargaftig B B 1988 Skin eosinophilia in atopic patients. Journal of Allergy and Clinical Immunology 81: 691–695

Hunter J A, Finkbeiner W E, Nadel J A, Goetzl E J, Holtzman M J 1985 Predominant generation of 15-lipoxygenase metabolites of arachidonic acid by epithelial cells from human trachea. Proceedings of the National Academy of Sciences USA 82: 4633–4637

Jeffery P K, Wardlaw A J, Nelson F C, Collins J V, Kay A B 1989 Bronchial biopsies in asthma: An ultrastructural, quantitative study and correlation with hyperreactivity. American Review of Respiratory Disease 140: 1745–1753

Joseph M, Tonnel A B, Tarpier G, Capron A 1983 Involvement of immunoglobulin E in the secretory process of alveolar macrophages from asthmatic patients. Journal of Clinical Investigation 71: 221–230

Kaye M G, Smith L J 1990 Effects of inhaled leukotriene D4 and platelet activating factor on airway reactivity in normal subjects. American Review of Respiratory Disease 141: 993–997

Kerrebijn K F, von Essen-Zandvliet E E M, Neijens H J 1987 Effect of long-term treatment with inhaled corticosteroids and beta-agonists on bronchial responsiveness in asthmatic children. Journal of Allergy and Clinical Immunology 79: 653–659

Kimani G, Tonnesen M G, Henson P G 1988 Stimulation of eosinophil adherence to human vascular endothelial cells in vitro by platelet activating factor. Journal of Immunology 140: 3161–3166

Kraan J, Koeter G H, van der Mark T W, Shuiter H J, de Vries K 1985 Changes in bronchial hyperactivity given by 4 weeks of treatment with antiasthmatic drugs in patients with asthma: a comparison between bulsomide and terbutaline. Journal of Allergy and Clinical Immunology 76: 628–636

Kraan J, Koeter G H, van der Mark T W et al 1988 Dosage and time effects of inhaled budesonide on bronchial hyperreactivity. American Review of Respiratory Disease 137: 44–48

Kroegel C, Yukawa T, Dent G, Venge P, Chung K F, Barnes P J 1989 Stimulation of degranulation from human eosinophils by platelet activating factor. Journal of Immunology 142: 3518–3526

Laitinen L A, Heino M, Laitinen A, Kava T, Haahtela T 1985 Damage of the airway epithelium and bronchial reactivity in patients with asthma. American Review of Respiratory Disease 131: 599–606

Metzger W J, Zavala D, Richerson H B et al 1987 Local allergen challenge and bronchoalveolar lavage of allergic asthmatic lungs. American Review of Respiratory Disease 135: 433–440

Moqbel R, Walsh G M, Nagakura T et al 1990 The effect of platelet-activating factor on IgE binding to, and IgE-dependent biological properties of, human eosinophils. Immunology 70: 251–277

O'Byrne P M, Hargreave F E, Kirby J G 1987 Airway inflammation and hyperresponsiveness. American Review of Respiratory Disease 136: 35–37

Paul-Eugene N, Dugas B, Picquot S, Lagente V, Mencia-Huerta J-M, Braquet P 1990 Influence of interleukin-4 and platelet activating factor on the FceRII/CD 23 expression on human monocytes. Journal of Lipid Medicine 2: 95–101

Persson C G A 1988 Plasma exudation and asthma. Lung 166: 1–23

Roberts N M, Page C P, Chung K F, Barnes P J 1988 The effect of a specific PAF antagonist, BN 52063, on antigen-induced cutaneous responses in man. Journal of Allergy and Clinical Immunology 82: 236–241

Roche W R, Beasley R, Williams J H, Holgate S T 1989 Subepithelial fibrosis in the bronchi of asthmatics. Lancet i: 520–524

Schleimer R P, Schulman E S, MacGlashan D W et al 1983 Effects of dexamethasone on mediator release from human lung fragments and purified human lung mast cells. Journal of Clinical Investigation 71: 1830–1835

Sekizawa K, Tamaoki J, Graf P D, Basbaum C B, Borson D B, Nadel J A 1987 Enkephalinase inhibitor potentiates mammalian tachykinin-induced contraction in ferret trachea. Journal of Pharmacology and Experimental Therapeutics 243: 1211–1217

Smith H 1989 Animal models of asthma. Pulmonary Pharmacology 2: 59–74

Smith L J, Geller S, Ebright L, Glass M, Tayrum P T 1990 Inhibition of leukotriene D4-induced bronchoconstriction in normal subjects by the oral LTD4 receptor antagonist ICI 204,219. American Review of Respiratory Disease 141: 988–992

Taylor K J, Luksza AR 1987 Peripheral blood eosinophil counts and bronchial responsiveness. Thorax 42: 452–456

Vathenen A S, Knox A J, Higgins B G, Britton J R, Tattersfield A E 1988 Rebound increase in bronchial responsiveness after treatment with inhaled terbutaline. Lancet i: 554–558

Wardlaw A J, Dunnette S, Gleich G J, Collins J V, Kay A B 1988 Eosinophils and mast cells in bronchoalveolar lavage in subjects with mild asthma. American Review of Respiratory Disease 88: 62–69

Wegner C D, Gundel R H, Reilly P, Haynes N, Letts L S, Rothlein R 1990 Intercellular adhesion molecule-1 (ICAM-1) in the pathogenesis of asthma. Science 247: 456–459

Yamaguchi Y, Hayashi Y, Sugara Y et al 1988 Highly purified murine interleukin 5 (IL-5) stimulates eosinophil function and prolongs in vitro survival. Journal of Experimental Medicine 167: 1737–1742

Yukawa T, Kroegel C, Dent G et al 1989 Effect of theophylline and adenosine on eosinophil function. American Review of Respiratory Disease 140: 327–333

Yukawa T, Read R C, Kroegel C et al 1990a The effects of activated eosinophils and neutrophils on guinea pig airway epithelium in vitro. American Journal of Respiratory Cell and Molecular Biology 2: 341–354

Yukawa T, Ukena D, Chanez P, Dent G, Chung K F, Barnes P J 1990b Beta-adrenergic receptors as eosinophils: Binding and functional studies. American Review of Respiratory Disease 141: 1446–1452

4

Problems with asthma care delivery

M. R. Partridge

Asthma is the only treatable condition in Western Europe that is increasing in frequency and severity. The condition cannot yet be cured but in most patients it can be controlled with a combination of relieving and preventative therapies. Understanding of the mechanisms behind the disease and the rationale behind treatment has improved significantly but there is evidence that the benefits of such knowledge are not reaching all asthmatics. How much this is due to deficiencies in health care services and how much is due to patient factors merits careful consideration.

THE SIZE OF THE PROBLEM

More than half of all asthma starts in childhood and at least a third before the age of 3 years. Prevalence rates vary according to diagnostic criteria but are unlikely to be less than 10% of the schoolchild population in the UK and in the USA (Lee et al 1983). One of the problems of interpretation of such epidemiological data is the likelihood that part of the apparent increase in asthma represents a change in doctors' habits with regard to diagnostic labelling. That this is not the whole explanation was shown by Burney et al (1990), who looked at the change in prevalence of reported 'persistent wheeze' (irrespective of diagnostic label) in children in the national study of health and growth between 1973 and 1986. They showed an approximate 5% per annum increase in the reporting of this symptom. Similarly in young adults a study of the prevalence of symptoms suggestive of asthma amongst those being considered for Finnish military service showed a 20-fold increase between 1961 and 1989 (Haahtela et al 1990). Nearly 70% of those with frequent wheezing at age 14 years will continue to have recurrent asthma into adult life (Kelly et al 1987) and the disease may of course first present at an older age. One study (Turner Warwick 1989) suggested that 43% of a general practice population of asthmatics had symptoms starting after the age of 20.

The change in prevalence of asthma is paralleled by increasing usage of health care facilities. The rate of consultations because of asthma in general practice has increased (most markedly in those aged under 4) and there has also been an increasing rate of admission to hospital for asthma (Khot et al

1984), with the rate for pre-school children having quadrupled over the past 10 years (Annual Report of the Chief Medical Officer of the DHSS 1986). Sadly the morbidity data are accompanied by an increase in mortality, with just over 2000 patients dying of asthma in the UK every year, or approximately one every 4 hours. This increase in death rate applies to every age group and is rising approximately 4.5% per annum in the 5–34 age group (Burney 1986). Almost 1 asthma death in every 10 involves people aged under 35 years whilst another 3 out of 10 are deaths among people of middle age (35–64 years). This picture of increasing suffering and increasing death rate is occurring at a time of increased use of anti-asthma drugs (Keating et al 1984).

WHY IS A TREATABLE CONDITION INCREASING IN FREQUENCY AND SEVERITY?

An almost parallel increase in mortality with usage of anti-asthma treatments raises some important questions. The possible explanations are speculative but include the following:

1. More deaths and more drugs reflect increased prevalence
2. Treatment is harmful
3. The disease is becoming more severe
4. There are problems with the delivery of asthma care (in the midst of plenty, some are receiving no or inappropriate treatment).

More deaths and more drugs reflect increased prevalence

If more people have a disease and the proportion dying from it remains the same then there will be a numerical increase in the number of deaths. As already discussed the prevalence of asthma has increased, and the similarity between the noted 5% per annum increase in the disease amongst junior school-children and the 4.5% increase per annum increase in death rate amongst those aged 5–34 years suggests that increasing prevalence may partly explain the increasing death rate. The reasons for the rising prevalence of the condition are unclear. The tendency to be atopic is inherited via a single gene (Cookson & Hopkin 1989) but not all with the tendency develop the disease. The genetic factors are unlikely to have altered over a short time period and so we must look for recent changes in the environment. Maternal smoking has increased as a habit over the same period that asthma has become commoner. The habit leads to increased umbilical cord immunoglobulin E (IgE) levels and an increased tendency for offspring to be asthmatic (Weitzman et al 1990). Over the same period changes in home environment (increased central heating, double glazing and fitted carpets) have increased children's exposure to house dust mite, and increased exposure may have led to an increase in sensitization and asthma (Sporie et al 1990). Finally, on the wider environmental issue the levels of a number of invisible pollutants such as oxides of nitrogen and ozone have increased over the last decade or so. These may give rise to attacks of asthma, but may also lead to damage to respiratory epithelium and easier entry for allergens. Further research is clearly needed to elucidate fully the reasons for the rising prevalence of asthma.

Is treatment harmful?

Whenever two variables move in the same direction over the same time period a cause and effect relationship must be questioned. Total sales of anti-asthma drugs have increased over the last two decades and there has been a significant increase in the use of nebulized bronchodilators over this time. Much of this increase is explained by hospital usage, but in the community there are fears that such usage may lead to a self-reliance on first aid nebulized therapy and a delay in the seeking of medical attention. (A similar situation was cited to explain the epidemic of asthma deaths in the early 1960s which coincided with the wider availability of metered-dose aerosols.) The dosages of bronchodilators used in a nebulizer can induce angina and arrythmias and can be considered less safe if given in the home without oxygen (Neville et al 1982). Their use may also detract from the prescription and use of regular preventative therapies for asthma.

However, despite these concerns there is no evidence that the switch to the nebulized route for bronchodilators in the UK is a factor in the increasing death rate. In New Zealand an earlier sudden rise in asthma deaths led to an evaluation of management of the disease in that country. Deaths were initially blamed on overuse of home nebulizers, a high usage of oral xanthines with β-agonists, more severe disease, poor medical care and poor patient compliance. A more recent explanation is the suggestion (Crane et al 1989) of a possible association between the use of the bronchodilator fenoterol and a risk of death in severe asthmatics. After initial criticisms the data have been re-evaluated, with similar conclusions (Pearce et al 1990), and there is now a UK recommendation to use alternative β-agonists (Drug and Therapeutics Bulletin 1990). Doubts must remain about the conclusions of these studies but they serve as a reminder that, whilst suffering from this disease is increasing, every possible cause must be examined. However, there is no current evidence that the commonly used UK treatments are responsible for the increasing death rate.

Is asthma becoming more severe?

Over the decade to 1982 there was a 16% rise in hospital admission rates for adults with asthma. However, there was no clear evidence that those being admitted to hospital had more severe asthma, the assumption being that this increased rate reflected a growing perception that hospital is a safer place to be during an attack of asthma. Similar changes in use of health care facilities without evidence of differences in severity of disease have been shown in Birmingham, where admission rates for Asians with asthma are significantly higher than for Caucasians whose asthma is of similar severity (Ayres 1986). Between 1980 and 1985 admissions to hospital of those aged under 4 years increased by 124% and in this age group the evidence is against the increase being due to an altered threshold for admission. Anderson (1990) has suggested that the trend is a consequence of more young children experiencing severe attacks requiring hospital admission. However, in the age range where most asthma deaths are occurring, there is no support for the hypothesis that increasing death rates reflect a change in type or severity of disease.

Problems with the delivery of care to the patient with asthma (in the midst of plenty, some are receiving no or inappropriate treatment)

Underdiagnosis

Until a patient has been diagnosed as having asthma they are unlikely to receive appropriate treatment. Such underdiagnosis is unlikely to account for the increasing death rate from asthma, as several studies have shown that those who die are usually diagnosed asthmatics with a long history of the condition (British Thoracic Association 1982). However, underdiagnosis may lead to morbidity and suffering despite the wider availability of treatments. Levy and Bell (1984) in a general practice audit showed that it required an average of 16–20 consultations with respiratory symptoms before a diagnosis of asthma was made. Speight et al (1983) showed a similar situation in children and the same pertains in adults, where two recent studies have shown delay and underdiagnosis of asthma (Banerjee et al 1987, Holgate & Dow 1988). In children a greater awareness that any respiratory symptom could be due to asthma is needed. Wheezing is common but coughing (especially at night or on exercise), chest tightness and exertional breathlessness are also likely symptoms. A simple asthma exercise test may confirm the diagnosis. In adults every patient with an unexplained cough should have asthma considered as a diagnosis, and in every patient with symptomatic airway narrowing asthma should be either confirmed or refuted by peak flow monitoring, reversibility trials with bronchodilators and if necessary by a diagnostic trial of oral steroids.

Inappropriate selection or use of inhaler devices

Both relieving bronchodilators, and preventative treatments are best taken by the inhaled route. This permits small quantities of drug to be delivered directly to the site of action. Whilst the metered-dose inhaler is the most commonly used device, some patients cannot coordinate activation with inspiration. For these and others with problems of manual dexterity, a dry powder inhaler, an auto-inhaler, or a spacer or chamber device is more appropriate. Correct selection of the device and instruction in its use are almost as important as selection of the correct treatment. However, the evidence suggests that insufficient attention is paid to this subject. Pedersen et al (1986) found an efficient inhaler technique in only 46% of children using a metered-dose inhaler. In another study of asthma in primary schools Storr et al (1987) found that 11 of 16 children were unable to use their inhalers, and the problem is also common in adults (Crompton 1982). A simple switch to an alternative device is not always a remedy, for in Storr's study 19 of the 48 children using a dry powder rotahaler system also had problems with that device. What is needed is careful preliminary selection of the best device for that patient, followed by careful instructions, follow-up and rechecking of technique.

Underuse of regular preventative therapy

The paradox of increasing suffering in the presence of increased usage of anti-asthma remedies may be explained by examination of the type of therapies being used. In 1970–1971, 89.4% of prescriptions were for bronchodilators (inhaled, nebulized and oral β-agonists, and oral xanthine preparations) (Hay & Higenbottam 1987). By 1981–1982 these relieving treatments were still accounting for 80.6% of total prescriptions. The more recent improved understanding of the inflammatory nature of asthma (see Chapter 3) has altered our perspective on treatment. Asthmatic airways are affected by infiltration of inflammatory cells (eosinophils and T-lymphocytes), by plasma exudation and oedema, by hypertrophy of smooth muscle and by shedding of epithelium. These changes are present even in those with mild asthma and negligible symptoms (Laitenen et al 1985, Jeffery et al 1989). If asthma is an inflammatory condition it follows that treatment should include anti-inflammatory medicines. The evidence suggests this is of benefit in reducing symptoms (Lorentzson et al 1990) and in reducing usage of oral steroids; one study (Brown et al 1984) suggests that more regular therapy reduces the risk of the airway narrowing becoming fixed and irreversible. In children Speight et al (1983) have shown that regular preventative treatment could lead to a tenfold reduction in disease-related school absenteeism. In adults Barnes (1989) has argued that anti-inflammatory treatments should be introduced much earlier in the course of the disease, but an audit of asthma in general practice showed that only a third of patients were receiving them and less than half of severely affected patients were so treated (Horn & Cochrane 1989). Another general practice study has more recently shown only 47% of adults with previously severe disease to be receiving inhaled steroids (Gellert et al 1990). In a later section (acute severe asthma) it will be seen how underuse of anti-inflammatory treatments leads to unnecessary hospitalization and death.

Poor patient expectation/stoicism

One of the consequences of airway inflammation is the induction of a state of bronchial hyperreactivity. This may be simply demonstrated by monitoring night-time and early morning peak flow readings. The larger the difference the greater the degree of bronchial hyperreactivity and the less good the control of the asthma. The associated symptom of night-time wakening due to cough and breathlessness is a clear marker of poorly controlled disease, and yet many patients accept these symptoms without seeking or demanding improved medication. Many doctors do not enquire regularly about nocturnal symptoms. Turner Warwick (1989) studied 7000 patients receiving repeat prescriptions for bronchodilators from their general practitioners. Seventy-three per cent of the patients reported that asthma caused them to wake during the night on at least one occasion per week. Thirty-nine per cent were awoken every night by their asthma. Another study of 454 patients by White et al (1989) showed that 30% were waking at least once a week with asthma. This represents not only interference with quality of life but significant risk. Symptoms also interfere with the life of the asthmatic in other ways, with 29% of patients in White's Study (1989) having four or more days off school or work in a 6-month period.

About a quarter of asthmatic children have some limitation to their participation in physical education and games at school (Anderson et al 1983). Martin et al (1982) have suggested that 20% of severe asthmatics have their choice of occupation limited by their disease. What is not clear is how much of this clinical picture and how much of the interference in activities of daily living could be improved by better management. The impression is that many asthmatics put up with symptoms, or adjust their life to avoid them, rather than seeking improved medical care. The reasons for such inaction are unclear. In a study of 210 adult asthmatics, Sibbald (1989) used interviews and questionnaires to assess a variety of patient characteristics and relationships. Given a variety of hypothetical symptoms it was shown that morbidity influenced behaviour in that those with the highest reported morbidity in the past 6 months were those who would delay longest before self-treating or seeking medical attention in the event of an acute attack. Twenty-five per cent of the patients felt stigmatized and pessimistic as a result of their asthma but this seemed to influence behaviour less than morbidity. This leads to the interesting speculation that chronicity of symptoms leads to complacency, or indifference or stoicism. Clearly further research is needed into the interrelationship between symptoms, stigma and response to disease, but the likelihood remains that many patients need to be encouraged to increase their expectations of what can be achieved with asthma treatment.

The problems of non-compliance

Making the correct diagnosis and prescribing the correct treatment will only reduce asthma suffering if the treatment is taken by the patient. To what extent do patients with asthma comply with medical advice?

Compliance is defined as the extent to which a patient's behaviour coincides with the doctor's advice. It may involve taking advice as to when to seek help in the event of deteriorating asthma or taking advice as to how and when to use certain medicines. With regard to therapy, we can assess degree of compliance by looking at how well a disease is controlled, by measuring blood or urine drug levels, by pill counting or aerosol weighing or by the use of microprocessors in the lid of bottles (Cramer et al 1989) or attached to inhalers (Spector et al 1986). In a variety of conditions (ranging from hypertension to epilepsy and tuberculosis) such tests have shown non-compliance rates of between 46% and 62% (Robbins 1980). In a similar study of patients with asthma Horn et al (1989) showed that only 60% of patients had urine salbutamol levels appropriate to the timing and dose of inhaled salbutamol which they claimed to be taking. Of the 40% who had probably not taken salbutamol as claimed, 13% had low levels and 27% had levels suggesting much greater prior use of salbutamol than was admitted.

Objective testing of drug levels may not always be needed. If the question is asked in an appropriate way, e.g. 'Can you tell me how often you remember to take the medicine?', then simple discussion with the patient may reveal non-compliance, although such methods will underestimate the size of the problem. Giving the patients questionnaires may also help. In an unpublished study just under 100 patients in my asthma clinic who had been exposed to written and video information about asthma were given a questionnaire and asked to tick which of several statements most closely approximated to their compliance with preventative treatments. Forty per cent claimed never to miss a dose. Twenty-nine per cent admitted that they 'stopped the treatment altogether when well' and the others were partial compliers to a varying degree. Interestingly the total non-compliers still had a need for a mean usage of 28.8 doses of bronchodilator per week, suggesting that resolution of asthma was not the main reason for not taking the preventive therapies. Reasons for non-compliance may include:

1. Misunderstanding
2. Lack of confidence in efficacy
3. Fear of side effects/dislike of drugs
4. Complacency
5. Rebellion
6. Difficulties with method of administration
7. Difficulties with timing of administration.

Difficulties with inhaler devices have been mentioned, and the need for patients to have clear instructions and information is discussed later.

However, it has been clearly shown that there is a direct relationship between the patient's satisfaction with the consultation and their subsequent compliance with treatment. In a non-asthma study Korsch & Negrete (1972) showed that, of a group of patients who were satisfied with the communication aspects of the interview, 54% complied totally with the prescribed treatment whereas the equivalent figure for the dissatisfied group was 16%. Compliance is also aided by simplifying therapeutic regimes; a move towards twice daily treatments for asthma prophylaxis should help, if the same applies to asthmatics as it does to those with epilepsy. In a study with a microprocessor in the lid of a bottle of anticonvulsants, compliance with treatment averaged 76% over 3428 patient days of observation — or 87% for once daily treatment, 81% for twice daily, and 77% for three times daily, but a mere 39% for doses four times a day (Cramer et al 1989).

Difficulties with the management of acute severe asthma

There have now been many studies of the circumstances surrounding death from asthma. Such studies are performed to shed light upon any patient or doctor actions which could be improved. The results of all of the studies are remarkably similar.

Macdonald et al (1976) studying 53 asthma deaths in hospital showed that the fatal attack usually persisted for several days before hospital admission and normally occurred in patients with a long history of asthma. The patient or doctor often underestimated the severity of the attack. On admission most patients were severely ill, peak flow and blood gases were rarely measured, steroids were underused and patients rarely received artificial ventilation before death. Fifty-three further deaths studied by Ormerod & Stableforth (1980) showed several avoidable factors. Recent discharge from hospital (16%), non-availability of aerosol bronchodilators (45%), underuse of corticosteroids (66%) and lack of objective measurements of airflow obstruction (100%) were found in asthma deaths occurring outside hospital. Inadequate initial assessment (50%), underuse of steroids (93%) and failure to monitor objectively were found in deaths in hospital.

The British Thoracic Association Study (1982) showed depressingly similar results. Steroids and bronchodilators were underprescribed, and inhaled steroids and cromoglycate had frequently not been used, and failure to recognize the severity of the asthma by patients, relatives and doctors often caused delay in starting appropriate treatment. The study concluded that there were potentially preventable factors contributing to the deaths in 86% of cases. Had the situation pertaining at the beginning of the decade improved by the end? A 1987 study of asthma deaths compared their management with those of a matched control group of patients who had survived an acute attack managed in the same hospital (Eason & Markowe, 1987). Inadequate monitoring and inadequate use of nebulized β-agonists occurred significantly more often in fatal cases. Use of sedation, inadequate steroid treatment, exposure to potentially toxic doses of aminophylline and inadequate clinical assessment were more common in cases than controls, but not significantly so. Failure to institute artificial ventilation contributed to seven deaths. Assessors considered important defects in management to have occurred in 83% of the cases and 40% of the controls.

A prospective audit of admissions with acute asthma to a Glasgow hospital (Bucknall et al 1988a) has confirmed that undersupervision and undertreatment of patients with asthma remains a common problem and is not confined to those dying of the condition. The survey revealed important differences depending upon whether or not the patient was admitted to a general ward or one with a specialist respiratory interest. If managed on a non-specialist ward, fewer patients were treated with oral steroids (67% versus 83%), had regular peak flow recordings (42% versus 73%) or were given follow-up appointments (50% versus 92%), and fewer had their inhaled therapy increased after discharge (28% versus 55%). As a result the non-respiratory group had more symptoms on follow-up, and 20% of first admissions in the non-specialist group were readmitted within the subsequent year, compared to 2% of the group treated on the wards with a respiratory interest (Bucknall et al 1988b). Whilst these temporally dissociated studies should not be regarded as a serial audit, they suggest the rather slow percolation of messages regarding good management to those other than respiratory physicians. An answer may be the greater use of protocols (e.g. British Thoracic Society statement 1990b) or provision of more specialist care in hospital.

Are all the current hospital admissions with asthma necessary? Many studies have suggested that acute severe asthma may be an inaccurate term. Asthma meriting hospitalization is usually severe but in many cases it is not acute. Retrospective questioning often reveals that control had been poor for some time and this can be elicited by asking about night-time symptoms. In a study of 75 serial admissions with severe asthma Blainey et al (1989, 1991) showed that 53% of patients were waking at least five nights per week in the week before admission. Thirty-five per cent had been waking this often for a month before admission. Only 37% were taking adequate doses of inhaled steroids. Fifty-four per cent of these patients had received medical advice in the week before admission but this had often involved prescriptions of antibiotics or more bronchodilators and only 15% had had appropriate changes in treatment, such as introduction or increase in inhaled or oral steroids.

It seems likely that better treatment of asthma in the community would reduce the numbers requiring admission to hospital. Those that continue to require hospitalization are likely to be those with more severe recurrent disease, and we need to ensure that on any one occasion the within-hospital management does not deter this group from reattending in the future. Deciding whether to seek medical attention involves the acutely ill asthmatic in a risk-versus-benefit analysis which will involve the use of information given to them (hopefully written and based on peak flow readings) but it will be modified by the patient's past experiences. Long waits in the accident and emergency department, repeated sampling of arterial blood gases by staff poorly trained in the technique, and a lack of knowledge by attending staff may deter the patient from prompt reattendance. If prompt hospital care by a specialist is not practical and care is provided by a non-respiratory team, then the patient should be managed by means of a protocol and be reviewed in an asthma clinic after discharge, (British Thoracic Society statement 1990a).

The paradox of rising asthma morbidity and mortality despite wider availability of asthma treatments is explained by an increasing prevalence of the disease coupled with deficiencies in the delivery of care to the patient. The increasing prevalence of asthma merits determined efforts to reduce smoking amongst females and further research into the environment, both within the home and outside. Problems with regard to delivery of asthma care require some concerted action by all health professionals but the way forward is becoming clearer.

THE WAY FORWARD

Guidelines for treatment

For some conditions there is controversy about the correct treatment, or there are multiple possibilities and conflicting evidence as to which is best. This is not the case for asthma, where two recent consensus conferences have produced clear guidelines as to the correct management of asthma in children and in adults. The former (Warner et al 1989) defines the problem, discusses diagnosis and outlines a clear rational prescribing policy for children with asthma. Whilst the main theme suggests β-agonists for mild episodic wheeze, cromoglycate for mild to moderate asthma, and inhaled steroids for moderate to severe disease, it also advises when to use xanthines, ipratropium bromide and oral steroids. Flow charts provide advice according to whether one is dealing with those aged under 1 year, 1–3 years, 3–5 years or 5–18 years, and they contain clear advice as to when specialist help should be sought. The statement also summarizes how to manage acute attacks and contains a section on the worrying problem of adolescents with asthma, this group accounting for most childhood asthma deaths. In this section is emphasized the need to enquire about smoking, the problem of non-compliance and aerosol abuse (with the need for prescription monitoring), and recognition of the problems of stigmatization and body image that may arise along with the physical consequences of severe disease delaying puberty and stunting growth. The development of adolescent clinics run jointly by paediatricians and adult chest physicians is encouraged.

The guidelines for the management of asthma in adults are divided into

P.SW   field disease = T.

notability   ? ubidilty
why

on show = likely of cure
. under diagnosis
. inappropriate selection / under
                        in both diseases
. unaware of preventative of
. poor pt expectation
. non compliance

(paradox of ↑ m·m despite ↑ availability of estimate
        → ↑ uv → defines in delting)
    The very forced.   of cure)

(can) in pt →   consensus guidelines
(?) out pt   step approach
                     information
                     self management plans

n

Biggest challenge shift in management
from district council   pt orientated
self management

two sections, dealing with chronic persistent asthma (British Thoracic Society 1990a) and acute severe asthma (British Thoracic Society 1990b). The former promote greater use of anti-inflammatory drugs, suggesting that inhaled steroids are needed in all adults needing a bronchodilator more than once daily or those with night-time symptoms. For those in whom such treatment does not lead to good control, compliance should be questioned and inhaler technique checked, and if not deficient the patient should be prescribed high-dose inhaled steroids preferably via a chamber device. Only if this does not lead to satisfactory control should oral bronchodilators, anticholinergic agents or high-dose inhaled bronchodilators be used. Guidelines for safe use of nebulizers are given and the need to reduce treatment as well as to increase it is emphasized, with advice as to how this should be done. The emphasis is on objective peak flow monitoring and greater participation of the patient in the management of asthma. The guidelines for the management of acute severe asthma re-emphasize the use of objective measurements of severity and are presented as a series of directions designed to help doctors manage patients in their home, in the accident and emergency department and as in-patients.

These consensus guidelines provide advice as to good management of asthma. They are educationally useful and provide an excellent basis for audit. However, as Rees (1990) has stressed, their lifespan may be limited and such guidelines must be regularly reviewed.

Improved information for patients

Patients are eager for information about their condition. User leaflets accompanying medicines have been studied extensively in hypertension and depression and in general practice in patients taking penicillin and non-steroidal anti-inflammatory drugs (George et al 1983). Such leaflets improve patient knowledge about their medicines, but have no detectable effect on compliance in those on long-term treatments, although they may improve compliance with short-term treatments such as antibiotics. These studies have recently been extended and in a controlled trial 1809 patients who received prescription leaflets knew more about their medicines, especially the side effects, and were significantly more satisfied than 1601 patients who were not given additional written information (Gibbs et al 1990).

How do we similarly provide patients with information about their asthma and its more general management, and does such information alter morbidity? In one study (Hilton et al 1986) one group of asthmatics underwent a maximum education programme (a booklet, and a subsequent treatment card and letter, followed by a consultation and audio tape, with three monthly follow-up appointments), whilst another group received only a treatment card and booklet by post, and a third group had no additional education and acted as a control group. Unfortunately only the maximal education group showed a significant improvement in knowledge of asthma, but in neither of the intervention groups was there any improvement in self-management ability or asthma morbidity. In another study (Partridge 1986), patients expressed a preference to receive information verbally from the doctor, but patients who had been exposed to leaflets, public meetings and watching videos stated that videos were the next most preferred method of receiving education. However, a study by Jenkinson et al (1988) showed that patient preference does not necessarily equate with effectiveness. Patients in this study were randomly allocated to be given a book, an audio tape, a book and tape or neither. Knowledge about the use of drugs was significantly increased 3 months later in the groups who received the material and this persisted after 12 months. Those given the book and the tape preferred the book but paradoxically learnt more from the tape. Again there was no demonstrable objective reduction in morbidity. Information leaflets, books and videos provide excellent information to enable the patient to pass an exam in asthma. They probably also increase patients' satisfaction with their therapy, but it is likely that they only have an impact on morbidity when *personalized* and coupled with self-management plans.

Improved doctor–patient communication

In a Mori poll, 1490 members of the National Asthma Campaign were asked about their reactions when they or their children were first diagnosed as having asthma (National Asthma Campaign 1990). Thirty-eight per cent were relieved to have a diagnosis, and this probably reflects the previously mentioned delays involved in making the diagnosis. Thirty-two per cent reported being extremely worried, 23% were frightened, 16% were bewildered, and 10% angry. Nearly two-thirds (62%) of the respondents lacked understanding of their asthma and 59% wanted more information. Only 22% felt they had had a good discussion with their doctor.

It is therefore likely that we are currently failing our patients with regard to the provision of suitable information, but we may also be overlooking their emotional reactions to having asthma. Such failure of communication may lead to non-compliance (Korsch & Negrette 1972). Communication involves three components: a sender, a message and a recipient. In this context the sender may be a doctor or a nurse, and the messages about asthma and its treatment need to be jargon free and provided in small quantities but repeated over time and by different means (e.g. leaflets, videos). However, exploration of the patients' fears and expectations of treatment is essential and we need to answer how far we may or may not be able to fulfil such expectations. Providing waiting patients with a sheet of paper and asking them to list what they are hoping to achieve from a consultation may prove useful. The patient who attends in the hope that they will be told what to avoid so that their asthma will go away will not be impressed if they instead receive, without explanation, an inhaler which they are told to take for ever. Fears about treatment are particularly common in those on steroid inhalers and these require an honest appraisal of the risk-versus-benefit analysis involved in each prescription. The pregnant asthmatic has a special need for reassurance about the relative safety of asthma therapies and their lack of effect upon the fetus.

Good communication is essential in all of medicine but it is especially important to establish a sympathetic and effective dialogue with the patient in the management of chronic conditions such as asthma, which involve long-term treatment. The training of doctors in communication skills has been shown to increase patient knowledge about their condition and to increase compliance (Ley 1976).

Regular supervision

Asthma is a chronic condition. Medical management in the past has often revolved around the care of acute attacks and exacerbations. More regular supervision would appear to have advantages. The numbers of asthmatics involved suggests that such supervision would have to be provided in the community and may need to be done by general practitioners in routine surgeries. However, the work may be shared with other health professionals and many practices now have nurse-run asthma clinics. In the UK the government's 1990 Contract for General Practitioners offers a financial inducement to those who organize clinics for the regular supervision of such diseases. Running a community asthma clinic involves firstly identifying all of a practice's asthmatics and maintaining a register. Depending upon the training undertaken by the nurse, further tasks then involve providing the patient with initial education and advice regarding symptoms, and teaching inhaler and peak flow techniques. Regular follow-up procedures are then established and the nurse can identify poor control through questioning about symptoms and lifestyle and by the review of peak flow charts. Doctor and nurse then need to establish referral procedures within the practice and develop clear protocols outlining changes that the nurse may make. Such clinics (and the associated self-management plan) may result in fewer calls for acute asthma attacks and fewer surgery visits from poorly controlled asthmatics (Charlton & Charlton 1990).

In hospital chest clinics and in paediatric departments there are advantages in patients with asthma returning to the same clinic on the same day of the week (although such grouping of patients should not lead to inflexibility and difficulties of attendance at other times as necessary). A hospital asthma clinic can maximize educational efforts by making appropriate leaflets readily available, and using video tapes on asthma in waiting areas (Partridge 1986). The patient may then see a nurse to have measurements of peak flow and for checking on good inhaler technique before seeing the doctor. Such arrangements provide an opportunity for reinforcement of messages and allow the necessarily limited doctor–patient time to be used most profitably. Grouping patients by condition into one clinic also has advantages for research studies and often provides patients with opportunities for exchange of views and mutual support.

Self-management plans

Self-management of asthma involves the patient being trained to manage their own treatment rather than being required to consult their doctor before making changes. To some extent all patients are involved in self-management for they use their bronchodilator as needed. More detailed plans may involve the patient in increasing their preventative treatment or in starting oral steroids. Such plans may be based upon subjective symptoms, for example 'Double your preventative treatment at the first hint of a cold and continue at that level for 5 days', or, increasingly such plans are based upon a combination of symptoms and objective measurements of peak flow.

The patient therefore has a basic need for:

1. Training in the use of inhalers and peak flow meters
2. Knowledge of the difference between relieving and preventative therapies
3. An ability to recognize signs of deteriorating asthma (especially nocturnal symptoms).

It is usually easiest to provide an individual self-management plan after obtaining a profile of a patient's asthma by a period of home peak flow monitoring. An adult, for example, may then be advised that if the usual peak flow is 500 and it falls to 400 it merits an increase in the preventative treatment, whilst a drop to 250 indicates the need for a course of oral steroids. A fall to less than 150–200 suggests the need to seek urgent medical advice. In another patient the threshold values may be quite different or may just involve the marking of the patient's peak flow meter with a red band to indicate the level below which they should call for medical help.

Beasley et al (1989) showed that such self-management plans based on the use of increased inhaled steroids and self-introduction of oral steroids lead to a significant improvement in control of symptoms of asthma and improvement in lung function. Interestingly, the benefits were obtained in the presence of a reduced overall requirement for oral steroids. This suggests either that the benefit is due to self-adjustment of inhaled steroid dosage or because the plans improve compliance or because of a combination of both. A further study of adults involving a similar mixture of education and self-management plans has shown a significant reduction in readmission rates to hospital of patients undergoing the programme (Mayo et al 1990). A review of programme usage in children suggests similar benefits (Klingelhofer & Gershwin 1988).

CONCLUSION

The prevalence of asthma is increasing. A cure is not yet available, but control of the condition is possible for the majority of patients. However, many are suffering unnecessarily because of delayed diagnosis, poor expectations and poor selection of treatments and inhaler devices. Some who are given the correct treatment do not take them and this often reflects inadequate information and poor communication between doctor and patient.

A reduction in suffering from asthma will follow completion of a jigsaw puzzle in which the key parts are likely to be guidelines on good management, better education, improved communication, regular supervision and personalization of advice to the individual enabling them to control their own disease.

REFERENCES

Anderson H R 1990 Trends and district variations in the hospital care of childhood asthma: Results of a regional study 1970–1985. Thorax 45: 431–437
Anderson H R, Bailey P A, Cooper J G, West S 1983 Morbidity and school absence caused by asthma and wheezing illness. Archives of Disease in Childhood 58: 777–784
Annual Report of the Chief Medical Officer of the DHSS 1986. HMSO, London
Ayres J G 1986 Acute asthma in asian patients: Hospital admissions and duration of stay in a district with a high immigrant population. British Journal of Diseases of the Chest 80: 242–248
Banerjee D K, Lee G S, Malik S R, Daly S 1987 Underdiagnosis of asthma in the elderly. British Journal of Diseases of the Chest 81: 23–29
Barnes P J 1989 A new approach to asthma therapy. New England Journal of Medicine 321: 1517–1527
Beasley R, Cushley M, Holgate S T 1989 A self management plan in the treatment of adult asthma. Thorax 44: 200–204
Blainey A D, Beale A, Lomas D, Partridge M R 1989 Acute preventable asthma: The cost of hospital admission. Thorax 44: 366P
Blainey A D, Beale A, Lomas D, Partridge M R 1991 Acute preventable asthma: The cost of hospital admission. Health Trends (in press)
British Thoracic Society, Research Unit of the Royal College of Physicians, Kings Fund Centre, National Asthma Campaign 1990a Guidelines for management of asthma in adults: I. Chronic persistent asthma. British Medical Journal 301: 651–653
British Thoracic Society, Research Unit of the Royal College of Physicians, Kings Fund Centre, National Asthma Campaign 1990b Guidelines for management of asthma in adults: II. Acute severe asthma. British Medical Journal 301: 797–800
British Thoracic Association 1982 Death from asthma in two regions in England. British Medical Journal 285: 1251–1255
Brown J P, Greville W, Finucane K E 1984 Asthma and irreversible airflow obstruction. Thorax 39: 131–136
Bucknall C E, Robertson C, Moran F, Stevenson R D 1988a Management of asthma in hospital: A prospective audit. British Medical Journal 296: 1637–1639
Bucknall C E, Robertson C, Moran F, Stevenson R D 1988b Differences in hospital asthma management. Lancet ii: 748–750
Burney P G J 1986 Asthma mortality in England and Wales: Evidence for a further increase, 1974–84. Lancet ii: 323–326
Burney P G J, Chinn S, Rona R J 1990 Has the prevalence of asthma increased in children? Evidence from the national study of health and growth 1973–1986. British Medical Journal 300: 1306–1310

Charlton I, Charlton G 1990 New perspective in asthma self management. Practitioner 234: 30–32

Cookson W O C M, Hopkin J M 1989 Dominant inheritance of atopic immunoglobulin-E responsiveness. Lancet ii: 86–89

Cramer J A, Mattson R H, Prevey M L, Scheyer R D, Ovellette V L 1989 How often is medication taken as prescribed? Journal of the American Medical Association 261: 3273–3277

Crane J, Pearce N, Flatt A et al 1989 Prescribed fenoterol and death from asthma in New Zealand, 1981–83: Case control study. Lancet i: 917–922

Crompton C K 1982 Problems patients have using pressurized aerosol inhalers. European Journal of Respiratory Diseases 63: 101–104

Drug and Therapeutics Bulletin 1990 Fenoterol and asthma deaths. Drug and Therapeutics Bulletin (Consumers Association) 28: 65–66

Eason J, Markowe H L J 1987 Controlled investigation of deaths from asthma in hospitals in the North East Thames Region. British Medical Journal 294: 1255–1258

Gellert A R, Gellert S L, Iliffe S R 1990 Prevalence and management of asthma in a London inner city general practice. British Journal of General Practice 40: 197–201

George C F, Waters W E, Nicholas J A 1983 Prescription information leaflets: A pilot study in general practice. British Medical Journal 287: 1193–1196

Gibbs S, Waters W E, George C F 1990 Communicating information to patients about medicine. Journal of the Royal Society of Medicine 83: 292–297

Haahtela T, Lindholm H, Bjorksten F, Koskenvuo K, Laitinen L A 1990 Prevalence of asthma in Finnish young men. British Medical Journal 301: 266–268

Hay I F C, Higenbottam T W 1987 Has the management of asthma improved? Lancet ii: 609–611

Hilton S, Sibbald B, Anderson H R, Freeling P 1986 Controlled evaluation of the effects of patient education on asthma morbidity in general practice. Lancet i: 26–29

Holgate S T, Dow L 1988 Airways disease in the elderly: An easy to miss diagnosis. Journal of Respiratory Disease 9: 14–22

Horn C R, Cochrane C M 1989 Management of asthma in general practice. Respiratory Medicine 83: 67–90.

Horn C R, Essex E, Hill P, Cochrane G M 1989 Does urinary salbutamol reflect compliance with aerosol regimen in patients with asthma? Respiratory Medicine 83: 15–18

Jeffrey P K, Wardlaw A J, Nelson F C, Collins J V, Kay A B 1989 Bronchial biopsies in asthma: An ultrastructural, quantitative study and correlation with hyperreactivity. Annual Review of Respiratory Disease 140: 1745–1753

Jenkinson D, Davison J, Jones S, Hawtin P 1988 Comparison of effects of a self management booklet and audiocassette for patients with asthma. British Medical Journal 297: 267–270

Keating G, Mitchell C A, Jackson R, Beaglehole R, Rea H H 1984 Trends in sales of drugs for asthma in New Zealand, Australia and the United Kingdom. British Medical Journal 289: 348–351

Kelly W J W, Hudson I, Phelan P D, Pain M C F, Olinsky A 1987 Childhood asthma in adult life: A further study at 28 years of age. British Medical Journal 294: 1059–1062

Khot A, Burn R, Evans N, Lenney C, Lenney W 1984 Seasonal variation and time trends in childhood asthma in England and Wales 1975–1981. British Medical Journal 289: 235–237

Klingelhofer E L, Gershwin M E 1988 Asthma self management programs: Premises, not promises. Journal of Asthma 25: 89–101

Korsch B M, Negrette V F 1972 Doctor patient communication. Scientific American 227: 66–72

Laitenen L A, Heino M, Laitinen A, Kava T, Haahtela T 1985 Damage of the airway epithelium and bronchial reactivity in patients with asthma. Annual Review of Respiratory Disease 131: 599–606

Lee D A, Winslow B R, Speight N P, Heyen L 1983 Prevalence and spectrum of asthma in childhood. British Medical Journal 286: 1256–1258

Levy M, Bell L 1984 General practice audit of asthma in childhood. British Medical Journal 289: 1115–1116

Ley P 1976 Towards better doctor–patient communications: Contributions from social and experimental psychology. In: Bennett A F (ed) Communications in medicine. Oxford University Press, for the Nuffield Provincial Hospital Trust, London

Lorentzson S, Bove J, Eriksson G, Persson G 1990 Use of inhaled corticosteroids in patients with mild asthma. Thorax 45: 733–735

Macdonald J B, Macdonald C T, Seaton A, Williams D A 1976 Asthma deaths in Cardiff 1963–74: 53 deaths in hospital. British Medical Journal 2: 721–723

Martin A J, Landau U, Phelan P D 1982 Asthma from childhood at age 21: The patient and his disease. British Medical Journal 284: 380–382

Mayo P H, Richman J, Harris H W 1990 Results of a program to reduce admissions for adult asthma. Annals of Internal Medicine 112: 864–871

National Asthma Campaign 1990 Mori Poll survey of members. Personal communication

Neville E, Corris P A, Vivian J, Nariman S, Gibson G J 1982 Nebulised salbutamol and angina. British Medical Journal 284: 796–797

Ormerod L P, Stableforth D E 1980 Asthma mortality in Birmingham 1975–7: 53 deaths. British Medical Journal 280: 689–690

Partridge M R 1986 Asthma education: More reading or more viewing? Journal of the Royal Society of Medicine 79: 326–328

Pearce N, Grainger J, Atkinson M et al 1990 Case control study of prescribed fenoterol and deaths from asthma in New Zealand, 1971-81. Thorax 45: 170–175.

Pedersen S, Frost L, Arnfred T 1986 Errors in inhalation technique and efficiency in inhaler use in asthmatic children. Allergy 41: 118–124

Rees P J 1990 Guidelines for the management of asthma in adults. British Medical Journal 301: 771–772

Robbins J A 1980 Patient compliance. Primary Care 7: 703–711

Sibbald B 1989 Patient self care in adult asthma. Thorax 44: 97–101

Spector S L, Kinsman R, Mawhinny H et al 1986 Compliance of patients with asthma with an experimental aerolized medication: Implications for controlled clinical trials. Journal of Allergy and Clinical Immunology 77: 65–70

Speight A N P, Lee D A, Hey E N 1983 Underdiagnosis and undertreatment of asthma in childhood. British Medical Journal 286: 1253–1256

Sporie R, Holgate S, Platts-Mills T A E, Cogswell J 1990 Exposure to house-dust mite allergen and the development of asthma in childhood. New England Journal of Medicine 323: 502–507

Storr J, Barrell T, Lenney W 1987 Asthma in primary schools. British Medical Journal 295: 251–252

Turner Warwick M 1989 Nocturnal asthma: A study in general practice. Journal of the Royal College of General Practitioners 39: 239–243

Warner J O, Götz M, Landau L I et al 1989 Management of asthma: A consensus statement. Archives of Disease in Childhood 64: 1065–1079

Weitzman M, Gortmakers S, Walker D R, Sobol A 1990 Maternal smoking and childhood asthma. Pediatrics 85: 505–508

White P T, Pharoah C A, Anderson H R 1989 Randomized controlled trial of small group education on the outcome of chronic asthma in general practice. Journal of the Royal College of General Practitioners 39: 182–186

5

Chronic obstructive pulmonary disease

T. L. Petty

The problem of chronic obstructive pulmonary disease (COPD), which encompasses the full spectrum between asthmatic bronchitis, chronic bronchitis and emphysema, continues to rise in the USA and in all industrialized nations where smoking is common. The Ninth International Classification of Disease, for the first time, designated COPD to refer to the full spectrum of chronic and irreversible air flow disorders. More specific 'labels' are also included, such as bronchitis, no. 490; asthma, no. 491; chronic bronchitis, no. 492, and emphysema, no. 493. COPD as its own designation is no. 496. For some unknown reason bronchiectasis is no. 494, and hypersensitivity pneumonitis (extrinsic allergic alveolitis) no. 495. These latter disease states are not common and do not materially influence the number of patients designated as COPD (no. 496), if all of these diagnoses are 'lumped together' as COPD in reporting (Feinleih et al 1989). Reversible asthma with episodes of normal air flow and non-obstructive chronic bronchitis, i.e. chronic cough and expectoration, but without air flow obstruction which carries a normal prognosis, should not be included in the COPD designation (Snider 1989).

The prevalence of COPD in North America has been variously estimated. When one adds together both symptomatic and early stages of disease, which are often only identified by spirometry, the true prevalence is probably 30 million individuals. In any case, COPD remains the fifth commonest cause of death in the USA in spite of recent advances in therapy. COPD was a direct or contributing cause for a total of 164 650 deaths in the USA in 1985 (Feinleih et al 1989), and COPD is the second most common cause of chronic disability in the USA. COPD deaths continue to rise in all developed countries, in contrast to the decline in deaths from many other causes (Thom 1989).

RISK FACTORS

COPD is a family clustering disease (Higgins 1984). The reason for this is not entirely known. One uncommon form of COPD, which can present as either an asthmatic or bronchitic syndrome, or with slowly developing and unrelenting dyspnoea, is due to the α_1-antitrypsin deficiency state. This hereditary disorder, however, accounts for only about 40 000 patients in North America (Brantly et al 1988). This type of COPD is important, however, because of the possibility of replacement therapy (see below), which could alter the natural course of disease.

By far the most important risk factor in COPD is smoking. The age, method and intensity of smoking, as well as years of exposure, all relate to the risk of developing COPD. It is a fact, however, that many patients who smoke do not develop COPD. This is probably because of tissue defence mechanisms which have yet to be discovered. The cessation of smoking can have the greatest impact on the course and prognosis of disease, particularly if instituted early.

Certain occupations also relate to risk. It is well known that in the Midwest of the USA non-smoking farmers can develop what is locally referred to as 'grain dust bronchitis'. The epidemiology of COPD associated with grain dust exposure is complex and includes the farming of grain, its storage and transport (Becklake 1980). This form of COPD is predominantly an inflammatory disorder of the conducting airways, with bronchospasm, inflammation and mucosal oedema, rather than due to loss of elastic recoil and destruction of alveolar walls (emphysema). This type of disease carries a better prognosis than the emphysematous form of COPD (see below). Although air pollution is also believed to be a risk factor, it is of relatively mild magnitude except in the most polluted areas of the world.

COURSE AND PROGNOSIS

The course of COPD covers 20–40 years. One might consider that it covers a lifetime, since the condition begins with conception in the susceptible individual. The oldest individuals, i.e. over the age of 85, will almost always develop some degree of emphysema. However, this is of little, if any, clinical significance because accompanying air flow is usually normal or only marginally reduced in the elderly.

Longitudinal studies by the Tucson group have shown striking differences in prognosis in different forms of COPD over a 10-year follow-up period (Burrows et al 1987a). Fig. 5.1 shows the relatively good survival in patients who have features of asthmatic bronchitis with little hyperinflation, and generally an intact air–blood interface as judged by carbon monoxide transfer (Burrows et al 1987a). By contrast, those patients who are hyperinflated, with a reduced transfer factor indicating emphysema, have the worst prognosis (group 3). Group 2, which is similar to group 3 in terms of prognosis, has features of both major types of COPD.

The course and prognosis relate to the degree of airflow obstruction, the presence or absence of reversibility, and the rate of decline of lung function while under treatment and observation. Thus, if patients have relatively mild air flow obstruction as judged by the forced expiration volume in 1 second (FEV_1) when first diagnosed, and they are successful in stopping

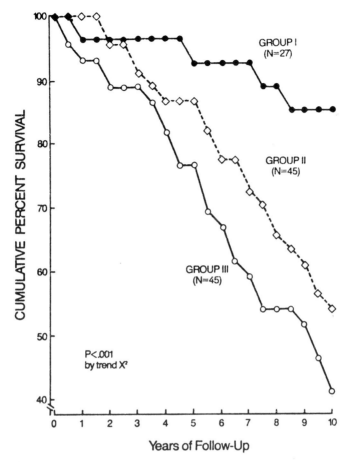

Fig. 5.1 Three survival curves in patients with different types of COPD. Group 1 patients have features of asthmatic bronchitis. Group 3 patients have features of emphysema with marked hyperinflation and a reduced transfer factor indicating an abnormality at the air–blood interface. Group 2 patients have features of both asthmatic bronchitis and emphysema. Note the striking survival differences.

smoking, their rate of ventilatory function deterioration becomes approximately parallel to the age-related rate in decline of FEV_1 (Peto et al 1983). Although the presence or absence of bronchospasm is defined as substantial air flow improvement in response to an inhaled bronchodilator, it has been shown to have a varying effect on prognosis, which is probably due to whether or not patients received systematic therapy over a lifetime (Kanner 1984, Ramsdell et al 1982, Ramsdale & Hargreave 1990). It is now known that reversibility of air flow obstruction with bronchodilators or corticosteroids is a favourable prognostic factor (Feinleih et al 1989, Petty et al 1970, Mendella et al 1982). This probably represents the long-term response to therapy for exacerbations of disease and the effect of maintenance management with bronchoactive drugs. In view of unexpected improvements in air flow with the use of bronchodilators and corticosteroids, COPD should be considered a potentially reversible disease until proven otherwise.

ASSESSMENT OF THE PATIENT

The most common presenting symptoms of COPD are cough, dyspnoea and wheeze. These are non-specific indicators of airway inflammation and bronchospasm, and abnormalities of air flow. The presence or absence of smoking and family history should be ascertained. The physical examination may be helpful if it shows hyperinflation and prolongation of the expiratory time. Hyperinflation alone does not mean air flow obstruction, but studies in fresh, whole, excised human lungs show that loss of elastic recoil is accompanied by hyperinflation in the mildest stages of disease (Petty et al 1987). Measuring the time of expiratory air flow can be a useful index of air flow disorders (Fig. 5.2) (Lal et al 1964). Measuring peak flow or carrying out spirometry should be part of the physical examination. Simple measures of volume over time will reveal air flow disorders. An FEV$_1$/FVC of less than 70% indicates patients who are at risk of developing premature loss of ventilatory function who will emerge into clinically detectable disease (Burrows et al 1987b).

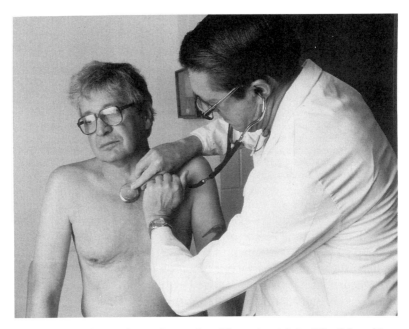

Fig. 5.2 Method of measuring expiratory time. The patient inhales fully, followed by a forceful exhalation in a manner similar to performing spirometry. The physician listens with his stethoscope over the manubrium and records the total time for expiration. Normal expiratory time is 6 seconds or less. A prolonged expiratory time is indicative of air flow obstruction.

A standard chest radiograph may show evidence of hyperinflation. However, unless it shows loss of alveolar tissue, which is hard to determine on standard films, the presence or absence of emphysema cannot be accurately determined. Use of high-resolution computed tomography (CT) scans can be helpful in identifying emphysema (Fraser et al 1989). Young patients with severe air flow disorders and patients with a strong family history of COPD should have measurements of the α_1-antitrypsin level (Brantly et al 1988).

MANAGEMENT

By far the most important approach to management is smoking cessation. The true impact of the physician's advice in smoking cessation is commonly underestimated. Serious advice to stop smoking may be successful in 5–10% of patients which each encounter. This is significant since 70% of smokers see a physician, often a primary care practitioner, every year for some disease state. Often this is a disease related to smoking. A full review of all of the pharmacological approaches used in smoking cessation is beyond the scope of this chapter. Nicotine replacement in the form of gum, transdermal patches or aerosols can be helpful (Prignot 1989). Formalized smoking cessation programmes are effective in selected individuals (Fiore et al 1990).

Bronchoactive drugs include β-agonists, anticholinergics, methylxanthines and corticosteroids. The β-agonists are most commonly given by the inhaled route via a metered-dose inhaler. Correct mastery of the technique is important. Anticholinergics seem to work at least as well as β-agonists, particularly in older individuals with COPD and incomplete reversibility (Braun et al 1989). Both inhaled β-agonists and anticholinergics are compatible. Indeed, they are available in the same metered-dose inhaler in many parts of the world but not in North America. Theophyllines are not potent bronchodilators. However, they appear to offer a global benefit, probably due in part to a favourable effect on respiratory muscle function (Hill 1988, Murciano et al 1989). Corticosteroids have been shown to be useful in exacerbations of COPD in a controlled clinical trial in patients requiring hospitalization, where greater improvement in FEV_1 was associated with corticosteroid use compared with placebo (Albert et al 1980). The role of corticosteroids in all stages of COPD has been recently reviewed (Hudson & Monti 1990). Uncontrolled evidence from the Netherlands suggests that long-term use of corticosteroids can retard the progress of disease (Postma et al 1985, 1988). Controlled clinical trials are underway to evaluate this possibility.

Mucolytic agents have previously been little used in North America. However, mucolytic drugs are in common usage in Europe (Pride et al 1989). A recent National Mucolytic Study in the USA which was a prospective, controlled and double-blind study, showed an improvement in mucus clearance. Statistically significant improvement was found in cough severity, chest discomfort, ease in bringing up sputum, and global symptoms in patients who received iodinated glycerol, compared with placebo (Petty 1990). The empirical use of oral antibiotics has been shown to shorten the course of exacerbations of chronic bronchitis in some but not all patients (Anthonisen et al 1987).

Whether or not any pharmacological agent, used alone or in combination, alters the course and prognosis of COPD has not yet been established. Controlled clinical trials which evaluate survival in any chronic disease state are difficult to design and almost impossible to conduct. However, it is now recognized that the age-specific death rate from COPD is rising into the late 60s or early 70s. This development strongly suggests a favourable effect of all forms of therapy, including smoking cessation and the use of oxygen, on the course and prognosis of COPD.

PULMONARY REHABILITATION

The techniques of pulmonary rehabilitation are methods of care which extend beyond pharmacological management. In brief, pulmonary rehabilitation involves patient and family education, as well as breathing retraining and physical reconditioning (Petty 1990a). Both university-oriented and community studies suggest a favourable effect on prognosis, and have documented the fact that most patients participating in the pulmonary rehabilitation programme can live into their late 60s or early 70s (Burns et al 1989). A clear-cut effect of pulmonary rehabilitation on long-term survival would be difficult to prove.

NUTRITIONAL THERAPY

One very adverse factor in the course and prognosis of COPD is involuntary weight loss. In fact, a 'malignant triad' of resting tachycardia, progressive dyspnoea and unrelenting weight loss is well known to experts in the field. When these three factors are present, survival beyond 1–2 years is unusual. Recent studies have focused on the hypermetabolic state of advanced COPD, and increased levels of catecholamine appear to be at least one of the mechanisms of hypermetabolism (Hofford et al 1990). Increased calorie expenditure from the increased work of breathing is also a factor. Nutritional replacement has been associated with weight gain and an apparent improvement in cell-mediated immunological defences (Fuenzalida et al 1990). Thus, nutritional repletion may offer another therapeutic strategy in advanced stages of disease.

OXYGEN

Two multicentre controlled clinical trials have shown that long-term oxygen therapy improves survival in chronic stable hypoxaemia associated with COPD. In brief, the British Medical Research Council (MRC) study showed an improvement in outcome in patients who received oxygen for 15 hours per day, compared to no oxygen (Medical Research Council Working Party 1981). The North American study, known as the nocturnal oxygen therapy trial (NOTT), showed markedly improved survival with continuous ambulatory oxygen therapy, compared with only nocturnal oxygen therapy from a stationary system (Nocturnal Oxygen Therapy Trial Group 1980). Taken together, these two studies showed that in selected patients with chronic stable hypoxaemia survival without oxygen was poor. Survival was better with oxygen given 12–15 hours per day. Survival was best in patients who could receive oxygen on an ambulatory basis for nearly 20 hours per day (Fig. 5.3). In general, oxygen is prescribed for patients with a chronic stable oxygen tension of less than 55 mmHg (7.3 kPa). This corresponds to an oxygen saturation of 88%. Patients with higher levels of oxygen tension and saturation, but with evidence of pulmonary hypertension, cor pulmonale and secondary erythrocytosis, are also candidates for long-term continuous oxygen. Improved exercise tolerance and better mental function with oxygen are additional indications for long-term continuous oxygen therapy. Three consensus conferences held in North America have concluded that

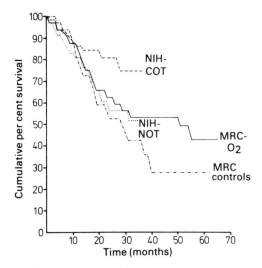

Fig. 5.3 The nocturnal oxygen therapy trial (NOTT) and the British Medical Research Council (MRC) studies demonstrated improved survival with oxygen therapy in patients with advanced COPD with chronic stable hypoxaemia. The NOTT group's patients received oxygen for 12 hours daily, including the hours of sleep. MRC patients received oxygen for 15 hours, including the hours of sleep. The best survival was in the NOTT patients who received continuous oxygen averaging 19.4 hours. A comparison group of patients under the MRC study received no supplemental oxygen. The conclusions from these two studies are that survival for chronic stable COPD with hypoxaemia is poor without oxygen. Survival is improved with oxygen given for about 50% of the time from a stationary source. Survival is best with continuous therapy given for nearly 20 hours per day from a portable source.

ambulatory oxygen, using a portable liquid system, has become the standard of care (Petty 1986, Petty & Snider 1988, O'Donohue & Petty 1990).

New developments in oxygen therapy include the transtracheal route of delivery (Christopher et al 1987). This offers improved comfort in patients who are having nasal congestion or other problems with the nasal cannulae such as painful ears. A reduced litre flow of more than 50%, and cosmetic advantages, make this form of therapy attractive in selected individuals. There is a suggestion of an altered pattern of the work of breathing while using transtracheal oxygen, which may explain the dramatic reduction in dyspnoea in some patients (Cousen & Make 1989). Further evaluation of the transtracheal method of oxygen administration is presently underway.

COPD AND LUNG CANCER

Several studies have now shown the interrelationship between the presence of COPD, as judged by simple measures of air flow obstruction, i.e. FEV_1, and a significantly higher risk of lung cancer than in age, gender and smoking-matched controls. One study compared the risk of lung cancer over a 10-year follow-up period in 113 individuals with air flow obstruction, compared with age, gender and smoking-matched individuals without air flow obstruction (Skillrud et al 1986). There were no occupational differences in the two groups. Nine patients with lung cancer emerged from the group with air flow obstruction, compared with only two patients without air flow obstruction. Also, an increased death rate from all causes was related to air flow obstruction, compared to normal air flow (Skillrud et al 1986). A much higher incidence of lung cancer also occurred in the Intermittent Positive Pressure Breathing Clinical Trial, compared to that expected from age and smoking alone (Tockman et al 1987). A similar increase in death rate occurred in the Johns Hopkins Neoplasm Research Study (Tockman et al 1987). Taken together, these two studies show a greatly increased risk of lung cancer when COPD is present. Thus, the question of early surveillance for lung cancer must be reopened in a targeted population with air flow obstruction. The use of new tumour markers, such as monoclonal antibodies, which identify a lung cancer transitional cell, may offer a new approach to finding lung cancer at a more treatable stage than when it is diagnosed by conventional methods (Hubbard & Crystal 1988). The presence of mucus hypersecretion also appears to be an independent risk factor for lung cancer mortality (Lange et al 1990).

FUTURE DIRECTIONS

Since COPD has readily identifiable risk factors and is easy to assess with simple spirometry, it seems astonishing that this disease state is most commonly diagnosed late in its natural history at a time when the patient's symptoms are disabling. It is now time for the primary care physician to take a leadership role in the early identification, assessment and treatment of patients with all forms of COPD. Any symptoms of cough, dyspnoea or wheeze should lead to simple spirometric measurements of air flow (FEV_1) and air volume (FVC). Any abnormality of flow, particularly when the FEV_1/FVC ratio is less than 70%, should call for aggressive therapy. By far the most important approach is smoking cessation. The systematic use of bronchodilators, under guidance with objective measurements by spirometry, should become the standard in the primary care physician's surgery. A preventive approach could rapidly reduce the premature morbidity and mortality which characterizes the course of COPD. Such an approach utilizing tools that are currently available could bring dramatic reductions in the necessity for hospital services, and the premature disability and termination of employment that characterize COPD.

PROLASTIN REPLACEMENT THERAPY

The human blood-derived α-antiprotease is now available for replacement therapy in patients with hereditarily determined deficiency state (Hubbard et al 1988). Weekly or monthly infusions have been demonstrated to raise the level of circulating antiprotease to the range of 80 mg%, believed to be protective (Hubbard et al 1988). The product is safe in terms of freedom from viruses, including hepatitis B virus and human immunodeficiency virus (HIV). A registry of patients with $α_1$-antitrypsin deficiency, including patients who are receiving prolastin therapy, as well as those who are not, are participating in a careful longitudinal evaluation of the outcome of patients with this deficiency state. This may shed additional light upon the possible impact of replacement therapy on the course and prognosis of COPD. Use of the inhaled route for delivery may offer economic and practical advantages in administration (Snider et al 1989). At the time of writing several synthetic antiproteases are under investigation and, in time, will be evaluated in the more common forms of COPD where the $α_1$-antitrypsin level is normal.

REFERENCES

Albert R K, Martin T R, Lewis S W 1980 Controlled clinical trial of methylprednisolone in patients with chronic bronchitis and acute respiratory insufficiency. Annals of Internal Medicine 92: 753–758
Anthonisen N R, Manfreda J, Warren C P, Hershfield E S, Harding G K, Nelson N A 1987 Antibiotic therapy in exacerbations of chronic obstructive pulmonary disease. Annals of Internal Medicine 106: 196–204
Becklake M R 1980 Grain dust and health: State of the art. In: Dosman J A, Cotton D J (eds) International symposium on grain dust and health, Saskatoon, Saskatchewan 1977. Academic Press, New York
Brantly M L, Paul L D, Miller B H, Falk R T, Wa M, Crystal R G 1988 Clinical features and history of the destructive lung disease associated with alpha-1-antitrypsin deficiency of adults with pulmonary symptoms. American Review of Respiratory Disease 138: 327–336

Braun S R, McKenzie W N, Copeland C, Knight L, Ellersieck M 1989 A comparison of ipratropium bromide and albuterol in the treatment of chronic obstructive airway disease. Archives of Internal Medicine 149: 544–547

Burns M R, Scherman B, Madison R, Kao D, Petty T L 1989 Pulmonary rehabilitation outcome. Respiratory Therapy 2: 25–30

Burrows B, Bloom J W, Traver G A et al 1987a The course and prognosis of different forms of chronic airways obstruction in a sample from the general population. New England Journal of Medicine 317: 1309–1314

Burrows B, Knudson R J, Camilli A E, Kyle S K, Lebowitz M D 1987b The 'horse-racing effect' and predicting decline in forced expiratory volume in one second from screening spirometry. American Review of Respiratory Disease 135: 788–793

Christopher K L, Spofford B T, Petrun M D, McCarty D C, Goodman J R, Petty T L 1987 A program for transtracheal oxygen delivery. Annals of Internal Medicine 107: 802–808

Cousen J E, Make B J 1989 Transtracheal oxygen decreases inspired minute ventilation. American Review of Respiratory Disease 139: 627–631

Feinleih M, Rosenberg H M, Collins J G, Delozier J E, Pokras R, Chevarley F M 1989 Trends in COPD morbidity and mortality in the United States. American Review of Respiratory Disease 140: S9–18

Fiore M C, Novotny T E, Pierce J P et al 1990 Methods used to quit smoking in the United States: Do cessation programs help? Journal of the American Medical Association 263: 2760–2765

Fraser R G, Pare' J A P, Pare' P D, Fraser R S, Genereax G P 1989 Diagnosis of diseases of the Chest, 3rd edn (Ch 11). Saunders, Philadelphia

Fuenzalida C E, Petty T L, Jones M J L et al 1990 The immune response to short term nutritional intervention in advanced chronic obstructive pulmonary disease. American Review of Respiratory Disease 142: 49–56

Higgins M 1984 Epidemiology of COPD: State of the art. Chest 85 (suppl 6): 3s–8s

Hill N S 1988 The use of theophylline in 'irreversible' chronic obstructive pulmonary disease: An update. Archives of Internal Medicine 148: 2579–2584

Hofford J M, Milakofsky L, Vogel W H, Sacher R S, Savage G J, Pell S 1990 The nutritional status in advanced emphysema associated with chronic bronchitis: A study of amino acid and catecholamine levels. American Review of Respiratory Disease 141: 902–908

Hubbard R C, Crystal R G 1988 Alpha-1-antitrypsin augmentation therapy for alpha-1-antitrypsin deficiency. American Journal of Medicine 84: 52–62

Hubbard R C, Sellers S, Czerski D, Stephens L, Crystal R G 1988 Biochemical efficacy and safety of monthly augmentation therapy for alpha-1-antitrypsin deficiency. Journal of the American Medical Association 260: 1259–1264

Hubbard R C, Brantly M L, Sellers S E, Mitchell M E, Crystal R G 1989 Anti-neutrophil-elastase defenses of the lower respiratory tract in alpha-1-antitrypsin deficiency directly augmented with an aerosol of alpha-1-antitrypsin. Annals of Internal Medicine 111: 206–212

Hudson L D, Monti C M 1990 Rationale and use of corticosteroids in chronic obstructive pulmonary disease. Medical Clinics of North America 74: 661–690

Kanner R E 1984 The relationship between airways responsiveness and chronic airflow limitation. Chest 86: 54–57

Lai S, Ferguson A D, Campbell E J M 1964 Forced expiratory time: A simple test for airways obstruction. British Medical Journal 1: 814–817

Lange P, Nyboe J, Appleyard M, Jensen G, Schnohr P 1990 Ventilatory function and chronic mucus hypersecretion as predictors of death from lung cancer. American Review of Respiratory Disease 141: 613–617

Medical Research Council Working Party 1981 Long term domiciliary oxygen therapy in chronic hypoxic cor pulmonale complicating chronic bronchitis and emphysema. Lancet i: 681–686

Mendella L A, Manfreda J, Warren C P, Anthonisen N R 1982 Steroid response in stable chronic obstructive pulmonary disease. Annals of Internal Medicine 96: 17–21

Murciano D, Auclair M H, Pariente R, Aubier M 1989 A randomized, controlled trial of theophylline in patients with severe, chronic obstructive pulmonary disease. New England Journal of Medicine 320: 1521–1525

Nocturnal Oxygen Therapy Trial Group 1980 Continuous or nocturnal oxygen therapy in hypoxemic chronic obstructive lung disease: A clinical trial. Annals of Internal Medicine 93: 391–398

O'Donohue W, Petty T L (co-chairmen) 1990 Third oxygen consensus conference report: New problems in supply, reimbursement and certification of medical necessity for long-term oxygen therapy. American Review of Respiratory Disease 142: 721–724

Peto R, Speizer F E, Cochrane A L et al 1983 The relevance in adults of air-flow obstruction, but not of mucus hypersecretion, to mortality from chronic lung disease: Results from 20 years of prospective observation. American Review of Respiratory Disease 128: 491–500

Petty T L (chairman) 1986 First oxygen consensus conference report: Problems in prescribing and supplying oxygen for Medicare patients. American Review of Respiratory Disease 134: 340–341

Petty T L 1990a The national mucolytic study: Results of a randomized, double-blind, placebo-controlled study of iodinated glycerol in chronic obstructive bronchitis. Chest 97: 75–83

Petty T L 1990b Pulmonary rehabilitation: Why, who, when, what and how? Journal of Respiratory Disease 11: 192–199

Petty T L, Snider G L (co-chairmen) 1988 Second oxygen consensus conference report: Further recommendations for prescribing and supplying long-term oxygen therapy. American Review of Respiratory Disease 138: 745–747

Petty T L, Brink G A, Miller M W, Consello P R 1970 Objective functional improvement in chronic airway obstruction. Chest 57: 216–223

Petty T L, Silvers W G, Stanford R E 1987 Mild emphysema is associated with reduced elastic recoil and increased lung size but not with air-flow limitation. American Review of Respiratory Disease 136: 867–871

Postma D S, Steenhuis E J, van der Weele L T H, Sluiter H J 1985 Severe chronic airflow obstruction: Can corticosteroids slow down progression? European Journal of Respiratory Disease 67: 56–64

Postma D S, Peters I, Steenhuis E J, Sluiter H J 1988 Moderately severe chronic airflow obstruction: Can corticosteroids slow down obstruction? European Respiration Journal 1: 22–26

Pride N B, Vermeire P, Allegra L 1989 Diagnostic labels applied to model case histories of chronic airflow obstruction: Responses to a questionnaire in 11 North American and Western European Countries. European Respiration Journal 2: 702–709

Prignot J 1989 Pharmacological approach to smoking cessation. European Respiration Journal 2: 550–560

Ramsdale E H, Hargreave F E 1990 Differences in airway responsiveness in asthma and chronic airflow obstruction. Medical Clinics of North America 74: 741–751

Ramsdell J W, Nachtwey F J, Moser K M 1982 Bronchial hyperreactivity in chronic obstructive bronchitis. American Review of Respiratory Disease 126: 829–832

Skillrud P M, Offord K P, Miller R D 1986 Higher risk of lung cancer in chronic obstructive pulmonary disease. Annals of Internal Medicine 105: 503–507

Snider G L 1989 Chronic obstructive pulmonary disease: A definition and implications of structural determinants of airflow obstruction for epidemiology. American Review of Respiratory Disease 140: S3–8

Thom T J 1989 International comparisons in COPD mortality. American Review of Respiratory Disease 140: S27–34

Tockman M S, Anthonisen N R, Wright E C, Donithan M G 1987 The intermittent positive pressure breathing trial group; and the Johns Hopkins Lung Project for the early detection of lung cancer: Airways obstruction and the risk for lung cancer. Annals of Internal Medicine 106: 512–518

6

Recent advances in venous thromboembolism

S. R. Benatar

Pulmonary embolism is a well-recognized (and much feared) cause of sudden death, especially in the postoperative period but also in debilitated and immobilized patients, in pregnancy and the puerperium. How commonly does this occur, which patients are most at risk and how often is pulmonary embolism the cause of death in patients not destined to die soon of other severe disease? How can non-fatal pulmonary emboli be accurately diagnosed so that treatment can be implemented early enough to prevent subsequent death from further embolus? Thrombosis in the deep veins of the legs, the usual source of pulmonary emboli, is often asymptomatic and unaccompanied by physical signs. How can deep venous thrombosis be accurately and safely diagnosed? Are there any differences in the natural history of symptomatic and asymptomatic deep venous thrombosis? How does treatment influence the natural history of deep vein thrombosis and pulmonary embolism? When is treatment with thrombolytics preferable to using heparin? What should be the duration of anticoagulant treatment? Does this differ from symptomatic deep vein thrombosis as compared with pulmonary embolism?

Asymptomatic calf vein thrombosis occurs in up to 50% of patients undergoing major surgery. Most resolve spontaneously with no short or long-term sequelae. A range of prophylactic measures are available which can reduce the incidence of postoperative deep calf vein thrombosis. But do these reduce the incidence of more dangerous proximally extending thrombi which give rise to significant pulmonary emboli? Should surgeons be using these prophylactic measures on a routine basis? Do they? If not, why not? If they did, what would be the costs and benefits?

These and other questions on venous thromboembolism remain controversial despite numerous studies during the last three decades which have contributed to advances in our understanding. The purpose of this chapter is to provide guidelines, based on current knowledge on the management of patients with venous thromboembolism. Historical aspects and details of therapy have been dealt with in greater detail in previous review (Hyers 1984, Benatar et al 1986).

EPIDEMIOLOGY AND NATURAL HISTORY

Venous thromboembolism may present either with symptoms in the region of thrombosis or with symptoms resulting from emboli to the lungs. Pulmonary embolism or deep vein thrombosis may be accompanied by 'silent' pathology at the other site and therefore both deep vein thrombosis and pulmonary embolism need to be considered in every patient, regardless of the clinical presentation.

The inaccuracy of clinical diagnosis of deep vein thrombosis and pulmonary embolism is now well recognized (Dalen et al 1971, Hull et al 1981, 1983a). This fact coupled with the knowledge that clinically recognizable deep vein thrombosis and pulmonary embolism are the tip of the venous thromboembolism iceberg, explains why only inaccurate estimates can be made of the size of the iceberg itself from studies which do not adequately sample the tip and which have not used accurate diagnostic methods. Controversy regarding many aspects of the epidemiology and natural history of thromboembolism results from lack of community studies, from difficulties in diagnosing deep vein thrombosis and pulmonary embolism and from the questionable validity of pulmonary embolism mortality rates derived from limited autopsy and death certification data (Benatar et al 1986).

Dalen and Alpert (1975) estimate that in the USA each year 630 000 people have a pulmonary embolus which is fatal in 200 000. Of these, pulmonary embolus is thought to be the sole cause of death in 100 000. These figures are based on the assumption that 15% of deaths in acute general hospitals, 25% of deaths in nursing homes or chronic care institutions and 5% of all non-cardiovascular, non-accidental deaths can be attributed to pulmonary emboli.

Goldhaber et al (1982) have contested this on the basis of a study of 1455 autopsies performed on 2372 consecutive patients (61% autopsy rate) who died at the Peter Bent Brigham Hospital between 1973 and 1977. This study showed that only 9 of 54 patients with a major pulmonary embolus suffered from diseases with a good prognosis. A review of death certification and hospital discharge data in a sample of acute care hospitals led to the conclusion that pulmonary embolism was an important event in only 0.4% of hospitalized patients (Goldhaber & Hennekins 1982). The potential flaws in the data are acknowledged by the authors but they raise the possibility that the estimates of Dalen and Alpert could be substantially inaccurate.

A retrospective hospital study of all autopsy reports and associated hospital records in Sheffield (autopsy rate 47%) showing that pulmonary embolism was the cause of death in 10% of patients (Sandler & Martin 1989) lends support to the assumptions made by Dalen and Alpert. Less than 15% of patients dying from pulmonary embolism were under 60 years old but only a third of patients had underlying carcinoma. Eighty-three per cent of patients with fatal pulmonary embolism had evidence of deep vein thrombosis at autopsy but the diagnosis was only suspected clinically in 19.5% and diagnosed objectively before death in 2.6%. Twenty-four per cent of patients who died from pulmonary embolism had undergone surgery a mean of 6.9 days previously.

Another similar study, however, supports the findings of Goldhaber. In an attempt to determine the accuracy of antemortem diagnosis of pulmonary embolism Rubinstein and colleagues reviewed 1276 autopsy records in an acute care, teaching hospital in Toronto (Rubinstein et al 1988). During the study period (1980–1984) the autopsy rate was 36.3%. Forty-four patients (3.4%) were identified in whom pulmonary embolism was the cause of death or a major contributing factor. The diagnosis was suspected before death in 14 (31.8%) and there were no distinctive features separating these patients from those in whom pulmonary embolism was not suspected before death.

There are many remaining gaps in our knowledge of the incidence of deep vein thrombosis and pulmonary embolism and the frequency with which they give rise to clinical episodes. It is, however, certain that many clinically significant episodes are not recognized before they are fatal and that a significant proportion occur in patients who might otherwise have a good prognosis.

AN APPROACH TO THE PATIENT WITH SUSPECTED PULMONARY EMBOLISM

When considering the diagnosis of pulmonary embolism in an individual patient, the major questions that need to be addressed are:

1. To what extent is the patient haemodynamically impaired and how much of this is due to pulmonary embolism as distinct from pre-existing cardiopulmonary disease?

2. Is it appropriate to pursue a definitive diagnosis of pulmonary embolism and its source in this patient by using pulmonary angiography and/or bilateral ascending venography?

3. If not, with what degree of confidence can the diagnoses of pulmonary embolism and deep vein thrombosis be made using lung scans and non-invasive venous studies?

4. Is there residual thrombus in the deep venous system which may pose risk of a further, perhaps fatal, pulmonary embolism?

5. Which of the therapeutic options should be chosen — embolectomy, fibrinolytic drugs or heparin?

6. How should progress be monitored and for how long should treatment continue?

7. What are the options if there are absolute contraindications to the use of thrombolytic or anticoagulant drugs?

Diagnosis of pulmonary embolism

The symptoms and signs of pulmonary embolism are dependent on the size and number of emboli, possible humoral and reflex mechanisms including pulmonary vasoconstriction, the patient's cardiopulmonary status, and the rapidity of clot fragmentation and lysis. Bedside diagnosis of pulmonary embolism is often difficult; pulmonary angiography has shown that clinical diagnosis is inaccurate in over 50% of patients (Dalen et al 1971, Poulose et al 1970). The classical triad of dyspnoea, pleuritic pain and haemoptysis is present in only 25% of patients and may occur with other chest diseases (Wenger et al 1972). Chest radiographic findings (useful in ruling out other disorders such as pneumothorax) and biochemical abnormalities such as increased lactic dehydrogenase, aspartate aminotransferase, bilirubin and fibrinogen degradation products are also non-specific for pulmonary emboli. ECG and blood gas abnormalities lack specificity as well as sensitivity and their interpretation may be further compounded by pre-existing cardiopulmonary disease.

Pulmonary angiography, the reference standard for the diagnosis of pulmonary embolism, requires considerable expertise both in its performance and interpretation (Goodman 1984). Diagnostic criteria include constant intraluminal filling defects in several films and sharp cut-offs in vessels greater than 2.5 mm in diameter. Reduced perfusion, peripheral pruning, oligaemia and loss of filling of small vessels are non-specific. Although in experienced hands both the morbidity and the mortality of pulmonary angiography are low, the invasive nature of angiography and the expense, time and expertise required are beyond the resources of many general hospitals. There has therefore been great interest in the development of non-invasive isotope lung-scanning techniques.

Lung scanning is a simple, safe and effective non-invasive technique for assessing regional pulmonary blood flow. However, it is not specific for pulmonary embolism because intraluminal vascular obstruction is not the only cause of reduction in blood flow. Other causes include reduced local ventilation due to airway obstruction, extraluminal vessel obstruction and bronchopulmonary anastomoses. The addition of four-view ventilation scanning, using krypton-81m, enhances diagnostic accuracy and is necessary to exclude areas of reduced ventilation as the cause of perfusion defects. Over 80% of patients with multiple segmental mismatches and almost 100% with multiple lobar mismatches have angiographically confirmed pulmonary emboli. However, this falls to less than 30% with single mismatches (Hull et al 1983a, Biello et al 1979, McNeil 1980, Cheely et al 1981, Polak & McNeil 1984, Branch & McNeil 1983). These predictions can be used in conjunction with clinical data to help make therapeutic decisions and to establish the need for definitive angiography in a small subset of patients (Benatar et al 1986) (Table 6.1). Some current recommendations regarding the use of lung scanning and angiography and the implications for treatment are summarized in Table 6.2. A recent large multicentre study emphasized that a normal ventilation perfusion scan virtually excludes the diagnosis of pulmonary embolism, whereas only a minority of patients with angiographically confirmed emboli had a high-probability scan. In addition, diagnostic accuracy of scans was reduced in patients with a history of previous pulmonary embolism. This study emphasizes the importance of careful interpretation of all positive scans in the light of the clinical context (PIOPED 1990).

In a prospective study of 173 consecutive patients presenting to emergency services with pleuritic pain, 36 (21%) had angiographic or autopsy-proven pulmonary embolism. Of patients with an abnormal perfusion scan, 50% had angiographically proven pulmonary emboli as compared with none of the patients in whom the perfusion scan was normal. Of patients with positive results on impedance plethysmography, 77% had pulmonary emboli as compared with 17% of those with negative impedance plethysmography. The use of ventilation scanning together with impedance plethysmography allowed a 50% reduction in the need for angiography (Hull et al 1988).

Table 6.1 Approximate percentage post-test probabilities of pulmonary embolism on the basis of combined clinical (pre-test) and scintigraphic (test) criteria (Havig 1977, Branch & McNeil 1983, McNeil 1980, Polak & McNeil 1984). Figures in parentheses relate to multiple scan defects in each category

Probability of pulmonary embolism on basis off lung scan	Clinical assessment of probability of pulmonary embolism		
	Low (%)	Medium (%)	High (%)
Perfusion scan			
Low-subsegmental defect(s)	1	2 (10)	10 (25)
Medium-segmental defect(s)	10	25 (75)	65 (85)
High-segmental defect(s)	25	55 (90)	85 (95)
Ventilation–perfusion scan			
Low-matched defect(s)	2	2	2
Medium-mismatched subsegmental defect(s)	1	3 (22)	40 (70)
High-mismatched segmental or lobar defect(s)	55	80 (95)	95 (100)

Table 6.2 Recommendations for ventilation–perfusion lung scanning based on diagnostic studies

• Normal six-view perfusion scan. Pulmonary embolism excluded

• Low-probability ventilation–perfusion scan. Either no treatment or proceed to definitive venous studies or pulmonary angiography before treatment, to avoid unnecessary anticoagulation

• High-probability ventilation–perfusion scan. Proceed with treatment

• If anticoagulants contraindicated, pulmonary angiography should be considered to confirm the diagnosis before undertaking vena cava interruption procedures

• Low-probability scans with positive venogram. Proceed with treatment

What is the origin of the pulmonary emboli and is there a risk of further embolization?

Deep vein thrombosis in the legs is the source of pulmonary emboli in over 90% of patients (Hull et al 1983a, Havig 1977). Deep vein thrombi have been demonstrated with venography in up to 70% of patients with angiographically proven pulmonary embolism in one series (80% of patients with deep vein thrombosis having no physical signs in the legs) (Hull et al 1983a) and in 87% of patients with high-probability pulmonary emboli in another (Corrigan et al 1974). A normal venogram does not exclude pulmonary embolism; the whole thrombus may have embolized or in some patients pelvic veins or upper limb veins may be the source of the embolus. If it is not possible to obtain appropriate investigations to verify the clinical diagnosis of pulmonary embolism, it is appropriate to try to make a definitive diagnosis of deep vein thrombosis, as the presence of the latter will provide the basis for treatment with anticoagulants. Bilateral ascending venography utilizing a well-established safe technique is the gold standard for diagnosing deep vein thrombosis (Rabinov & Paulin 1972). The demonstration of deep vein thrombosis will provide not only the evidence required to institute therapy but may also influence the decision whether to use anticoagulants or fibrinolytics. In patients presenting with pulmonary embolism, anticoagulants should be given even if thrombus is confined to the calf on venogram, as the proximal portion may have embolized and proximal extension may occur if no treatment is given. The treatment of symptomatic deep vein thrombosis in the absence of clinical pulmonary emboli is discussed below.

What are the therapeutic options and which should be chosen?

Acute massive pulmonary embolism often leads to death within an hour or two of the event, before effective therapy can be instituted. In those who survive long enough to receive medical attention, therapeutic options include pulmonary embolectomy, fibrinolytic drugs and heparin. While in the past embolectomy has been recommended as the treatment of choice for patients surviving in a shocked state for more than 2 hours, accumulating experience with fibrinolytic therapy has shown a survival rate of 75% — a rate which compares favourably with embolectomy (Miller et al 1977). Fibrinolytics have the advantage of being less traumatic for the patient, more widely applicable, less expensive and effective in lysing both pulmonary emboli and deep vein thrombi, thus reducing the risk of recurrent embolization. Embolectomy should therefore probably be reserved for those patients in whom there is a contraindication to thrombolytic therapy or for situations where the facilities and expertise make embolectomy the ideal procedure.

Inferior vena cava procedures

Many techniques are available to occlude or compartmentalize the inferior vena cava, and so prevent recurrent pulmonary emboli. The role of these procedures remains controversial (Greenfield 1984, Bomalski et al 1982). In some countries, such as the UK, they have never been popular, while in the USA they have been extensively used in the past. Reduction in their use is largely the result of better use of heparin and fibrinolytic drugs. When inferior vena cava interruption is necessary the transvenous use of a Greenfield filter is generally preferred (Kanter & Moser 1988). The experience of the operator is possibly more critical in determining the choice of procedure and the outcome than the device used.

AN APPROACH TO THE PATIENT WITH SUSPECTED DEEP VEIN THROMBOSIS

Diagnosis

When a patient presents with pain, swelling and tenderness in the lower limb, deep vein thrombosis must be considered. Thrombosis of the deep calf veins and proximal extension of non-occlusive thrombus seldom produces symptoms or signs above the knee, and clinical diagnosis is notoriously inaccurate if the symptoms are confined to the calf (Hull et al 1981, Browse et al 1988). Occlusive proximal thrombosis produces oedema of the whole leg and can be more confidently diagnosed clinically. Venography, which confirms the clinical diagnosis is less than 50% of all clinically suspected cases, is the gold standard against which all other techniques must be judged. [125]I isotope scanning is a cheap, simple and accurate means of diagnosing asymptomatic calf vein thrombi in the postoperative period. The delay required for the isotope to be incorporated into the developing thrombus and the insensitivity of the technique to proximal thrombi make it unsuitable for diagnosing symptomatic deep vein thrombosis. Other available methods to diagnose deep vein thrombosis (Browse et al 1988) have not been as widely adopted as impedance plethysmography, which is gaining popularity as a simple, safe and reliable means of diagnosing clinically significant proximal deep vein thrombosis. Its use in the out-patient clinic allows a definitive diagnosis to be made in up to 95% of patients with proximal deep vein thrombosis. Although less than 30% of calf thrombi are detected by impedance plethysmography unless these extend (which can be detected by serial impedance plethysmography) they pose little risk. The out-patient use of this diagnostic procedure can obviate unnecessary admission and anticoagulant therapy. An approach to the diagnosis of deep vein thrombosis (Hull et al 1983b) and recurrent deep vein thrombosis (Huisman et al 1986) using impedance plethysmography is illustrated in Figs 6.1 and 6.2.

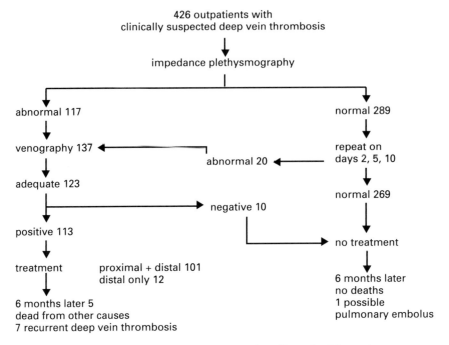

Fig. 6.1 Impedance plethysmography in the out-patient diagnosis of deep vein thrombosis. (Huisman et al 1986.)

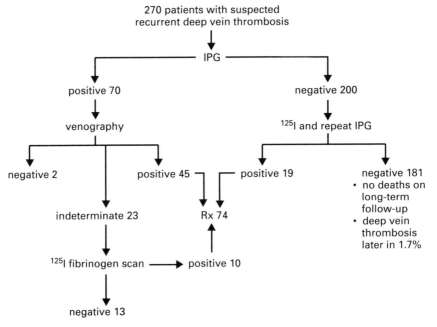

Fig. 6.2 Investigation of patients with suspected recurrent deep vein thrombosis. IPG, impedance plethysmography. (Hull et al 1983b.)

Why did the patient develop a deep vein thrombosis?

Well-established risk factors for thromboembolic disease are shown in Table 6.3 (Benatar et al 1986). When there is no obvious risk factor, an important consideration is whether to search for an underlying abnormality in the coagulation process. A wide variety of disorders of coagulation have been described in which the risk of venous thrombosis and embolism is increased (Table 6.4). Careful search for these abnormalities in selected patients with no other apparent risk factor is necessary to identify families at risk. It has been suggested that one of these abnormalities may be detected in up to 15% of patients with otherwise unexplained venous thromboembolism (Moser 1990).

Treatment

Asymptomatic calf deep vein thromboses developing in the postoperative

Table 6.3   Risk factors for venous thromboembolism

Previous episodes of venous thromboembolism

Underlying cardiac disease

Carcinoma

Trauma — including surgery

Pregnancy, puerperium, oral contraceptives, oestrogens

Immobility

Obesity

Blood group A

Gram-negative sepsis

Myeloproliferative disorders

Ulcerative colitis, Cushing's disease, homocystinuria, Behcet's syndrome

Table 6.4   Coagulation disorders predisposing to venous thrombosis

Deficiency of
    antithrombin III
    protein C
    protein S

Defective
    plasminogen
    release of plasminogen activator

Increased
    circulating coagulation protein factors 5, 7

Hyperreactive
    platelets

period have a benign natural history without therapy. It has commonly been thought that this may also apply to symptomatic calf vein thrombi. While the embolic risk from deep veins of the calf is less than from more proximal thrombi, a controlled trial has shown that treatment of symptomatic calf vein thrombosis for 3 months favourably influences the natural history by preventing propagation of the thrombus and reducing the frequency of pulmonary embolism (Lagerstedt et al 1985). Standard initial therapy for deep vein thrombosis comprises i.v. or s.c. heparin to prolong the activated partial thromboplastin time (APTT) to twice normal for approximately 7 days, and 5 days of overlap with a coumarin derivative. As occlusive iliofemoral deep vein thrombosis often leads to troublesome post-thrombotic symptoms which may be reduced in frequency if venous damage is reduced by early thrombolysis, fibrinolytic therapy is increasingly being considered appropriate therapy for this subgroup of patients (Rogers & Lutcher 1990).

MONITORING PROGRESS AND DURATION OF TREATMENT

Angiographic and lung scan evaluation of the rate of resolution of pulmonary emboli have shown that the rate and degree of resolution are related to the underlying cardiopulmonary status, and to the size and age of the emboli (Goldhaber et al 1982, Sasahara & Hyers 1973, Tow & Simon 1975). Ten to twenty per cent improvement in perfusion occurs within the first 24 hours and complete resolution can occur in 2 weeks, but is more commonly delayed for up to several weeks or even months (Sasahara & Hyers 1973). Scan abnormalities may persist for up to one year (MacIntyre & Sasahara 1975). Haemodynamic abnormalities resolve in proportion to improvement in the lung scan (Sasahara & Hyers 1973, MacIntyre & Sasahara 1975).

Resolution of emboli, assessed angiographically, is more rapid in patients treated with fibrinolytics than with heparin, but the advantage is largely confined to more rapid resolution within the first 24 hours, with later results being similar in patients treated with fibrinolytics or heparin (Sasahara & Hyers 1973, Tow & Simon 1975).

When fibrinolytic drugs are used, these are given for 48–72 hours and it is rational to monitor therapy both to ensure an adequate lytic state and to prevent haemorrhage. Measurement of the thrombin time and its maintenance at two to four times normal is probably the most widely available suitable laboratory investigation. In many centres, however, monitoring is not attempted and standard doses of fibrinolytics are used (Benatar et al 1986). On completion of 48 or 72 hours of thrombolytic therapy, heparin should be started without a loading dose 4 hours later or when the thrombin time has fallen to less than twice the normal value. For optimum effect the dose of heparin should be adjusted to achieve an APTT at 1.5–2.5 times the control value. This is most safely achieved using a constant i.v. infusion. Seven days is an adequate duration of i.v. heparin therapy, with coumarin derivatives overlapping for at least 5 days prior to stopping heparin.

The need for continued anticoagulation in order to prevent recurrent thromboembolism is well established (Hull et al 1979, O'Sullivan 1972). This is most conveniently achieved using oral warfarin sodium, although adjusted s.c. heparin therapy is also effective (Hull et al 1982). The recommended duration of anticoagulation ranges from a minimum of 3 months in uncomplicated first episodes of deep vein thrombosis or pulmonary embolism with a definite non-recurrent precipitating cause, to indefinite treatment in patients with recurrent life-threatening thromboembolism (Lagerstedt et al 1985, O'Sullivan 1972).

Both the short and long-term prognosis following major pulmonary embolism have been studied by several groups. Approximately 8–20% of patients with a confirmed diagnosis of pulmonary embolism die early in the course of the disease, with 20–50% of these deaths being due to the embolus itself. There is a late mortality of 15–30% following discharge from hospital, with most deaths being due to other underlying disease rather than to recurrent pulmonary emboli or thromboembolic pulmonary hypertension (MacIntyre & Sasahara 1975, Paraskos et al 1973, Hall et al 1977, MacIntyre et al 1982).

In a study of 60 patients (mean age 59) with acute, angiographically confirmed emboli, 58 survived hospital admission. During a 1–7-year follow-up period (mean 29 months) 19 patients died, 18 due to underlying disease (usually cardiac) and one from chronic cor pulmonale. Thirty-nine patients were long-term survivors. Recurrent embolism was suspected during follow-up in 3 patients, but confirmed in only one. Lung scans in the survivors showed complete resolution in 65%. Persistent unresolved emboli were present in only 5 patients at postmortem, including the patient with chronic cor pulmonale. Of the 60 patients in this study 40 had been subjected to inferior vena cava interruption procedures and 10 treated with long-term anticoagulants (Paraskos et al 1973). These results contrast with a large British series of 56 patients surviving acute massive pulmonary embolism (in none of whom were vena cava procedures performed) and followed up for 1–9 years, with 23% taking long-term anticoagulants. Of 46 patients without underlying cardiopulmonary disease, 67% were asymptomatic and only one patient had suffered recurrent pulmonary embolism. Patients with underlying cardiopulmonary disease had a poorer long-term prognosis (Hall et al 1977). MacIntyre has reported 53 patients who had acute pulmonary embolism without underlying cardiopulmonary disease and were followed for 5–9 years after the acute event. Of these patients with an initial predisposing factor for pulmonary embolism (e.g. surgery, leg injury, immobilization), 24% died during the follow-up period as compared with 55% of patients in whom no predisposing factor was identified (60% of these died of malignant disease) (Macintyre et al 1982).

It is evident that the long-term prognosis is worst in those patients with underlying severe cardiopulmonary disease which, rather than recurrent emboli, is the cause of death in many. The prognosis is also poor for those patients without a definitive, transient predisposing cause such as surgery or immobilization, and who may have an occult malignancy or defective coagulation mechanism. An extensive work-up for malignancy in patients with unexplained deep vein thrombosis or pulmonary embolism is not, however, productive (Griffin et al 1987), but close follow-up is justified, especially in patients under the age of 50 years (Goldberg et al 1987).

Recurrent pulmonary embolism leading to chronic pulmonary hypertension and cor pulmonale is relatively uncommon and probably occurs in less than 2% of patients following pulmonary embolism (Dalen & Alpert 1975, Paraskos et al 1973, Benotti et al 1983, Sutton et al 1977, Riedel et al 1982). A recent advance in the management of these patients has been the development of late embolectomy or endarterectomy, which in carefully selected patients have produced promising results. Moser (1990) has seen more than 200 patients with chronic thromboembolic pulmonary hypertension since 1970 and has subjected many to pulmonary thromboendarterectomy. Diagnosis and management of such patients have been documented in several reports (Chitwood et al 1985, Moser et al 1987).

Criteria for offering thromboendarterectomy are the presence of significantly raised pulmonary vascular resistance at rest (>300 dynes/sec cm^{-5}), evidence of thrombus in main, lobar or segmental arteries, no other serious coexisting disease and sufficient disability for patients to justifiably be willing to undergo the procedure, which carries significant mortality and morbidity rates. Bilateral phrenic nerve palsy, reperfusion pulmonary oedema and psychiatric disturbance have been the most common postoperative complications.

PREVENTION OF DEEP VEIN THROMBOSIS AND PULMONARY EMBOLISM IN SURGICAL PATIENTS

The recognition that calf vein thrombosis is a common postoperative event and that its incidence can be reduced by a variety of prophylactic measures has led to the hope that these same measures may reduce the frequency with which thrombi extend into the proximal portions of the deep venous system, from which they may embolize and cause sudden death in the postoperative period. Because proximal venous thrombosis is present in only 25% of patients with postoperative calf vein deep vein thrombosis and only a proportion of these give rise to significant pulmonary emboli, very large numbers of patients need to be studied to show a statistically significant effect of any prophylactic regimen. The conflicting results from many published trials have led to the performance of meta-analysis (Collins et al 1988), the results of which need to be interpreted cautiously. Collins et al have pointed out that, while only 500 patients would need to be studied in order to demonstrate a reduction in the incidence of postoperative deep vein thrombosis from 20% to 10%, 5000 patients would need to be studied to show a reduction in the incidence of postoperative pulmonary embolism from 3% to 1.5%, and 20 000 patients would have to be studied to show a reduction in postoperative death due to pulmonary embolism from 0.8% to 0.4%. In their review of more than 70 randomized trials involving almost 16 000 patients, the perioperative use of low-dose s.c. heparin reduced death attributed to pulmonary embolism from 55 out of 7486 controls to 19 out of 8112 patients (Collins et al 1988). This 50% reduction in mortality from pulmonary embolism is to a considerable extent (42%) accounted for by the International Multicentre Trial (which contributed only 27% of patients in the meta-analysis) in which, despite a 100% reduction in fatal pulmonary emboli, there was no reduction in total mortality and the methodology employed attracted criticism (Sherry 1975). The dilemma facing the practising surgeon is illustrated by clearly spelling out the logistics involved in prophylaxis. Assuming a 0.5% incidence of fatal postoperative pulmonary embolism and that a prophylactic agent could reduce this by 50%, then the routine use of this agent in 1000 general surgical patients could result in preventing fatal pulmonary embolism in 2 or 3 patients. As a significant proportion of fatal pulmonary emboli occur in patients with metastatic malignant disease, the net saving of patients who would otherwise have recovered may be as low as one or two patients. The remaining 998 patients would have received unnecessary prophylaxis. If prophylaxis were of proven value, inexpensive, easily applied and devoid of side effects, then such a policy could be justified. Side effects, however, remain a matter of concern even if their incidence is low, and thus the benefit-to-risk equation for routine prophylaxis remains doubtful. These observations account for the fact that low-dose s.c. heparin or other prophylactic regimens have not become well established in routine clinical practice (Collins et al 1988, Sherry 1975, Terblanche et al 1982).

A promising area for future research would be the development of predictive indices to identify patients at greatest risk, with a view to limiting effective prophylaxis (which may comprise a combination of agents) to this group, or to routinely using non-invasive techniques such as impedance plethysmography to make an early postoperative diagnosis of proximal deep vein thrombosis and then instituting full anticoagulation.

An exception to the above is the well-established fact that the incidence of clinically significant thromboembolism following hip surgery can be reduced using warfarin anticoagulation perioperatively. This form of prophylaxis is, however, not suitable for patients undergoing abdominal surgery.

VENOUS THROMBOEMBOLISM IN PREGNANCY

The risk of deep vein thrombosis in pregnant or puerperal woman has been estimated to be about $5^{1}/_{2}$ times the risk in control females who are not taking oral contraceptives (Vessey & Doll 1968), and in a community study venous thromboembolism was clinically diagnosed in 1 : 200 pregnancies (Coon et al 1973). Obstetric complications and previous venous thromboembolism characterize up to a third of patients with postpartum thromboembolism (Aaro & Jurgens 1974). Some of the increased risk during the puerperium may be attributable to the (previous) use of oestrogens to suppress lactation (Vessey 1980). Death from pulmonary embolism occurs rarely, 1–2 per 100 000 pregnancies, but is always a tragic event (Vessey & Doll 1968).

Treatment of venous thromboembolism in pregnancy remains problematic. Untreated, almost 20% of patients with deep vein thrombosis develop pulmonary embolism, and of these nearly 30% are fatal (Villasanta 1965). Although heparin does not cross the placental barrier (and cause embryopathy like warfarin) a review of the world literature led to the conclusion that its use was nevertheless associated with a similar (30%) chance of an adverse infant outcome (Hall et al 1980). A more recent retrospective review of 100 pregnancies, in which heparin was given in 43 for treatment of venous thromboembolism, in 55 for prophylaxis and in 2 for prosthetic heart valves (mean duration of treatment 18 weeks), has provided much more encouraging data (Ginsberg et al 1989). The rates of prematurity, abortions, stillbirths, neonatal deaths and congenital abnormalities were similar to those in the normal population. The study of unselected consecutive patients reduced the potential for selection bias, one of the deficiencies inherent in the study of a historical cohort. Although the risk of heparin-associated osteoporosis was not studied and this remains of major concern, this study provides information which reduces the uncertainties involved in managing venous thromboembolism in pregnancy.

CONCLUSIONS

Major strides have been made in the accurate non-invasive diagnosis of deep vein thrombosis and pulmonary embolism. The invasive techniques of pulmonary angiography and bilateral ascending venography have been used to establish the accuracy of non-invasive tests such as ventilation–perfusion scanning and impedance plethysmography in the diagnosis and serial evaluation of progress and resolution of these disorders. Although our knowledge of the natural history of venous thromboembolism remains incomplete it is now possible to plan therapy and monitor progress more rationally than in the past.

Although asymptomatic postoperative deep vein thrombosis can be prevented using a variety of prophylactic techniques, the incidence of significant thromboembolic events is so low that the use of prophylactic regimens to reduce (but not prevent) these has not yet reached the level of clinical applicability on a wide scale. Despite improvements in understanding the hypercoagulable state, no cause can be identified in a large proportion of such patients, and much remains to be learned about why some patients are more prone than others to venous thromboembolism.

REFERENCES

Aaro L A, Jurgens J L 1974 Thrombophlebitis and pulmonary embolism as complications of pregnancy. Medical Clinics of North America 58: 829–834
Benatar S R, Immelman E J, Jeffery P 1986 Pulmonary embolism. British Journal of Diseases of the Chest 80: 313–334
Benotti J R, Ockene I S, Alpert J S, Dalen D E 1983 The clinical profile of unresolved pulmonary embolism. Chest 84: 669–678
Biello D R, Mattar A G, McKnight R C, Siegal B A 1979 Ventilation–perfusion studies in suspected pulmonary embolism. American Journal of Radiology 133: 1033–1037
Bomalski J S, Martin G J, Hughes R L, Yao J S T 1982 Inferior vena cava interruption in the management of pulmonary embolism. Chest 82: 767–774
Branch W T Jr, McNeil B 1983 Analysis of the differential diagnosis and assessment of pleuritic chest pain in young adults. American Journal of Medicine 75: 671–679
Browse N L, Burnand K G, Thomas M L 1988 Diseases of the veins: Pathology, diagnosis and treatment. Edward Arnold, London, pp 475–499
Cheely R, McCartney W H, Perry J R et al 1981 The role of non-invasive testing versus pulmonary angiography in the diagnosis of pulmonary embolism. American Journal of Medicine 70: 17–22
Chitwood W Jr, Lyerly H K, Sabiston K D C Jr 1985 Surgical management of chronic pulmonary embolism. Annals of Surgery 201: 11–26.
Collins R, Scrimgeour A, Yusuf S, Peto R 1988 Reduction in fatal pulmonary embolism and venous thrombosis by peri-operative administration. New England Journal of Medicine 318: 1162–1173
Coon W W, Willis P W, Keller J B 1973 Venous thromboembolism and other venous diseases in the Tecumseh community health study. Circulation 48: 839–846
Corrigan T P, Fossard D P, Spindler J et al 1974 Phlebography in the management of pulmonary embolism. British Journal of Surgery 61: 484–488
Dalen J E, Alpert J S 1975 Natural history of pulmonary embolism. Progress in Cardiovascular Diseases 17: 259–270
Dalen J, Brooks H L, Johnson L W, Meister S G, Szucs M M, Dexter L 1971 Pulmonary angiography in acute pulmonary embolism: Indications, techniques and results in 367 patients. American Heart Journal 81: 175–185
Ginsberg J S, Kowalchuk G, Hirsh J, Brill-Edwards P, Burrows R 1989 Heparin therapy during pregnancy: Risks to the fetus and mother. Archives of Internal Medicine 149: 2233–2236
Goldsberg R J, Seneff M, Gore J M et al 1987 Occult malignant neoplasm in patients with deep venous thrombosis. Archives of Internal Medicine 147: 251–253
Goldhaber S Z, Hennekens C H 1982 Time trends in hospital mortality and diagnosis of pulmonary embolism. American Heart Journal 104: 305–306
Goldhaber S Z, Hennekens C H, Evans D A, Newton C E, Godleski J J 1982 Factors associated with correct ante mortem diagnosis of major pulmonary embolism. American Journal of Medicine 73: 822–826
Goodman P C 1984 Pulmonary angiography. Clinics in Chest Medicine 5: 465–478
Greenfield L J 1984 Vena caval interruption and pulmonary embolectomy. Clinics in Chest Medicine 5: 495–505
Griffin M R, Stanson A W, Brown M L et al 1987 Deep venous thrombosis and pulmonary embolism: Risk of subsequent malignant neoplasms. Archives of Internal Medicine 147: 1907–1911

Hall J G, Pauli R M, Wilson K M 1980 Maternal and fetal sequelae of anticoagulation during pregnancy. American Journal of Medicine 68: 122–140

Hall R J C, Sutton G C, Kerr I H 1977 Long term prognosis of treated acute massive pulmonary embolism. British Heart Journal 39: 1128–1134

Havig O 1977 Source of pulmonary emboli. Acta Chirurgica Scandinavica (suppl) 478: 42–47

Huisman M V, Buller H R, Ten Cate J, Vreeken J 1986 Serial impedance plethysmography for suspected deep venous thrombosis in outpatients. New England Journal of Medicine 314: 823–828

Hull R, Delmore T, Genton E et al 1979 Warfarin sodium versus low-dose heparin in the long term treatment of venous thrombosis. New England Journal of Medicine 301: 855–858

Hull R, Hirsch J, Sackett D L et al 1981 Clinical validity of a negative venogram in patients with clinically suspected venous thrombosis. Circulation 64: 622–625

Hull R, Delmore T, Carter C et al 1982 Adjusted subcutaneous heparin versus warfarin sodium in the long term treatment of venous thrombosis. New England Journal of Medicine 306: 189–194

Hull R D, Hirsch J, Carter C J et al 1983a Pulmonary angiography, ventilation lung scanning and venography for clinically suspected pulmonary embolism with abnormal perfusion scan. Annals of Internal Medicine 98: 891–899

Hull R, Carter C, Jay R et al 1983b The diagnosis of acute recurrent deep vein thrombosis. A diagnostic challenge. Circulation 67: 901–906

Hull R D, Raskob G E, Carter C J et al 1988 Pulmonary embolism in outpatients with pleuritic pain Archives of Internal Medicine 148: 830–844

Hyers T M (ed) 1984 Pulmonary embolism and hypertension. Clinics in chest medicine, vol 5, no 3. Saunders, Philadelphia

Kanter B, Moser K M 1988 The Greenfield vena cava filter. Chest 93: 170–175

Lagerstedt C L, Olsson G C, Fagher B O, Oqvist B W, Albrechtson U 1985 Need for long term anticoagulant treatment in symptomatic calf vein thrombosis. Lancet ii: 515–518

MacIntyre D, Moran F, Banham S W 1982 Pulmonary embolism: A long term follow-up. Postgraduate Medical Journal 58: 222–225

MacIntyre K M, Sasahara A A 1975 Haemodynamic and ventricular responses to pulmonary emboli. Progress in Cardiovascular Diseases 17: 175–190

McNeil B J 1980 Ventilation–perfusion studies and the diagnosis of pulmonary embolism. Journal of Nuclear Medicine 21: 319–323

Miller G A H, Hall R J C, Paneth M 1977 Pulmonary embolectomy, heparin and streptokinase: Their place in the treatment of acute massive pulmonary embolism. American Heart Journal 93: 568–574

Moser K M 1990 Venous thrombo-embolism. American Review of Respiratory Disease 141: 235–249

Moser K M, Daily P O, Peterson K L et al 1987 Thrombo-endarterectomy for chronic, major vessel thrombo-embolic pulmonary hypertension in 42 patients: Immediate and long term results. Annals of Internal Medicine 107: 560–565

O'Sullivan E F 1972 Duration of anticoagulant therapy in venous thrombo-embolism. Medical Journal of Australia 2: 1104–1107

Paraskos J A, Adelstein S J, Smith R E et al 1973 Late prognosis of acute pulmonary embolism. New England Journal of Medicine 289: 55–58

PIOPED Investigators 1990 Value of the ventilation/perfusion scan in acute pulmonary embolism: Results of the prospective investigation of pulmonary embolism diagnosis (PIOPED). Journal of the American Medical Association 263: 2753–2759

Polak J F, McNeil B J 1984 Pulmonary scintigraphy and the diagnosis of pulmonary embolism. Clinics in Chest Medicine 5: 457–464

Poulose K P, Reba R C, Gilday D C, Deland F H, Wagner H N 1970 Diagnosis of pulmonary embolism: A correlative study of the clinical, scan, and angiographic findings. British Medical Journal 3: 67–71

Rabinov K, Paulin S 1972 Roentgen diagnosis of venous thrombosis in the leg. Archives of Surgery 104: 134–139

Riedel M, Stanek V, Widimsky J, Prerovsky I 1982 Long term follow-up of patients with pulmonary thrombo-embolism: Late prognosis and evolution of haemodynamic and respiratory data: Chest 81: 151–158

Rogers L Q, Lutcher C L 1990 Streptokinase therapy for deep vein thrombosis: A comprehensive review of the English literature. American Journal of Medicine 88: 389–395

Rubinstein I, Murray D, Hoffstein V 1988 Fatal pulmonary embolism in hospitalised patients. Archives of Internal Medicine 148: 1425–1426

Sandler D A, Martin J F 1989 Autopsy proven pulmonary embolism in hospital patients: Are we detecting enough deep vein thrombosis? Journal of the Royal Society of Medicine 82: 203–205

Sasahara A A, Hyers T M (co-chairmen) 1973 The urokinase pulmonary embolism trial: A national co-operative study. Circulation 47 (suppl 2): II1–108

Sherry S 1975 Low-dose heparin prophylaxis for post-operative venous thrombo-embolism. New England Journal of Medicine 293: 300–302

Sutton G C, Hall R J C, Kerr I H 1977 Clinical course and late prognosis of treated subacute massive, acute minor and chronic thrombo-embolic pulmonary hypertension. British Heart Journal 39: 1135–1152

Terblanche J, Benatar S R, Immelman E J 1982 Prophylaxis against fatal post-operative pulmonary embolism. Surgery 91: 534–536

Tow D E, Simon A L 1975 Comparison of lung scanning and pulmonary angiography in the detection and follow-up of pulmonary embolism: Urokinase pulmonary embolism trial experience. Progress in Cardiovascular Diseases 17: 239–245

Vessey M P 1980 Female hormones and vascular disease: Epidemiologic overview. British Journal of Family Planning 6 (suppl): 1–12

Vessey M P, Doll R 1968 Investigation of relationship between use of oral contraceptives and thromboembolic disease. British Medical Journal 2: 199–205

Villasanta U 1965 Thromboembolic disease in pregnancy. American Journal of Obstetrics and Gynecology 93: 142–160

Wenger N K, Stein P D, Willis P W 1972 Massive acute pulmonary embolism: The deceivingly non-specific manifestations. Journal of the American Medical Association 220: 843–844

7

Community-acquired pneumonia

J. T. Macfarlane

The last 10 years have seen a reawakening of interest in pneumonia in terms of its incidence, aetiology, epidemiology, outcome and management. New pathogens have been identified, the importance of older 'pathogens' has been clarified and a bewildering array of potent new antibiotics is now available.

Fortunately the current understanding and knowledge of community-acquired pneumonia permits a relatively simple and logical approach to the investigation and management of such patients. This chapter aims to review the current state of knowledge and to emphasize how this knowledge can be translated into practical management.

INCIDENCE AND OCCURRENCE

Limited community studies in England suggest that the incidence of community-acquired pneumonia is between one and three adults per 1000 population (Macfarlane 1987), being higher in the very young and elderly. In a recent British Thoracic Society multicentre study (1987), 29 participating physicians investigated 450 adults admitted to hospital with community pneumonia over one year, making an average of 15 new patients per physician annually. The patient being admitted to hospital with pneumonia represents the tip of a pyramid. A GP group practice will treat 1000 adults with antibiotics for a chest infection each year. Between 50 and 100 of these patients will have radiographic evidence of pneumonia, only 10–20 will be admitted to hospital and one will die. Studies have shown that only 7–20% of adults with pneumonia are admitted to hospital (Bartlett 1989, Woodhead et al 1987a).

EPIDEMIOLOGY

The last 10 years have seen a considerable improvement in the understanding of the epidemiology of community-acquired pneumonia. This has important practical implications as the microbiological cause of any particular pneumonia is not known at presentation, when the clinician has to decide upon a 'best guess' antibiotic based on the likely pathogen, which in turn may rely on epidemiological clues (Fig. 7.1). Unfortunately no infection has a sufficiently distinct presentation to allow an accurate clinical aetiological diagnosis (Fig. 7.1) (Pennington 1988, Woodhead & Macfarlane 1987).

The incidence of some respiratory pathogens is seasonal (Noah 1989). Influenza A virus infections occur in variable epidemics in the first 4 months of the year and at the same time there is usually a significant rise in reports of staphylococcal (Woodhead et al 1987b), pneumococcal,

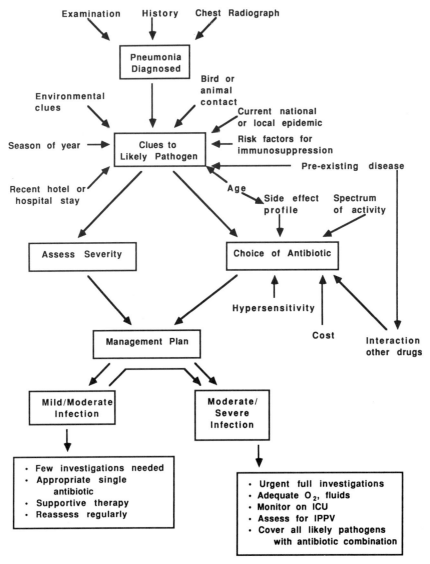

Fig. 7.1 Factors to consider when assessing the cause and management of community-acquired pneumonia. (ICU, intensive care unit; IPPV, intermittent positive pressure ventilation; O_2, added inspired oxygen therapy.)

Haemophilus and *Branhamella* lower respiratory tract infections (Mannion 1987). *Haemophilus influenzae* infections also show a summer peak. *Legionella* infection is significantly more common in the summer and early autumn, in Britain partly explained by infection acquired during summer foreign holiday travel (PHLS Communicable Disease Surveillance Centre 1988). Respiratory syncytial virus (RSV), very common in children under the age of 1 year, causes winter epidemics and almost disappears in the summer and autumn, as does parainfluenza strains 1 and 2, whereas parainfluenza 3 virus is prevalent between June and September.

In contrast, whooping cough and mycoplasma have 4-yearly cycles (Lind & Bentzon 1988, Noah 1989). In between epidemics, mycoplasma infection is unusual (Woodhead 1988) although there is normally a small rise in numbers of cases the winter before the epidemic starts (Fig. 7.2).

A knowledge of the ways in which respiratory pathogens are transmitted is also helpful to the clinician. Although most infections, including those caused by viruses, are transmitted by person-to-person contact on droplet transmission, more unusual modes of transmission also occur. *Legionella* bacteria can contaminate and multiply in water systems. Outbreaks are most commonly associated with infected mists from wet cooling towers, showers and spray taps fed from domestic warm-water systems and even mists over whirlpool spas fed by natural water supplies (Bartlett et al 1986, Goldberg et al 1989). Enquiry into a recent hotel or hospital stay or a knowledge of an outbreak of pneumonia in a locality is therefore important in assessment. Recent reports of an outbreak of pneumonia in canoeists were traced back to excess levels of algae in a lake, illustrating another hazard from water-associated pathogens (Turner et al 1990).

Zoonotic transmission of respiratory pathogens is illustrated by tularaemia, psittacosis and Q fever. A recent large review of psittacosis from Australia recorded contact with birds in 85% of 135 patients (Yung & Grayson

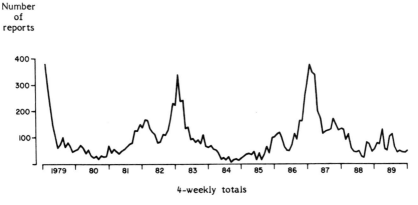

Fig. 7.2 Laboratory reports of *Mycoplasma pneumoniae* infection in England and Wales showing 4-yearly epidemics. (Reproduced with permission of PHLS Communicable Disease Surveillance Centre.)

1988). It has been suggested that *Chlamydia pneumoniae* (strain TWAR) infection may be implicated in some cases without bird contact (see later section). Q fever is a zoonotic infection carried by a wide range of domestic and wild animals and birds. Infection is transmitted by tick bites or faeces gaining entry through a skin abrasion or inhalation. In Nova Scotia, where tick fever has become endemic, stray cats are recognized as a major source of infection (Marrie et al 1985). In the USA up to two-thirds of cattle, sheep and stray dogs have serological evidence of infection. Being very resistant to drying, infected material can disseminate widely and obscure any link between outbreaks of Q fever and animal contact.

AETIOLOGY OF COMMUNITY-ACQUIRED PNEUMONIA

Recent studies confirm that pneumococcal infection remains the most common cause (Table 7.1) and probably accounts for many of the cases where no pathogen can be identified, diagnosis being hampered by prior antibiotics or incomplete specimen collection (British Thoracic Society 1987). *Mycoplasma pneumoniae* is the second most common pathogen, although the incidence varies considerably depending on whether studies were performed during epidemic periods or not (Woodhead 1988). Influenza A is the most important viral pathogen, not because of primary viral pneumonia but because of secondary bacterial superinfection, particularly

Table 7.1 Spectrum of pathogens causing adult community-acquired pneumonia (CAP). Data from studies of severe infection managed by intensive care included

	CAP (%) (2384 patients)	Severe CAP (%) (233 patients)
Strep. pneumoniae	32	27
No cause found	38	33
Mycoplasma pneumoniae	10	2.3
Haemophilus influenzae	8.5	5
Influenza virus	8	2.3
Legionella ssp.	4.5	17
Psittacosis/Q fever	3	1
Other viruses	2.7	8[a]
Staph. aureus	3.9	< 1
Gram-negative bacilli	1.6	2

CAP data based on various European studies.

Severe CAP data from various intensive care unit based studies which showed an overall mortality of 39%.

[a] Four of these 17 patients had varicella pneumonia.

by *Staphylococcus, Pneumococcus* and *Haemophilus*. The other atypical infections such as *Legionella*, Q fever and psittacosis account for less than 5% of cases, although there are marked geographical variations, with Q fever and *Legionella* infection being much commoner in some parts of Europe than others (Bartlett 1986, Woodhead & Macfarlane 1990).

Other bacterial infections are unusual. Staphylococcal pneumonia is associated with proven influenza virus infection in over half of cases (Woodhead et al 1987). From the therapeutic point of view, it is important to note that Gram-negative bacillary infections are unusual except in the debilitated elderly (Verghese & Berk 1983) and alcoholics (Moore et al 1977).

Newer pathogens

Chlamydia pneumoniae (TWAR)

This pathogen was first described as a cause of pneumonia in 1985, and subsequent studies have suggested that it may account for between 4% and 12% of all pneumonias (Glynn & Jones 1990). Population studies over a wide geographical area show a sero prevalence of around 40% in adults, with primary infection occurring in early adulthood and reinfection in later life (Grayston et al 1989). Direct human-to-human transmission is postulated and epidemics of pneumonia have been seen amongst military recruits in Finland over a number of years (Kleemola et al 1988). The clinical, laboratory and radiographic features are indistinguishable from other atypical pneumonias. The serological diagnosis is made by diagnostic changes in TWAR microimmunofluorescence antibody titres. The species-specific chlamydia complement-fixing antibodies rise in primary infection but, apparently, not in secondary reinfection. Tetracycline appears to be of some value in therapy. Until further studies are reported, it is difficult to know how widespread the problem is with this new pathogen.

Branhamella catarrhalis

This organism is an old pathogen under a new guise. It is an oropharyngeal commensal, previously classified as a *Neisseria* species. However, evidence for a pathogenic role in pneumonia is based not only on sputum isolation but also isolation from transtracheal aspirate, blood culture and by detecting an antibody response (Bartlett 1989). Isolation rates from expectorated sputum in unselected patients have varied from 1.3% to 4% in various large series (Bartlett 1989). Of nearly 4000 sputum specimens reported from Brighton, UK, 4% yielded *Bran. catarrhalis*, compared with a 10% yield for *H. influenzae* (Mannion 1987). The majority of reported infections occur in older patients with underlying chronic lung disease who either have exacerbations of bronchitis or bronchopneumonia (Hager et al 1987, McLeod et al 1983). Pneumonia is uncommon. Only 2 cases of *Bran. cattarhalis* infection were found in a recent large study of 588 cases of community-acquired pneumonia (Marrie et al 1989). It is of practical importance to note that over 50% of strains of *Bran. cattarhalis* now produce β-lactamase and are resistant to amino-penicillins. Effective antibiotics include second and third-generation cephalosporins, erythromycin, chloramphenicol, co-amoxyclav and co-trimoxazole (even though trimethoprim resistance is usual). The production of β-lactamase may result in indirect pathogenicity by protecting other strains that would otherwise be sensitive to ampicillins. Of relevance, co-infections with *H. influenzae* and *Strep. pneumoniae* occur in a percentage of patients (Mannion 1987).

Mixed infections

Community-acquired pneumonia caused by dual infections has received little attention but has important practical implications. Whereas a concurrent viral infection will have little influence on the choice of antibiotic when treating with a bacterial pneumonia, the possibility of multiple bacterial infections prompt caution against use of narrow-spectrum antibiotics such as benzylpenicillin for pneumococcal pneumonia. Simultaneous infection with *Strep. pneumoniae* and other aerobic bacteria has been reported for many years (Esposito 1988). Motte et al (1987) described a patient with pneumococcal pneumonia who did not improve with penicillin due to the presence of a β-lactamase-producing *Bran. catarrhalis*. Mixed infections were reported in 13% of cases where a pathogen was identified in one large series (British Thoracic Society 1987). Our own studies have identified mixed infections in 20–25% of proven cases (Macfarlane et al 1982, Woodhead et al 1987). *Legionella* pneumonia has been associated with mixed infection in 10% of cases (Woodhead & Macfarlane 1986), staphylococcal pneumonia with other bacterial pathogens in 16% of cases (Woodhead et al 1987b) and mycoplasma pneumonia with evidence of concurrent pneumococcal infection in 12–50% of cases (British Thoracic Society 1987, Macfarlane et al 1979). Mannion (1987) reported dual bacterial infection in 8% patients with chest infections, the majority of these including either *H. influenzae* or *Bran. catarrhalis*, both capable of producing protective β-lactamase.

Dual infections should be considered if a patient does not improve as expected with antibiotics directed at the initially identified pathogen or when deciding on antibiotic cover for anyone with severe pneumonia of unknown cause.

Pneumonia at extremes of age

The patterns of pneumonia at the extremes of age show important differences (Macfarlane 1990). In neonates, streptococcal, staphylococcal, Gram-negative and chlamydial pneumonias are seen, and in children under 2 years the major respiratory pathogen is respiratory syncytial virus (RSV). At school age, mycoplasma and pneumococcal infections are most usual, although *H. influenzae* pneumonia can occur (Kinnear 1989).

Acute pneumonia in the elderly is common and carries a high mortality ranging from 24% to 31% (Verghese & Berk 1983, Venkatesan et al 1990). Reports from the USA record *Strep. pneumoniae* to be common and Gram-negative bacilli to account for 6–36% of infections (Verghese & Berg 1983). A recent review from Britain reported a pattern very similar to younger adults, apart from a higher incidence of *H. influenzae* infection (perhaps due to an increased incidence of chronic lung disease) and a lower incidence of *Legionella* and other atypical infections (Venkatesan et al 1990). Gram-negative bacillary infections were uncommon.

DIAGNOSTIC METHODS

Although there has been much research in recent years on developing new or improving old methods for the rapid aetiological diagnosis of severe nosocomial pneumonia, and pneumonia in immunocompromised individuals, there has been relatively little practical change in guidelines for the investigation of community-acquired pneumonia. This is because the majority of patients improve with empirical antibiotic therapy which is rarely influenced by the results of routine microbiological and serological investigations. Also aggressive and invasive investigations do not influence the outcome of severe community-acquired pneumonia (Sorensen et al 1989). Sputum and blood culture remain the most commonly requested investigations but both have their limitations. Blood cultures are positive in less than a quarter of cases of pneumococcal and other community bacterial pneumonias, and sputum culture is often unrewarding if prior antibiotics have been given (British Thoracic Society 1987). Gram stain of sputum remains a rapid and specific test for bacterial pneumonia but has a low sensitivity of around 10% for pneumococcal infection if antibiotics have already been given (British Thoracic Society 1987). Other studies have shown a higher diagnostic yield from Gram stains at 65% in previously untreated pneumococcal pneumonia (Lehtomaki et al 1988). A similarly high yield from sputum Gram stain is found with staphylococcal pneumonia (Woodhead et al 1987b), emphasizing that urgent sputum Gram stain should be available in hospitals admitting patients with pneumonia. However, only two-thirds of patients will have spontaneous sputum production on admission and antibiotics should not be delayed for this reason. The rapid technique of transtracheal injection of saline (Macfarlane & Ward 1984) is highly successful in inducing sputum and is simpler to perform than inducing sputum by inhalation of nebulized hypertonic saline, a technique gaining popularity for the diagnosis of pneumocystis pneumonia in AIDS patients (Manresa 1989).

Invasive diagnostic techniques are not routinely used for community-acquired pneumonia. However, studies have shown value from protected specimen brush and bronchoalveolar lavage specimens obtained at bronchoscopy (Sorensen et al 1989) and from transthoracic needle aspiration (Barnes et al 1988, Dorca et al 1988). In the study by Dorca et al (1988) transthoracic needle aspiration produced a specificity of 100% and sensitivity of 56.6% in 173 cases of community-acquired pneumonia, with very little morbidity. Transtracheal aspiration is rarely performed nowadays.

The detection of pneumococcal polysaccharide antigen in respiratory samples has been shown to be a rapid and reliable diagnostic method (Ausina 1989, British Thoracic Society 1987, Macfarlane et al 1982), providing evidence of pneumococcal aetiology in up to 90% of cases confirmed by other methods (Lehtomaki et al 1988). Antigen may remain detectable in sputum, serum, concentrated urine and pleural fluid for several days or occasionally weeks after starting antibiotics (Venkatesan et al 1990). Antigen detection is not necessary on a routine basis but is helpful in problem cases. False-positive tests can occur in sputum but are rare for urine, blood or pleural fluid. Antigen detection can also be used for diagnosing *H. influenzae* type B infection, but as most *H. influenzae* causing adult respiratory infections are non-typable antigen detection is of limited diagnostic value here (Ausina 1989).

Legionella infection is diagnosed by recovery of the organism in culture, detection of its antigens or nucleic acids in clinical specimens or demonstration of an antibody response. The latter is commonly used but is least satisfactory as seroconversion may take 4–8 weeks or longer and sometimes may not occur at all (Monforte et al 1988). Although both culture and direct detection of legionellae in clinical specimens by immunofluorescent staining are both highly specific, the sensitivity is low (Ausina 1989). Neither has a routine place in the investigation of community-acquired pneumonia except where there is a suspicion of *Legionella* infection in a patient with severe pneumonia.

On most occasions the diagnosis of atypical and viral infections requires the detection of antibody responses in serum. The detection of mycoplasma-specific immunoglobulin M (IgM) is a useful and early indication of current infection (British Thoracic Society 1987, Glynn & Jones 1990) but is not widely available.

Viral respiratory tract infections are a major cause of morbidity in infants and children, and rapid diagnostic tests for viral infections are now used extensively for identifying RSV and are being developed for other respiratory viruses, including influenza, parainfluenza types 1 and 3 and adenovirus. Immunofluorescence tests for viral antigen in exfoliated nasopharyngeal cells produce varying sensitivities for different viruses, being highest for RSV (90–95%), followed by parainfluenza type 1 (63%), influenza virus (42%), parainfluenza type 3 (31%) and adenovirus (28%) (Kauffman 1988, Ray & Minnich 1987).

MANAGEMENT

Assessing severity of infection

This is an essential early part of the management of any patient with pneumonia, whether at home or in hospital. Recent studies by the British Thoracic Society (1987) and others (Macfarlane 1983, Marrie et al 1989, Woodhead et al 1985) have identified useful pointers to severe pneumonia (Table 7.2). Patients identified as having potentially severe pneumonia should be transferred early to a high dependency unit or intensive care unit where they can be closely monitored and if necessary receive assisted ventilation for advancing respiratory failure.

Assisted ventilation in community-acquired pneumonia

Assisted ventilation saves lives in community-acquired pneumonia, with

Table 7.2   Recognition and initial management of severe community-acquired pneumonia of unknown cause

Pointers to severe infection

- Confusion
- Respiratory rate > 30/min
- Diastolic BP < 60 mmHg
- Atrial fibrillation

- Blood urea > 7 mmol/l
- White cell count < $4 \times 10^9/l$
- Serum albumin < 25 g/l
- Arterial oxygen < 8 kPA
- Multilobe involvement

Initial management

- Cefuroxime 1.5 g i.v. 8-hourly
  plus
  erythromycin lactobionate 1 g i.v. 6-hourly
- Alter appropriately if pathogen identified
- Consider adding rifampicin to cover *Legionella* infection if deteriorating and no pathogen identified

- Correct hydration
- Adequate oxygen therapy
- Monitor on intensive care unit
- Assisted ventilation if needed

Initial Investigations

- Blood culture. Gram stain and culture of sputum or pleural fluid if available
- Serological tests for viral, atypical and *Legionella* antibodies. Mycoplasma IgM antibody
- Pneumococcal antigen detection in urine/blood/sputum
- Sample bronchoalveolar secretions (if obtainable) for Gram stain, culture and fluorescent staining for *Legionella*, viruses and *Pneumocystis*

various studies showing survival rates of between 46% and 78% in patients who presumably would otherwise have perished (British Thoracic Society 1987, Sorensen et al 1989, Woodhead et al 1985, Woodhead 1990). Transfer to the intensive care unit was precipitated by an 'unexpected' cardiorespiratory arrest in a proportion of cases, suggesting that important pointers to the severity of the pneumonia were missed. Generally, if a previously fit adult with pneumonia cannot maintain an arterial oxygen tension (PaO_2) of 8 kPA (60 mmHg) by oxygen mask he will probably require assisted ventilation. If ventilation is required this is likely to be within the first 3 days of admission for the majority of cases but may be required urgently with progressive staphylococcal or pneumococcal pneumonia. The majority of patients that die do so during the first 7–9 days of ventilation from progressive multi-organ failure, whereas those that eventually survive may require ventilation for many days or even weeks, emphasizing the importance of not giving up hope after the first week or so (Macfarlane 1987).

Choice of antibiotic

The small number of common microbiological causes of community-acquired pneumonia makes a logical antibiotic choice relatively easy. In many cases oral therapy is appropriate, i.v. antibiotics being reserved for those with moderate or severe infection. Whichever antibiotic is chosen, it must cover pneumococcal infection effectively as this is by far the commonest cause.

Aminopenicillins

Aminopenicillins remain the first choice for treating community-acquired pneumonia in most circumstances. Amoxycillin remains the best choice for oral administration, being well absorbed from the intestinal tract, in contrast to ampicillin, which is affected by concurrent food. Levels achieved in the respiratory tract are usually sufficient to treat sensitive bacteria such as pneumococci and most *H. influenzae*. Side effects such as diarrhoea or rashes occur in less than 3% of cases and other toxic effects or important drug interactions are rare.

Co-amoxyclav is a good choice when ampicillin-resistant *Haemophilus influenzae* or *Bran. catarrhalis* are likely. *Staph. aureus* will normally be sensitive, making this antibiotic a good choice for treating mild lower respiratory infections complicating influenza. Diarrhoea occurs more often than with amoxycillin.

Cephalosporins

Oral cephalosporins such as cephalexin and cephradine are ineffective against *H. influenzae* and inappropriate for treating pneumonia. Newer oral agents including cefaclor, cefixime and cefuroxime axetil are more effective for *H. influenzae* but are expensive, and the latter two can cause diarrhoea. They may be indicated in situations similar to those for co-amoxyclav mentioned before. Cefixime can be given once daily.

Generally parental third-generation cephalosporins are not appropriate for community-acquired infections. Cefuroxime has a place in the treatment of severe community-acquired pneumonia (see later, and Table 7.2).

Macrolides

Erythromycin is well established as a valuable antibiotic for treating community-acquired pneumonia because its spectrum of activity covers atypical infections, including *Legionella*, but it has troublesome side effects. Absorption by the oral route is very variable but levels achieved in the respiratory tract are usually adequate for pneumococci but less so for eradicating *H. influenzae*. Rashes are rare but gastrointestinal intolerance can occur in up to 20% of patients. Treatment may need to be stopped on account of severity in some cases. Drug interactions can occur with digoxin, theophyllines, oral contraceptives, carbamazepine and warfarin. Erythromycin is a useful alternative to an aminopenicillin, particularly in younger patients, where *H. influenzae* infection would be unusual and mycoplasma infection relatively more likely.

Intravenous erythromycin is a valuable drug for the treatment of *Legionella* infections and also severe community-acquired pneumonia of unknown cause (see later), but is expensive, causes phlebitis and is often prescribed unnecessarily.

Tetracyclines

Variable absorption and respiratory tract penetration, side effects and pneumococcal resistance of up to 30% make tetracycline a poor choice for pneumonia except for atypical infections such as psittacosis (Yung & Grayson 1988). Of the different preparations doxycycline has the best absorption and side-effect profile.

Cotrimoxazole

The absorption, respiratory tract penetration and spectrum of activity of this combination antibiotic is very good. Trimethoprim is actively concentrated in the lung. Cotrimoxazole has been recommended for first-line treatment in childhood pneumonia in developing countries (Campbell et al 1988). The main concern is with severe skin rashes in up to 8% of cases, bone marrow suppression particularly in older patients, and drug interactions with anticonvulsants, anticoagulants and hypoglycaemic agents.

Although trimethoprim alone is much safer than cotrimoxazole and can be used for treating infective bronchitis, it would rarely be used alone for pneumonia.

Quinolones

Quinolones such as ciprofloxacin have recently become established as extremely valuable antibiotics for treating a wide range of infections. Potential advantages of these agents include good absorption with oral administration, a low incidence of side effects (rash in 1%, gastrointestinal intolerance in 4–8%) and a broad spectrum of activity against most common respiratory bacteria including legionellae and other atypical infections. However, the real concern is that some of these agents are relatively inactive in vitro against *Strep. pneumoniae*. They are also expensive. Studies have suggested that quinolones are effective for treating lower respiratory tract infections (Bartlett 1989), although it is surprising that in one large multicentre trial involving 667 patients with lower respiratory tract infections eradication of *Strep. pneumoniae* infection following treatment was only assessed in 19 cases, suggesting that this might not be a truly representative study (Grassi et al 1987). At present these potent new antibiotics are rarely indicated for the initial treatment of community-acquired pneumonia. Potentiation of serum theophylline levels can be a problem with ciprofloxacin.

Changes in antibiotic resistance patterns

This is becoming a clinical problem in some parts of Europe and clinicians should be kept informed of local resistance patterns by their microbiological colleagues. Although the majority of pneumococcal isolates remain penicillin sensitive, resistance is a growing problem throughout the world, particularly in South Africa and in Spain, where up to 50% of isolates are penicillin resistant (Editorial 1988, Esposito 1988). A particularly worrying development has been the increase in *H. influenzae* resistance to ampicillin. In the UK the overall prevalence of ampicillin resistance has changed from 1.6% in 1977 to 6.2% in 1981 and 7.8% in 1986 (Bartlett 1989). The frequency of β-lactamase production by *H. influenzae* isolates in the USA is 5–15% for non-typable strains (the usual pathogens in adult community acquired-pneumonia) and 20–30% for typable strains (Doern et al 1988, Wallace et al 1988). A recent European study has shown sharp differences in resistance patterns between countries, probably explained by different antibiotic policies (Machka et al 1988) (Fig. 7.3). Rising levels of erythromycin-resistant *H. influenzae* are being reported. In one Swedish study resistance rose from 4.6% to 66.5% of isolates between 1980 and 1985 (Malmborg 1986). The problem of β-lactamase production by *Bran. catarrhalis* has already been mentioned.

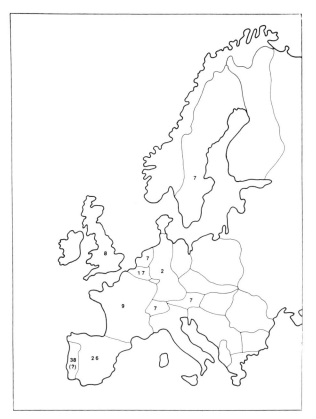

Fig. 7.3   Percentage incidence of ampicillin-resistant *H. influenzae* isolates from different European countries. (Adapted from Machka et al 1988.)

The management of severe community-acquired pneumonia of unknown cause

When faced with a patient with severe community-acquired pneumonia of unknown cause, antibiotics will have to be started pending the results of invasive investigations and laboratory examination of respiratory secretions, blood cultures and serological tests. Antibiotic choice must cover the likely causes of severe infection in this setting, which include *Strep. pneumoniae*, *H. influenzae*, *Staph. aureus*, *Legionella pneumophila*, as well as on occasions mycoplasma and psittacosis (Table 7.1). A suggested policy is summarized in Table 7.2.

MORTALITY

Hospital-based studies have generally shown a mortality of around 10–15%, although the British Thoracic Society (1987) multicentre study in Britain recorded a surprisingly low mortality of 5.7%. The age range (15–74 years) may have contributed to this low mortality, as factors associated with increasing mortality include advancing age, pre-existing disease and the cause of the pneumonia. Pneumococcal bacteraemia carries a poor prognosis, particularly if serotype 3 is involved. Mortality rates of 25–45% are still reported (Bartlett 1989). The combination of staphylococcal and influenza virus infection is frequently fatal even in previously fit young persons (Woodhead et al 1987b).

PREVENTION

The length of this review does not allow discussion of this important subject and readers are referred to recent reviews of immunization strategies for the prevention of influenza (Glezen 1990) and pneumococcal infection (Finch 1988).

CONCLUSIONS

A knowledge of the epidemiology of community-acquired pneumonia is important for the clinician. Only a few pathogens commonly cause community-acquired pneumonia, making a logical choice of antibiotic relatively easy. The antibiotic chosen must cover *Strep. pneumoniae*, by far the commonest pathogen. Most cases of pneumonia will recover with simple therapy and minimal investigations, but severe infection must be identified early and managed aggressively.

REFERENCES

Ausina V 1989 Rapid laboratory diagnostic methods in respiratory infections. Current Opinion Infectious Diseases 2: 541–546

Barnes D J, Naraqi S, Igo J D 1988 Community acquired acinetobacter pneumonia in adults in Papua New Guinea. Reviews of Infectious Diseases 10: 636–639

Bartlett C L R, Macrae A D, Macfarlane J T 1986 Legionella infections. Edward Arnold, London

Bartlett J G 1989 Community acquired bacterial infections. Current Opinion in Infectious Diseases 2: 521–525

British Thoracic Society, Public Health Laboratory Service 1987 Community acquired pneumonia in adults in British hospitals in 1982–83: A survey of aetiology, mortality, prognostic factors and outcome. Quarterly Journal of Medicine 239: 195–200

Campbell H, Byass P, Forgie I M et al 1988 Trial of cotrimoxazole versus procaine penicillin with ampicillin in treatment of community acquired pneumonia in young Gambian children. Lancet ii: 1182–1183

Doern GV, Jorgensen J H, Thornsberry C et al 1988 National collaborative study of the prevalence of antimicrobial resistance among clinical isolates of *Haemophilus influenzae*. Antimicrobial Agents and Chemotherapy 32: 180–185

Dorca J, Boada J, Verdaguer R et al 1988 Transthoracic aspiration with ultra thin needle in the diagnosis of bacterial pulmonary infection. European Respiration Journal 1 (suppl 2): 264S

Editorial 1988 Penicillin resistant pneumococci. Lancet i: 1142–1143

Esposito A L 1988 Pneumococcal pneumonia. Current Opinion in Infectious Diseases 1: 566–570

Finch R 1988 Is pneumococcal infection a preventable disease? Journal of Infection 17: 95–98

Glezen W P 1990 Influena: Epidemiology, prevention and treatment. Current Opinion in Infectious Diseases 3: 166–168

Glynn J R, Jones A C 1990 Atypical respiratory infections, including *Chlamydia TWAR* infection and legionella infection. Current Opinion in Infectious Diseases 3: 169–175

Goldberg D J, Collier P W, Fallon R J 1989 Lochgoilhead fever: Outbreak of non-pneumonic legionellosis due to *Legionella micdadei*. Lancet i: 316–318

Grassi C, Grassi G G, Mangiarotti P 1987 Clinical efficacy of ofloxacin in lower respiratory tract infections: A multicentre study. Drugs 34 (suppl 1): 80–82

Grayston J T, Wang S P, Kuo C C, Campbell L A 1989 Current knowledge on *Chlamydia pneumoniae*, strain TWAR, an important cause of pneumonia and other acute respiratory diseases. European Journal of Clinical Microbiology and Infectious Diseases 8: 191–202

Hager H, Verghese A, Alvarez S, Berk S L 1987 *Branhamella catarrhalis* respiratory infections. Research in Infectious Diseases 9: 1140–1149

Kauffman R S 1988 Viral respiratory infections. Current Opinion in Infectious Diseases 1: 575–579

Kinnear G C 1989 Childhood respiratory infections. Current Opinion in Infectious Diseases 2: 531–535

Kleemola M, Saikku P, Visakorpi P et al 1988 Epidemics of pneumonia caused by TWAR, a new Chlamydia organism, in military trainees in Finland. Journal of Infectious Diseases 157: 230–236

Lehtomaki K, Leinonen M, Takala A et al 1988 Etiological diagnosis of pneumonia in military conscripts by combined use of bacterial culture and serological methods. European Journal of Clinical Microbiology and Infectious Diseases 7: 348–354

Lind K, Bentzon M W 1988 Changes in the epidemiological pattern of *Mycoplasma pneumoniae* infections in Denmark. Epidemiology and Infection 101: 377–386

Macfarlane J T 1983 Adverse prognostic factors in pneumonia. Thorax 38: 231

Macfarlane J T 1987 Community acquired pneumonia. British Journal of Diseases of the Chest 81: 116–127

Macfarlane J T 1990 Pneumonia. Medicine International (in press).

Macfarlane J T, Ward M J 1984 Transtracheal injection of saline in the investigation of pneumonia. British Medical Journal 288: 974–975

Macfarlane J T, Adegboye D S, Warrell M J 1979 Mycoplasma pneumonia and the aetiology lobar pneumonia in Northern Nigeria. Thorax 34: 713–719

Macfarlane J T, Ward M J, Finch R G, Macrae A D 1982 Hospital study of adult community acquired pneumonia. Lancet ii: 255–257

Machka K, Bravendy I, Dabernat H et al 1988 Distribution and resistance patterns of *Haemophilus influenzae*: A European co-operative study. European Journal of Clinical Microbiology and Infectious Diseases 7: 14–24

Malmborg A S 1986 The renaissance of erythromycin. Journal of Antimicrobial Chemotherapy 18: 293–299

Mannion P T 1987 Sputum microbiology in a district general hospital: The role of *Branhamella catarrhalis*. British Journal of Diseases of the Chest 81: 391–396

Manresa F 1989 Rapid clinical diagnostic methods in respiratory infections. Current Opinion in Infectious Diseases 2: 536–540

Marrie T J, Haldane E V, Faulkner R S et al 1985 The importance of *Coxiella burnetii* as a cause of pneumonia in Nova Scotia. Canadian Journal of Public Health 76: 233–236

Marrie T J, Durant H, Yates L 1989 Community acquired pneumonia requiring hospitalisation: 5 years prospective study. Reviews of Infectious Diseases 11: 586–599

McLeod D T, Ahmed F, Power J T et al 1983 Bronchopulmonary infection due to *Branhamella catarrhalis*. British Medical Journal 287: 1146–1147

Monforte R, Estruch R, Vidal J et al 1988 Delayed seroconversion in legionnaires disease. Lancet ii: 513

Moore M A, Merson M H, Charache P, Shepard R H 1977 The characteristics and mortality of outpatient acquired pneumonia. Johns Hopkins Hospital Journal 140: 9–14

Motte S, Serruys E, Thys J P 1987 Therapeutic failure due to *Branhamella catarrhalis* in pneumococcal pneumonia. Chest 92: 382

Noah N D 1989 Cyclical patterns and predictability in infection. Epidemiology and Infection 102: 175–190

Pennington J E 1988 Community acquired pneumonia and acute bronchitis. In: Pennington J E (ed) Respiratory infections: Diagnosis and management. Raven Press, New York, pp 159–170

PHLS Communicable Disease Surveillance Centre 1988 Legionnaires' disease. British Medical Journal 296: 778–779

Ray C G, Minnich L L 1987 Efficiency of immunofluorescence for rapid detection of common respiratory viruses. Journal of Clinical Microbiology 25: 355–357

Sorensen J, Forsberg P, Hakanson E et al 1989 A new diagnostic approach to the patient with severe pneumonia. Scandinavian Journal of Infectious Diseases 21: 33–41

Turner P C, Gammie A J, Hollinrake K, Codd G A 1990 Pneumonia associated with contact with cyanobacteria. British Medical Journal 300: 1440–1441

Venkatesan P, Gladman J, Macfarlane J T et al 1990 A hospital study of community acquired pneumonia in the elderly. Thorax 45: 254–258

Verghese A, Berk S L 1983 Bacterial pneumonia in the elderly. Medicine (Baltimore) 62: 271–285

Wallace R J, Steele L C, Brooks D L et al 1988 Ampicillin, tetracycline and chloramphenicol resistant *Haemophilus influenzae* in adults with chronic lung disease: Relationship to resistance to prior antimicrobial therapy. American Review of Respiratory Disease 137: 695–699

Woodhead M A 1988 Atypical infections and legionella. Current Opinion in Infectious Diseases 1: 548–554

Woodhead M A 1990 BTS study of severe community acquired pneumonia in the intensive care unit. Thorax 45: 305P

Woodhead M A, Macfarlane J T 1986 Legionnaires disease: A review of 79 community acquired cases in Nottingham. Thorax 41: 635–640

Woodhead M A, Macfarlane J T 1987 Comparative clinical and laboratory features of legionella with pneumococcal and mycoplasma pneumonias. British Journal of Diseases of the Chest 81: 133–139

Woodhead M A, Macfarlane J T 1990 The management of pneumonia in the community. Respiratory Disease in Practice April: 17–22

Woodhead M A, Macfarlane J T, Rodgers F G et al 1985 Aetiology and outcome of severe community acquired pneumonia. Journal of Infection 10: 204–210

Woodhead M A, Macfarlane J T, McCracken et al 1987a Prospective study of the aetiology and outcome of pneumonia in the community. Lancet i: 671–674

Woodhead M A, Radvan J, Macfarlane J T 1987b Adult community acquired staphylococcal pneumonia in the antibiotic era: A review of 61 cases. Quarterly Journal of Medicine 245: 783–790

Yung A P, Grayson M L 1988 Psittacosis: A review of 135 cases. Medical Journal of Australia 148: 228–232

8

Pulmonary complications of AIDS

D. M. Mitchell

In 1983 the association between infection with the human immunodeficiency virus (HIV) and the development of AIDS was established (Barre-Sinoussi et al 1983, Gallo et al 1984). AIDS is the final phase of this chronic viral infection and is characterized by the presence of certain major opportunist infections or neoplasms (Morbidity and Mortality Weekly Reports 1987). HIV-induced damage to the immune system leads to profound depression of cell-mediated immunity, which results in a characteristic spectrum of opportunist infections, with the lung being commonly affected. In addition to opportunist infections, HIV-infected individuals may also develop a range of other complications including neurological disease, a progressive wasting disease (slim disease), skin disorders, neoplastic diseases of which Kaposi sarcoma is the most common, and, in the lung, lymphocytic interstitial pneumonitis and non-specific interstitial pneumonitis, the aetiology of which remains undetermined. There is an asymptomatic phase when individuals infected with HIV have only a minor degree of compromised immunity. During this phase there is an increased risk of developing tuberculosis or severe pneumococcal infection. At this stage of HIV infection there are opportunities for antiretroviral therapy with Zidovudine to delay symptomatic disease and for prophylaxis against tuberculosis, *Pneumocystis* pneumonia and possibly pneumococcal infection as well. The purpose of this chapter is to review the current diagnostic and therapeutic approaches to the pulmonary complications of HIV infection.

SPECTRUM OF LUNG DISEASE

Pulmonary diseases associated with HIV infection are listed in Table 8.1. In an early series 41% of AIDS patients had pulmonary complications (Murray et al 1984). Of these 85% had pneumocystis pneumonia, 17% cytomegalovirus infection, 17% infection with *Mycobacterium avium intracellulare*, 4% had tuberculosis, 4% legionnaires' disease and 2% pyogenic bacterial infection. A further 8% also had Kaposi sarcoma. Infection with fungi, herpes simplex, *Nocardia* and *Toxoplasma gondii* were rare. Since then *Pneumocystis* pneumonia has remained the main opportunist infection seen in AIDS patients in Europe and North America, being the AIDS-defining

Table 8.1 Pulmonary complications of HIV infection

Infections	
Viruses	Cytomegalovirus
	Herpes simplex
	Varicella zoster
	Epstein–Barr?
	Adenovirus
Bacteria	*Strep. pneumoniae*
	Haemophilus influenzae
	Staph. aureus
	Branhamella catarrhalis
	Gram-negative bacteria
	Mycoplasma
	Nocardia
Mycobacteria	*M. tuberculosis*
	M. avium intracellulare
	M. xenopi/kansasii, etc.
Fungi	*Candida* spp.
	Aspergillus spp.
	Coccidiodes immitis
	Cryptococcus neoformans
	Histoplasma capsulatum
Parasites	*Pneumocystis carinii*
	Cryptosporidia
	Strongyloides stercoralis
	Toxoplasma gondii

Malignancies
Kaposi sarcoma
Non-Hodgkin's lymphoma
Bronchogenic carcinoma?

Other conditions
Non-specific interstitial pneumonitis
Lymphocytic interstitial pneumonitis
Alveolar proteinosis
Pulmonary drug reactions

diagnosis in 64% of cases and occurring in up to 80% of all AIDS cases at some stage (Murray et al 1987); it is, however, far less common in Africa, where TB is a major opportunist infection. The annual incidence of *Pneumocystis* pneumonia in AIDS patients was about 35% (Polsky et al 1986), and its tendency to relapse has resulted in widespread use of prophylaxis to prevent recurrence or even to prevent first episodes. Also serious pneumonia due to pyogenic bacteria and tuberculosis have been increasingly identified as of major importance in HIV infection, whereas cytomegalovirus, although often cultured from the lung, is now thought only rarely to cause significant pneumonitis. *Mycobacterium avium intracellulare* and occasionally other mycobacteria are frequently isolated from the lung, whereas fungal and parasitic infections other than *Pneumocystis* remain relatively rare. Non-specific interstitial pneumonitis and lymphocytic interstitial pneumonitis (Murray et al 1984, Allen & Curran 1985) continue to be reported in small numbers, whereas Kaposi sarcoma, which is seen mainly in homosexual and bisexual AIDS patients, can result in extensive pulmonary involvement (Allen & Curran 1985, Meduri et al 1986).

CLINICAL PRESENTATION

Patients who present with a respiratory complication of HIV infection may already be known to be HIV seropositive or to belong to a high-risk group for infection. Some may already have AIDS. Others present without obvious risk factors, denying them or being unaware of them (e.g. blood transfusion). This makes enquiry regarding risk factors mandatory for any unusual respiratory illness. Most pulmonary illness in AIDS patients presents with a background of several weeks or months of ill health, with weight loss, fatigue or fever. A patient with *Pneumocystis* pneumonia characteristically presents with a several week history of dry cough, fever with sweats, exertion dyspnoea and a feeling of difficulty breathing in (Engelberg et al 1984, Kovacs et al 1984). Sputum production, chest pain and sudden onset are less usual but do occur, making distinction from bacterial pneumonia difficult. All the other pulmonary diseases associated with AIDS can present in a similar manner to *Pneumocystis* pneumonia. Physical examination is more likely to reveal markers of HIV infection itself rather than helpful diagnostic features of chest illness. Lymphadenopathy, cutaneous Kaposi sarcoma or evident weight loss may be seen. Examination of the mouth may reveal oral candidiasis, hairy leukoplakia or Kaposi sarcoma, whereas examination of the skin may show seborrhoeic dermatitis, molluscum contagiosum and folliculitis, which should prompt enquiry into the possibility of HIV infection (Hollander 1988). A rapid respiratory rate, pyrexia and tachycardia are common in *Pneumocystis* pneumonia, whereas crackles or signs of pleural effusion are unusual and suggest an alternative diagnosis. Cyanosis is seen in advanced respiratory disease. Asthma, bronchitis and upper respiratory infections probably occur as frequently in HIV-infected persons as in normal individuals, whereas bacterial pneumonia is more frequent and severe (Polsky et al 1986).

DIAGNOSTIC EVALUATION

As *Pneumocystis* pneumonia is by far the most common problem seen in AIDS, the diagnostic work up is heavily weighted towards establishing the presence or absence of *Pneumocystis* pneumonia as well as identifying the other pulmonary complications of HIV infection. Every effort should be made to make a definitive diagnosis to allow the correct therapy to be given. An empirical approach to therapy is appropriate only for those patients too ill for diagnostic procedures at presentation or while awaiting results of diagnostic tests (Mitchell 1989).

Laboratory investigations

The presence of HIV infection can be established by detecting specific serum antibodies to the virus by screening tests (ELISA), positive results being confirmed by Western blot. A low CD4-positive lymphocyte count correlates with the severity of immunosuppression and the tendency to develop opportunist infections (Fahey et al 1990, Phair et al 1990). In addition to routine blood count and biochemistry, blood cultures should be done in any ill patient as bacteraemia is common in HIV infection (Krumholz et al 1989). Antibody tests for the diagnosis of *Pneumocystis* pneumonia are not helpful (Pifer et al 1978), nor are currently available tests for *Pneumocystis* antigen (Young 1987, Walzer 1988), but the introduction of DNA probes and use of the polymerase chain reaction to detect the presence of *Pneumocystis* in lung tissue or bronchial washings has resulted in encouraging initial reports, and further evaluation is underway (Tanabe et al 1988, Wakefield et al 1990). Serum lactate dehydrogenase levels are increased in *Pneumocystis* pneumonia but lesser increases occur in HIV-positive patients with other pulmonary diseases. The absolute level of lactate dehydrogenase does, however, have prognostic significance (Smith R L et al 1988, Zaman & White 1988).

Chest radiograph

Between 5% and 15% of HIV-seropositive patients subsequently found to have *Pneumocystis* pneumonia have a normal chest X-ray at presentation (Rankin et al 1988, Suster et al 1986, Goodman & Gamsu 1987, Golden & Sollitto 1988), so that it is important not to ignore symptoms on account of a normal chest X-ray. The radiographic changes of the pulmonary complications of AIDS are neither specific to any particular infection or neoplasm nor to AIDS itself. The most frequent change seen in *Pneumocystis* pneumonia is bilateral perihilar haze, which can be minimal and easily missed. More severe cases show diffuse interstitial perihilar shadows with sparing at the apices and bases, and severe cases have extensive alveolar filling with air bronchograms (Fig. 8.1). These changes can also be seen in bacterial pneumonia, mycobacterial infection, Kaposi sarcoma and lymphocytic interstitial pneumonitis (Ognibene et al 1985, Goodman et al 1984, Pitchenik & Robinson 1985, Solal-Celigny et al 1985). About 5–10% of cases of *Pneumocystis* pneumonia have various atypical features, including cysts (DeLorenzo et al 1987) and upper zone shadows (Milligan et al 1985). Evolution of changes in *Pneumocystis* pneumonia may be rapid, so that an initially normal chest X-ray may be grossly abnormal after a few days, whereas resolution of changes may be slow and may never return to

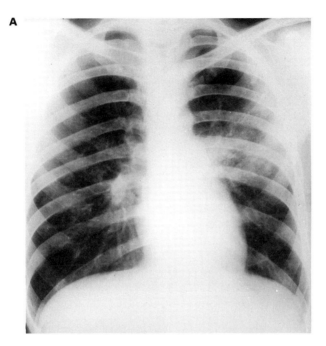

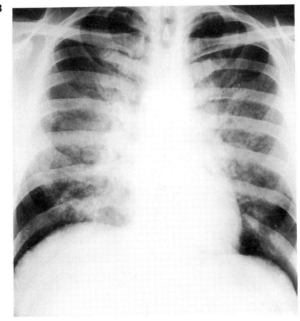

C

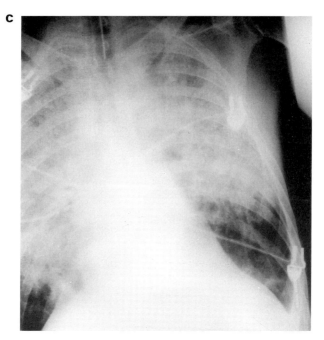

Fig. 8.1 Chest radiograph appearances of *Pneumocystis* pneumonia: **A** mild; **B** moderate; **C** severe.

normal. Focal consolidation is more likely to be due to bacterial pneumonia but can occur with *Pneumocystis* or mycobacterial disease (Stover et al 1985, Naidich et al 1987). Tuberculosis can present with both upper zone shadowing or atypical features (Pitchenik & Robinson 1985). Coarse nodular shadows suggest Kaposi sarcoma (Ognibene et al 1985, Naidich et al 1987). Hilar or mediastinal adenopathy is very unusual in *Pneumocystis* pneumonia and suggests the presence of tuberculosis, *Mycobacterium avium intracellulare*, lymphoma or Kaposi sarcoma, whereas an effusion suggests one of these four diagnoses or the presence of empyema (Meduri et al 1986, Pitchenik & Robinson 1985). Other imaging techniques such as gallium citrate scanning and computed tomography add little in the routine investigation of these patients (Millar & Mitchell 1990).

Arterial blood gases and oximetry

Blood gas measurement allows determination of the degree of respiratory failure and calculation of the alveolar arterial oxygen gradient. Only 8% of patients with *Pneumocystis* pneumonia have a normal alveolar arterial oxygen gradient at rest (Orenstein et al 1986). Exercise-induced arterial oxygen desaturation detected by oximetry has been advocated as a sensitive index for the presence of *Pneumocystis* pneumonia. Twenty of 24 patients with *Pneumocystis* pneumonia and normal oxygen tensions at rest developed oxygen desaturation on exercise, whereas only 2 of 19 patients with other AIDS-related respiratory problems did so (Smith D E et al 1988).

Pulmonary function tests

Routine pulmonary function tests are a quick and readily available way of screening HIV-positive patients for pulmonary disease (Coleman et al 1984, Shaw et al 1988). A reduction in the transfer factor (DLCO; Diffusing Capacity for Carbon Monoxide) is the most sensitive measurement for the presence of *Pneumocystis* pneumonia but lacks specificity, reduced values of below 70% of predicted normal being seen in some patients with all other forms of AIDS-related lung disease, and also in HIV-seropositive patients without respiratory symptoms (Shaw et al 1988, Mitchell et al 1988). This reduction in DLCO in these patients is independent of smoking or i.v. drug abuse, and may relate to the presence of lymphocytic alveolitis or subclinical interstitial pneumonitis which have been described in these patients (Suffredini et al 1987, Guillon et al 1988). Despite this lack of specificity, the DLCO is a useful screening test, particularly when sequential measurements are made. A sudden fall in DLCO associated with new respiratory symptoms nearly always represents the presence of respiratory disease and the need for further investigation. In one study 12 of 13 patients with *Pneumocystis* pneumonia had a DLCO of less than 70% of predicted normal with a mean value of 50% of predicted normal, which improved to 63% on recovery. By contrast the mean DLCO (percentage of predicted normal) for patients with AIDS-related complex was 77%, for patients with non-pulmonary Kaposi sarcoma 70% and patients with AIDS but without overt lung disease 70% (Shaw et al 1988).

Investigations to establish an aetiological diagnosis

From the above discussion it is clear that the non-invasive investigations described are of value in establishing the presence and extent of organic pulmonary disease and monitoring its progress. They all share roughly equivalent sensitivity, but all lack specificity in providing a definitive diagnosis. As many diseases affect the lung in HIV-positive patients and as most have specific and effective treatments, it is important to make a definite diagnosis. This is usually possible by performing fibreoptic bronchoscopy with bronchoalveolar lavage (BAL) or transbronchial lung biopsy (TBB). The recent introduction of induced sputum in some centres has allowed only those with a negative test to proceed to bronchoscopy.

Induced sputum

This technique involves the patient inhaling an aerosol of hypertonic saline from an ultrasonic nebulizer. This results in the patient coughing up mucoid material containing *Pneumocystis*, which can be identified by staining techniques. An early comparative study showed that 11 of 20 (55%) patients, who all had a positive bronchoscopy diagnosis of *Pneumocystis* pneumonia, also had a positive induced sputum using silver methionine stain to outline the pneumocysts (Pitchenik et al 1986). In another study 14 of 25 (56%) patients who had *Pneumocystis* pneumonia diagnosed at bronchoscopy had positive induced sputum using Giemsa stain to identify the trophozoites of pneumocystis (Bigby et al 1986). Induced sputum is now in widespread use in centres that have developed it. Other centres have experienced difficulties which relate either to sample acquisition or laboratory processing. Examination of samples of induced sputum requires more skill and time than the examination of BAL. Liquefaction of sputum samples by dithiothreitol, followed by centrifugation and concentration of alveolar casts containing *Pneumocystis*, increases the diagnostic yield (Zaman et al 1988). Immunofluorescent staining of induced sputum using monoclonal antibodies to *Pneumocystis* gives a higher diagnostic yield than ordinary staining. A recent study (Kovacs et al 1988) showed a diagnostic yield of 80% with routine staining (toluidine blue O) and 92% with immunofluorescence. The development of *Pneumocyst*-specific DNA probes should further increase the sensitivity (Wakefield et al 1990, Tanabe et al 1988).

Bronchoscopy

A large early series showed that 91% of all pulmonary infections in AIDS were diagnosed by a combination of BAL and TBB via fibreoptic bronchoscopy (Murray et al 1984). In a further study diagnostic yields were 88% for TBB and 85% for BAL, with a combined yield of 94% (Stover et al 1984). Diagnostic yields are so good from BAL for *Pneumocystis* that most groups now recommend that TBB can be omitted routinely (Ognibene et al 1984, Golden et al 1986, Griffiths et al 1989). This greatly simplifies and shortens the procedure and removes the morbidity of haemorrhage and pneumothorax associated with TBB. However, as prophylaxis for *Pneumocystis* is now widespread, this policy may need revision as the incidence of *Pneumocystis* declines or its manifestations become increasingly atypical, for example giving rise to a low cyst count on BAL. BAL alone, however, will miss other diagnoses such as non-specific interstitial pneumonitis and lymphocytic interstitial pneumonitis, and so TBB still has a place for selected cases (Morris et al 1987, Oldham et al 1989, Ognibene et al 1988). Endobronchial Kaposi sarcoma may be seen at bronchoscopy as flat or raised erythematous patches on the bronchial mucosa (Meduri et al 1986, Ognibene et al 1985), and as there are nearly always Kaposi sarcoma lesions at other sites, such as the skin, biopsy is rarely necessary. Antimicrobial therapy for *Pneumocystis* pneumonia can be started before bronchoscopy is performed, as cysts of *Pneumocystis* persist for days or weeks following therapy, so that the diagnosis will not be lost (DeLorenzo et al 1985, Shelhamer et al 1984). Patients with *Pneumocystis* pneumonia are often severely hypoxaemic and have very irritable airways. Premedication with nebulized 4% lignocaine, a short-acting benzodiazepine (e.g. midazolam) and supplemental oxygen given by mask or nasal cannulae monitored by oximetry allows safe, comfortable bronchoscopy in the majority of patients.

Open lung biopsy and fine needle aspirate

Open lung biopsy provides a high diagnostic yield in interstitial lung disease (Sattersfield & McLaughlin 1979, Venn et al 1985) with low morbidity and a high diagnostic yield in non-AIDS immunocompromised patients with *Pneumocystis* pneumonia (Michaelis et al 1976, Rosen et al 1975). It is only very rarely required in AIDS patients because of the high diagnostic yield from bronchoscopy (Fitzgerald et al 1987). In a series of 18 patients with negative bronchoscopy and transbronchial biopsy, open lung biopsy yielded treatable infection as a cause of illness in only 5 patients (Fitzgerald et al 1987). Percutaneous fine needle aspiration can give rapid diagnosis of pulmonary infection in children and adults (Mimica et al 1971, Palmer et al 1980). In patients with AIDS, however, there has been a high incidence of complications and it cannot be recommended (Craddock et al 1987).

TREATMENT OF PNEUMOCYSTIS PNEUMONIA

Mortality for *Pneumocystis* pneumonia is now less than 10% per episode (Kales et al 1987, Brenner et al 1987) but is over 90% in patients requiring mechanical ventilation (Wachter et al 1986, Schein et al 1986, Rosen et al 1986). Before widespread introduction of prophylaxis for *Pneumocystis*, the relapse rate after one episode was about 35% by 6 months and 60% by one year (Fischl 1988). Several antimicrobials are effective against *Pneumocystis* pneumonia (Table 8.2), but co-trimoxazole in high dose remains the treatment of choice. The recommended dose for trimethoprim is 15–20 mg/kg per day, and for sulphamethoxazole 75–100 mg/kg per day given intravenously. Serum concentration of trimethoprim should be between 5 and 8 µg/ml. Treatment failure has been reported with levels below 5 µg/ml (Fischl 1988). Side effects (which are common in AIDS patients) occur in 50–80% (Sattler et al 1988), the most common being nausea, vomiting and skin rash. These usually occur during the first week of treatment and can often be controlled with antihistamines and antiemetics. Bone marrow suppression is common and can be minimized by dose reduction. Some authorities suggest adding folinic acid (Sattler et al 1988, Wharton et al 1986, Gordin et al 1984). Treatment should continue for 3 weeks, and as co-trimoxazole is well absorbed oral treatment can often be started after a few days if nausea is controlled and when the temperature settles. Mild cases can be treated orally from the outset.

Table 8.2 Antimicrobial
agents for *Pneumocystis*
pneumonia

First-line therapy
Co-trimoxazole
Pentamidine
Dapsone–trimethoprim

Second-line therapy
Nebulized pentamidine
Clindamycin–primaquine
Trimetrexate
Difluoromethylornithine
Piritrexim

Unlike co-trimoxazole, pentamidine must be given intravenously, the dose being 4 mg/kg per day (Fischl 1988). Adverse reactions are common and may be severe. They include nausea, vomiting, rash, tachycardia, hypertension, hypoglycaemia, hyperglycaemia, pancreatitis, nephrotoxicity and hepatotoxicity (Sattler et al 1988, Wharton et al 1986, Gordin et al 1984). In a randomized prospective study of the efficacy of co-trimoxazole and pentamidine for *Pneumocystis* pneumonia in AIDS patients (Wharton et al 1986) there was no detectable difference between the two treatments, but over half the patients had changed to the alternative treatment because of side effects. In a second randomized prospective study (Sattler et al 1988) all patients received 3 weeks of treatment and did not cross over to alternative therapy if side effects occurred. All side effects were managed symptomatically or by dose reduction. Co-trimoxazole therapy resulted in more rapid improvement and lower mortality (14%) than pentamidine (39%). Co-trimoxazole has an additional advantage over pentamidine, as being a broad-spectrum antibiotic it will often be effective against concomitant bacterial infection, which is common.

The combination of dapsone and trimethoprim is as effective (Leoung et al 1986) as co-trimoxazole for mild and moderate *Pneumocystis* pneumonia, with the advantage of fewer side effects (Medina et al 1990), and is useful for patients who previously developed serious side effects with co-trimoxazole or pentamidine. Newer drugs and combination of drugs are currently under evaluation. Clindamycin with primaquine has been successfully used in patients unresponsive or intolerant to first-line therapy (Toma et al 1989). Trimetrexate, an analogue of methotrexate, has also been used for second-line therapy (Allegria et al 1987). The patients who responded had a high subsequent relapse rate. Difluoromethylornithine, a polyamine synthesis inhibitor (Golden et al 1984), has also been employed for salvage therapy with less encouraging results, whereas the newer agent piritrexim is under evaluation (Falloon et al 1990). Drug toxicity following i.v. pentamidine prompted investigation of pentamidine delivered directly to the lung via nebulized aerosol for the therapy of *Pneumocystis* pneumonia. Thirteen of

15 patients (87%) with mild to moderate *Pneumocystis* pneumonia improved following 600 mg of nebulized pentamidine daily for 3 weeks (Montgomery et al 1987). There were no systemic side effects, cough occurred in 12 patients and serum pentamidine concentrations were extremely low. In a further study, 9 of 13 similarly treated patients (70%) improved (Conte et al 1987). Cough and bronchospasm were noted as side effects and 3 patients had an early relapse. The nebulizer used must deliver particles of small enough size to allow good deposition of drug within the lung. The initial study (Montgomery et al 1987) used the Respirgard II nebulizer, which produced small particles of a Mass Median Aerodynamic Diameter (MMAD) of 0.8 μm with a Geometric Standard Deviation (GSD) of 1.5 μm (Miller et al 1989). Very similar devices have now been evaluated and are also suitable. These include the Acorn System 22 Miser (O'Doherty et al 1988, Simmonds et al 1989). Subsequent experience with nebulized pentamidine has shown overall response rates for mild and moderate *Pneumocystis* pneumonia of about 70%, but relapse after nebulized pentamidine is relatively frequent. Nebulized pentamidine should probably be reserved for mild *Pneumocystis* pneumonia or for patients who have had serious side effects on parenteral therapy (Armstrong & Bernard 1988). A recent large comparative study of nebulized pentamidine with co-trimoxazole for the treatment of mild *Pneumocystis* pneumonia showed that nebulized pentamidine was as effective as co-trimoxazole, with fewer side effects, but response rates were slower (Montgomery et al 1990).

Management of deterioration

At least 85% of patients with *Pneumocystis* pneumonia will start to improve on therapy between 2 and 6 days. If no improvement is seen by the sixth day, the diagnosis should be reviewed and other causes of deterioration considered (e.g. incorrect diagnosis, pneumothorax, left ventricular failure, anaemia, drug side effects, other AIDS illness). This may require consideration of further bronchoscopy in search of a co-pathogen (e.g. mycobacterial or bacterial infection). If *Pneumocystis* pneumonia remains the main problem, alternative antimicrobial therapy should be considered (although 90% of patients who fail on i.v. co-trimoxazole will also fail to respond to i.v. pentamidine) (Murray et al 1984), and if the patient has deteriorated with worsening respiratory failure additional support measures should be considered.

Although evidence is conflicting, there would seem little doubt that corticosteroids have a useful role to play in *Pneumocystis* pneumonia complicated by respiratory failure. An early study showed that 9 of 10 patients with *Pneumocystis* pneumonia in respiratory failure treated with methylprednisolone 40 mg 6-hourly for 7 days improved, whereas only 2 of 8 patients not treated survived (MacFadden et al 1987). However, a prospective double-blind study of 41 patients with *Pneumocystis* and respiratory failure showed no benefit within the treatment group given 60 mg of methylprednisolone four times daily in reducing schedule for 8 days (Clement et al 1989). A further large controlled randomized study (Bozzette et al 1990) examined the 12-week outcome of patients with *Pneumocystis* pneumonia treated with corticosteroids in addition to antimicrobial therapy, and showed that corticosteroid treatment reduced respiratory failure and death.

Patients with severe *Pneumocystis* pneumonia are likely to become fluid overloaded. Review of fluid balance and i.v. diuretics will often produce temporary improvement in patients with worsening respiratory failure.

Nasal continuous positive airway pressure (CPAP) ventilation has been used in spontaneously breathing patients remaining severely hypoxaemic despite supplemental oxygen to good effect in patients with *Pneumocystis* pneumonia (Kesten & Rebuck 1988), thus avoiding the need for mechanical ventilation.

The prognosis for AIDS patients with *Pneumocystis* pneumonia admitted to intensive care units for intermittent positive pressure ventilation is in excess of 95% (Schein et al 1986, Rosen et al 1986, Steinbrook et al 1985, Wachter et al 1988), although recently improvements in these figures have been reported (El-Sadr & Simberkoff 1988, Friedman et al 1989, Wachter et al 1989, Luce et al 1988). The decision to provide mechanical ventilation to patients with *Pneumocystis* pneumonia is complex and must include considerations of the patients' overall prognosis, the presence of other AIDS-related complications, the wishes of the patients and relatives and the problems of managing AIDS patients on the ITU (Miller & Mitchell 1990).

Prevention of *Pneumocystis* pneumonia

As *Pneumocystis* pneumonia is a relapsing condition with a significant mortality, prophylaxis should be offered on recovery. Furthermore, as *Pneumocystis* pneumonia is the commonest opportunist infection in AIDS, but tends to occur relatively late in the natural history of HIV infection, primary prophylaxis can be offered to all HIV-seropositive individuals when their CD4 lymphocyte count falls below 0.2 to 0.3×10^9 per litre, at which level of immunosuppression *Pneumocystis* pneumonia becomes increasingly likely (Phair et al 1990). Various prophylactic agents are available, and are not only effective in greatly reducing the incidence of *Pneumocystis* pneumonia but have also been shown to increase survival (Fischl et al 1988, Leoung et al 1989). Co-trimoxazole is effective in prophylaxis, but carries the problem of side effects (Fischl et al 1988). Some authorities prefer to use dapsone or Fansidar, which are both effective for prophylaxis (Metroka et al 1989, Fischl & Dickinson 1986), thus holding co-trimoxazole in reserve for episodes of *Pneumocystis* pneumonia. There has been major interest in nebulized pentamidine given in various dosage regimes for prophylaxis.

Generally 300 mg given every 2 weeks affords good protection (Leoung et al 1989, Leoung et al 1990), and nebulized pentamidine has now been adopted by many centres in view of its efficacy and low toxicity.

Bacterial pneumonia

HIV-infected individuals have an increased incidence of bacterial pneumonia and bacteraemia. Although the available data are sparse, one study reported an annual attack rate for pneumococcal pneumonia of 18 per 1000 HIV-infected patients, the rate being approximately 3–4 per 1000 in the general population (Simberkoff et al 1984, Polsky et al 1986, Chaisson 1989, Selwin et al 1988). In AIDS patients most pulmonary bacterial infections are due to *Streptococcus pneumoniae, Haemophilus influenzae* and *Branhamella catarrhalis*. Severe infection due to *Staphylococcus aureus* and Gram-negative bacteria also occur, particularly in the later stages of AIDS. The increased susceptibility to capsulated organisms in AIDS patients is thought to relate to the inability to mount normal antibody responses. Bacterial pneumonia and bacteraemia may occur with rapid onset and are usually severe in AIDS patients, so the possibility should always be considered in the differential diagnosis. Most bacterial infections respond to appropriate antibiotics, although there is a tendency to relapse following treatment. In view of the frequency and severity of pneumococcal infection, the US CDC recommends that all HIV-infected individuals over 2 years of age should be immunized with pneumococcal polyvalent vaccines (Immunization Practices Advisory Committee 1989), although there are no data currently available to support the efficacy of this policy.

Viral infections

Cytomegalovirus (CMV) is a major opportunist pathogen in AIDS, causing choroidoretinitis, colitis, hepatitis, adrenalitis, radiculitis and oesophagitis. It is frequently isolated from saliva, sputum and BAL of AIDS patients, but probably causes pneumonitis on rare occasions only. This is in contrast to allograft recipients where CMV is a common cause of pneumonitis. CMV infection is almost universal in homosexual HIV-seropositive patients, and is isolated in between 30% and 40% of AIDS patients undergoing bronchoscopy for pneumonia of all causes (Murray et al 1984, Broaddus et al 1985). If CMV pneumonitis is diagnosed in AIDS it is normally by a process of exclusion, i.e. following treatment of other infective causes and exclusion of non-infective processes such as Kaposi sarcoma. CMV responds to Ganciclovir, which has to be administered intravenously. Maintenance treatment is required to prevent relapse. Herpes simplex and varicella zoster may very occasionally cause pneumonitis in AIDS patients (Murray et al 1984, Suster et al 1986, Cohen et al 1988).

Mycobacterial infection

Both tuberculosis and atypical mycobacterial infection are seen with increased frequency in HIV-seropositive individuals (see also Chapter 9). The incidence of TB in HIV-infected individuals reflects the background prevalence of tuberculosis in the community, where the individual lives or has lived. In the majority of cases TB is the result of endogenous reactivation rather than fresh infection (Selwin et al 1989). The increased incidence of TB results from reactivation of latent infection as cell-mediated immunity declines. It has also been suggested that TB occurring in an HIV-seropositive individual speeds up the natural history of HIV disease, as mycobacteria are potent activators of CD4-positive lymphocytes, resulting in further HIV proliferation. TB may often be the first serious infection to be seen in patients with progressive HIV disease (Sunderam et al 1986, Chaisson et al 1987, Pitchenik et al 1984). TB developing in a non-pulmonary site in an HIV-positive individual is now regarded as an AIDS-defining diagnosis (Morbidity and Mortality Weekly Reports 1987). Patients with AIDS who develop tuberculosis frequently have false-negative tuberculin skin test responses (Sunderam et al 1986) and may present with atypical clinical and radiograph features. Sputum is frequently negative for acid-fast bacilli and the clinical course may be rapid, resembling primary rather than post-primary disease. These features all add to diagnostic difficulties (Sunderam et al 1986, Chaisson et al 1987, Pitchenik et al 1984, Pitchenik & Rubinstein 1985). TB in European AIDS cases occurs in approximately 5–10% of cases (Helbert et al 1990). TB in patients with HIV infection generally responds well to conventional antituberculous chemotherapy with three or four drugs (rifampicin, isoniazid, pyrazinamide and ethambutol) given for 9 months (Sunderam et al 1986, Chaisson et al 1987, Pitchenik et al 1984). Relapse after chemotherapy has been described but is relatively rare (Sunderam et al 1987). In the USA it is now recommended that all tuberculin test positive HIV-seropositive individuals should receive isoniazid chemoprophylaxis (American Thoracic Society and Centers for Disease Control 1986).

Mycobacterium avium intracellulare infection

Disseminated infection with *Mycobacterium avium intracellulare* (MAI) is common in the terminal phase of AIDS, occurring in up to 50% of patients (Wong et al 1985). Although MAI infection is common in AIDS patients, the extent to which it contributes to clinical disease varies. Many of these patients are unwell because of numerous concomitant infections or tumours rather than because of MAI. Many clinicians therefore would not attempt routine treatment, as treatment even if successful may not prolong survival (Wong et al 1985, Hawkins et al 1986, Helbert et al 1990). However, there are undoubtedly cases where MAI is accountable for significant clinical illness and warrants treatment. MAI is resistant to all first-line drugs in vitro and shows variable resistance patterns to many of the other drugs available. Various combinations have been employed with various and generally poor results. A four-drug regime consisting of rifampicin, ethambutol, amikacin and ciprofloxacin has produced the most consistent benefits (Murray & Mills 1990).

Other non-tuberculous mycobacterial infections

Infections with mycobacteria other than TB and MAI are extremely rare but do occur, and include *M. xenopi, M. kansasii* and *M. gordonae. M. kansasii* is likely to respond to isoniazid, rifampicin and ethambutol given for a minimum of 18 months. Ciprofloxacin has good activity in vitro against *M. xenopi* and should probably be included in the treatment regime (Helbert et al 1990, Young et al 1987).

Non-specific interstitial pneumonitis and lymphocytic interstitial pneumonitis

Lymphocytic interstitial pneumonitis (LIP) is common in childhood AIDS and also occurs in adults. It is characterized by lymphocytic alveolitis, with an increase in CD8-positive lymphocytes, and it probably represents a diffuse lymphoproliferative process. The clinical course is usually indolent, with anecdotal reports of steroid responsiveness. The aetiology remains obscure. Both Epstein–Barr virus (EBV) and HIV have been implicated (Andiman et al 1985, Ziza et al 1985). Non-specific interstitial pneumonitis (NIP) largely remains a diagnosis of exclusion of infectious and other conditions, and is characterized histologically by a chronic interstitial pneumonitis (Suffredini et al 1987, Solal-Celigny et al 1985).

Kaposi sarcoma

Kaposi sarcoma can affect pulmonary parenchyma, pleura, hilar and mediastinal lymph nodes and pericardium as well as producing the endobronchial lesions seen at bronchoscopy (O'Brien 1989, Ognibene et al 1985, Meduri et al 1986). When significant pulmonary disease is present, there is nearly always extensive involvement at other sites such as the skin and lymph nodes. Extensive pleural and parenchymal disease can result in respiratory failure, whereas extensive endobronchial involvement can occasionally produce air flow obstruction. Recurrent pleural effusions usually respond to bleomycin pleurodesis. In severe cases of Kaposi sarcoma with pulmonary disease, respiratory distress and failure will usually respond to combination chemotherapy with etoposide and vincristine (Kaplan et al 1986). More aggressive disease may respond to doxorubicin, bleomycin and vincristine with a partial response rate of about 50% (Kaplan et al 1986, Gill et al 1988). Overall prognosis is very poor.

CONCLUSION

Pneumocystis pneumonia remains the most important cause of pneumonia in patients with AIDS in Europe and North America. The treatment of choice is co-trimoxazole, although other effective treatments are available and newer agents are under evaluation. The response to treatment for *Pneumocystis* pneumonia is excellent, with a mortality for first episodes of less than 10%. Prophylaxis for *Pneumocystis* pneumonia is effective and should be offered to all patients following an episode of *Pneumocystis* pneumonia, and probably also to patients with low CD4 lymphocyte counts before they develop an episode. The other common treatable causes of respiratory disease in HIV-seropositive individuals are bacterial pneumonias and tuberculosis, where results from therapy are also very good and where there are also possibilities for prophylaxis. The value of treatment for MAI remains uncertain. Other forms of pulmonary disease in HIV infection are on the whole refractory to treatment and carry a poor prognosis. It is important to establish a definite diagnosis as quickly as possible after presentation so that appropriate therapy can be given.

REFERENCES

Allegria C J, Chabner B A, Tuazon C U et al 1987 Trimetrexate for the treatment of *Pneumocystis carinii* pneumonia in patients with acquired immunodeficiency syndrome. New England Journal of Medicine 317: 978–985

Allen J R, Curran J W 1985 Epidemiology of the acquired immunodeficiency syndrome. In: Gallin J I, Fauci A S (eds) Advances in host defence mechanisms, vol 5. Acquired immunodeficiency syndrome. Raven Press, New York, pp 1–17

American Thoracic Society and Centers for Disease Control 1986 Treatment of tuberculosis and tuberculosis infection in adults and children. American Review of Respiratory Disease 134: 355–363

Andiman W A, Martin K, Rubinstein A et al 1985 Opportunistic lymphoproliferations associated with the Epstein–Barr viral DNA in infants and children with AIDS. Lancet ii: 1390–1393

Armstrong D, Bernard E 1988 Aerosol pentamidine. Annals of Internal Medicine 109: 852–854

Barre-Sinoussi F, Chermann J C, Rey F et al 1983 Isolation of a T-lymphotropic retrovirus from a patient at risk for immunodeficiency syndrome (AIDS). Science 220: 868–871

Bigby T, Margolskee D, Curtis J et al 1986 The usefulness of induced sputum in the diagnosis of *Pneumocystis carinii* pneumonia in patients with the acquired immunodeficiency syndrome. American Review of Respiratory Disease 133: 515–518

Bozzette S A, Sattler F, Chin J et al 1990 Corticosteroids in pneumocystis pneumonia: 12 weeks outcome of a controlled randomised trial. Sixth International Conference on AIDS, San Francisco, vol 3, S B 17: p 100

Brenner M, Ognibene F P, Lack E E et al 1987 Prognostic factors and life expectancy of patients with acquired immunodeficiency syndrome and *Pneumocystis carinii* pneumonia. American Review of Respiratory Disease 136: 1199–1206

Broaddus V C, Dake M D, Stulbarg M S et al 1985 Bronchoalveolar lavage and transbronchial biopsy for the diagnosis of pulmonary infections in the acquired immunodeficiency syndrome. Annals of Internal Medicine 102: 747–752

Centres for Disease Control. General Recommendations on immunization 1989. Morbidity and Mortality Weekly Report 38: 205–282

Chaisson R E 1989 Bacterial pneumonia in patients with human immunodeficiency virus infection. Seminars in Respiratory Infection 4: 133–138

Chaisson R E, Schecter G F, Theuer C P et al 1987 Tuberculosis in patients with the acquired immunodeficiency syndrome: Clinical features, response to therapy and survival. American Review of Respiratory Disease 136: 570–574

Clement M, Edison R, Turner J et al 1989 Corticosteroids as adjunctive therapy in severe *Pneumocystis carinii* pneumonia: A prospective placebo controlled trial (abstract). American Review of Respiratory Disease 139: A250

Cohen P R, Beltrani V P, Grossman M E et al 1988 Disseminated herpes zoster in patients with human immunodeficiency virus infection. American Journal of Medicine 84: 1076–1080

Coleman D L, Dodek P M, Golden J A 1984 Correlation between serial pulmonary function tests and fibreoptic bronchoscopy in patients with *Pneumocystis carinii* pneumonia and the acquired immune deficiency syndrome. American Review of Respiratory Disease 129: 491–493

Conte J E, Hollander H, Golden J A 1987 Inhaled or reduced dose intravenous pentamidine for *Pneumocystis carinii* pneumonia: A pilot study. Annals of Internal Medicine 1007: 495–498

Craddock C, Pastvol G, Bull R et al 1987 Cardiorespiratory arrest and autonomic neuropathy in AIDS. Lancet ii: 16–18

DeLorenzo L J, Maguire G P, Wormser G P et al 1985 Persistence of *Pneumocystis carinii* pneumonia in the acquired immunodeficiency syndrome: Evaluation of therapy by follow-up transbronchial lung biopsy. Chest 88: 79–83

DeLorenzo L J, Huang C T, Maguire G P et al 1987 Roentgenographic patterns of *Pneumocystis carinii* pneumonia in 104 patients with AIDS. Chest 91: 323–327

El-Sadr W, Simberkoff M S 1988 Survival and prognostic factors in severe *Pneumocystis carinii* pneumonia requiring mechanical ventilation. American Review of Respiratory Disease 137: 1264–1267

Engelberg L A, Lerner C W, Tapper M L 1984 Clinical features of pneumocystic pneumonia in the acquired immune deficiency syndrome. American Review of Respiratory Disease 130: 689–694

Fahey J L, Taylor J M G, Detels R et al 1990 The prognostic value of cellular and serologic markers in infection with the human immunodeficiency virus type I. New England Journal of Medicine 322: 166–172

Falloon J, Kovacs J, Allegra C et al 1990 A pilot study of piritrexim with leucovorin for the treatment of pneumocystis pneumonia. Sixth International Conference on AIDS, San Francisco, vol 1, Th B 399: p 221

Fischl M A 1988 Treatment and prophylaxis of *Pneumocystis carinii* pneumonia. AIDS 2 (suppl 1): S 143–150

Fischl M A, Dickinson G M 1986 Fansidar prophylaxis of *Pneumocystis carinii* pneumonia in the acquired immunodeficiency syndrome. Annals of Internal Medicine 105: 629

Fischl M A, Dickinson G M, La Voie L 1988 Safety and efficacy of sulfamethoxazole and trimethoprim chemoprophylaxis for *Pneumocystis carinii* pneumonia in AIDS. Journal of the American Medical Association 259: 1185–1189

Fitzgerald W, Bevelaqua F A, Garay S M et al 1987 The role of open lung biopsy in patients with the acquired immunodeficiency syndrome. Chest 91: 659–661

Friedman Y, Franklin C, Rackow E C et al 1989 Improved survival in patients with AIDS, *Pneumocystis carinii* pneumonia and severe respiratory failure. Chest 96: 862–866

Gallo R C, Salahuddin S Z, Popovic M et al 1984 Frequent detection and isolation of cytopathic retroviruses (HTLV-III) from patients with AIDS and at risk from AIDS. Science 224: 500–503

Gill P, Krailo M, Slater L et al 1988 Results of randomised trial of ABV (adriamycin, bleomycin and vincristine) vs an inadvanced epidemic Kaposi's sarcoma [abstract]. Proceedings of IVth International Conference on AIDS, Stockholm, p 323

Golden J A, Sollitto R A 1988 The radiology of pulmonary disease: Chest radiography, computed tomography, and gallium scanning. In: White D A, Stover D E (eds) Pulmonary effects of AIDS. Clinics in Chest Medicine 9: 481–495

Golden J A, Sjoerdsma A, Santi D V 1984 *Pneumocystis carinii* pneumonia treated with alpha-difluoromethylornithine. Western Journal of Medicine 141: 613–623

Golden J A, Hollander H, Stubarg M S et al 1986 Bronchoalveolar lavage as the exclusive diagnostic modality for *Pneumocystis carinii* pneumonia. Chest 90: 18–22 ·

Goodman P C, Gamsu G 1987 Pulmonary radiographic findings in the acquired immunodeficiency syndrome. Postgraduate Radiology 7: 3–15

Goodman P C, Broaddus V C, Hopewell P C et al 1984 Chest radiographic patterns in the acquired immune deficiency syndrome. American Review of Respiratory Disease 130: 689–694

Gordin F M, Simon G L, Wofsy C B et al 1984 Adverse reactions to trimethoprim–sulfamethoxazole in patients with the acquired immunodeficiency syndrome. Annals of Internal Medicine 100: 495–499

Griffiths M M, Kocjan G, Miller R F et al 1989 Diagnosis of pulmonary disease in human immunodeficiency virus infection: Role of transbronchial biopsy and bronchoalveolar lavage. Thorax 44: 554–558

Guillon J M, Autran B, Denis M et al 1988 Human immunodeficiency virus related lymphocytic alveolitis. Chest 94: 1264–1270

Hawkins C C, Gold J W M, Whimbey E et al 1986 Treatment of disseminated *Mycobacterium avium intracellulare* infections in patients with the acquired immunodeficiency syndrome. Annals of Internal Medicine 105: 184–188

Helbert M, Robinson D, Buchanan D et al 1990 Mycobacterial infection in patients infected with the human immunodeficiency virus. Thorax 45: 45–48

Hollander H 1988 Work-up of the HIV-infected patient: Practical approach. Infectious Disease Clinics of North America 2: 353–358

Immunization Practices Advisory Committee, Centers for Disease Control 1989 Pneumococcal polysaccharide vaccine. Morbidity and Mortality Weekly Report 38: 64–76

Kales C P, Murron J R, Torres R A et al 1987 Early predictors of in-hospital mortality for *Pneumocystis carinii* pneumonia in the acquired immunodeficiency syndrome. Archives of Internal Medicine 147: 1413–1417

Kaplan L, Abrams D, Volberding P A 1986 Treatment of Kaposi's sarcoma in acquired immunodeficiency syndrome with an alternating vincristine–vinblastine regimen. Cancer Treatment Reports 70: 1121–1122

Kesten S, Rebuck A S 1988 Nasal continuous positive airway pressure in *Pneumocystis carinii* pneumonia. Lancet ii: 1414–1415

Kovacs J A, Heimenz J W, Macher A M et al 1984 *Pneumocystis carinii* pneumonia: A comparison between patients with the acquired immunodeficiency syndrome and patients with other immunodeficiency. Annals of Internal Medicine 100: 663–671

Kovacs J A, Ng V L, Masur H et al 1988 Diagnosis of *Pneumocystis carinii* pneumonia: Improved detection in sputum with use of monoclonal antibodies. New England Journal of Medicine 318: 589–593

Krumholz H, Sande M A, Lo B 1989 Community-acquired bacteremia in patients with acquired immunodeficiency: Clinical presentation, bacteriology and outcome. American Journal of Medicine 86: 776–779

Leoung G S, Feigal D W, Montgomery A B et al 1990 Aerosolised pentamidine for prophylaxis against *Pneumocystis carinii* pneumonia: The San Francisco community prophylaxis trial. New England Journal of Medicine 323: 769–775

Leoung G S, Mills J, Hopewell P C et al 1986 Dapsone–trimethoprim for *Pneumocystis carinii* pneumonia in the acquired immunodeficiency syndrome. Annals of Internal Medicine 105: 45–48

Leoung G S, Montgomery A B, Abrams D J et al 1989 Aerosol pentamidine for *Pneumocystis carinii* prophylaxis: A 3 arm randomized trial. Abstracts of the 5th International Conference on AIDS 196

Luce J M, Wachter R M, Hopewell P C 1988 Intensive care of patients with the acquired immunodeficiency syndrome: Time for a reassessment? American Review of Respiratory Disease 137: 1261–1263

MacFadden D K, Edelson J D, Hyland R H et al 1987 Corticosteroids as adjunctive therapy in treatment of *Pneumocystis carinii* pneumonia in patients with acquired immunodeficiency syndrome. Lancet i: 1477–1479

Medina I, Mills J, Leoung G et al 1990 Oral therapy for *Pneumocystis carinii* pneumonia in the acquired immunodeficiency syndrome. New England Journal of Medicine 323: 776–782

Meduri G U, Stover D E, Lee M et al 1986 Pulmonary Kaposi sarcoma in the acquired immunodeficiency syndrome: Clinical radiologic and pathologic manifestations. American Journal of Medicine 81: 11–18

Metroka C E, Jacobus D, Lewis M 1989 Successful chemoprophylaxis for pneumocystis with dapsone or bactrim. Abstracts of the Fifth International Conference on AIDS 196

Michaelis L L, Leight G S, Powell R D et al 1976 *Pneumocystis pneumonia*: The importance of early open lung biopsy. Annals of Surgery 183: 301–306

Millar A B, Mitchell D M 1990 Non-invasive investigation of pulmonary disease in patients positive for the immunodeficiency virus. Thorax 45: 57–61

Miller R F, Mitchell D M 1990 Management of respiratory failure in patients with the acquired immunodeficiency syndrome and *Pneumocystis carinii* pneumonia. Thorax 45: 140–146

Miller R F, Godfrey-Faussett P, Semple S J G et al 1989 Nebulised pentamidine as treatment for *Pneumocystis carinii* pneumonia in the acquired immune deficiency syndrome. Thorax 44: 565–569

Milligan S A, Stulbarg M S, Gamsu G et al 1985 *Pneumocystis carinii* pneumonia radiographically simulating tuberculosis. American Review of Respiratory Disease 132: 1124–1126

Mimica I, Omoso E, Howard J E et al 1971 Lung puncture in the aetiological diagnosis of pneumonia: A study of 543 infants and children. American Journal of Diseases of Children 122: 278–282

Mitchell D M 1989 Diagnostic problems in AIDS and the lung. Respiratory Medicine 83: 9–14

Mitchell D M, Shaw R J, Roussak C et al 1988 Abnormalities of pulmonary function in human immunodeficiency virus (HIV) infected patients. American Review of Respiratory Disease 137: 120

Montgomery A B, Edison R E, Sattler F et al 1990 Aerosolised pentamidine vs trimethoprim/sulfamethoxazole for acute *Pneumocystis carinii* pneumonia. A randomised double blind trial. Sixth International Conference on AIDS, San Francisco, vol 1, Th B 395: p 220

Montgomery A M, Luce J M, Turner J et al 1987 Aerosolised pentamidine as sole therapy for *Pneumocystis carinii* pneumonia in patients with acquired immunodeficiency syndrome. Lancet ii: 480–483

Morbidity and Mortality Weekly Reports 1987 Revision of the CDC surveillance case definition for acquired immunodeficiency syndrome. Morbidity and Mortality Weekly Reports 36 (suppl): 3–155

Morris J C, Rosen M J, Marcheosky et al 1987 Lymphocytic interstitial pneumonia in patients at risk for the acquired immune deficiency syndrome. Chest 91: 63–67

Murray J F, Mills J 1990 Pulmonary infectious complications of human immunodeficiency virus infection. American Review of Respiratory Disease 141: 1356–1372

Murray J F, Felton C P, Garay S et al 1984 Pulmonary complications of the acquired immunodeficiency syndrome: Report of a National Heart, Lung and Blood Institute workshop. New England Journal of Medicine 310: 1682–1688

Murray J F, Garay S M, Hopewell P C et al 1987 NHLBI workshop summary: Pulmonary complications of the acquired immunodeficiency syndrome. An update. American Review of Respiratory Disease 135: 504–509

Naidich D P, Garay S M, Lutman B S et al 1987 Radiographic manifestations of pulmonary disease in the acquired immunodeficiency syndrome (AIDS). Seminars in Roentgenology 22: 14–30

O'Brien R F 1989 Pulmonary and pleural Kaposi's sarcoma in the acquired immune deficiency syndrome. Seminars in Respiratory Medicine 10: 12–20

O'Doherty M J, Page C, Bradbeer C et al 1988 Differences in relative efficiency of nebulisers for pentamidine administration. Lancet ii: 1283–1286

Ognibene F P, Shelhamer J, Gill V et al 1984 The diagnosis of *Pneumocystis carinii* pneumonia in patients with acquired immunodeficiency syndrome using subsegmental bronchoalveolar lavage. American Review of Respiratory Disease 129: 929–932

Ognibene F P, Stels R G, Macher A M et al 1985 Kaposi's sarcoma causing pulmonary infiltrates and respiratory failure in the acquired immunodeficiency syndrome. Annals of Internal Medicine 102: 471–475

Ognibene F P, Masur H, Rogers P et al 1988 Non-specific interstitial pneumonitis without evidence of *Pneumocystis carinii* in asymptomatic patients infected with human immunodeficiency virus (HIV). Annals of Internal Medicine 109: 874–879

Oldham S A A, Castino M, Jacobson F L et al 1989 HIV associated lymphocytic interstitial pneumonia: Radiologic manifestations and pathologic correlation. Radiology 170: 83–87

Orenstein M, Weber C A, Cash M et al 1986 Value of broncho-alveolar lavage in the diagnosis of pulmonary infection in acquired immune deficiency syndrome. Thorax 41: 345–349

Palmer D L, Davidson M, Lusk R 1980 Needle aspiration of the lung in complex pneumonias. Chest 78: 16–21

Phair J, Munoz A, Detels R et al 1990 The risk of *Pneumocystis carinii* pneumonia among men infected with human immunodeficiency virus type 1. New England Journal of Medicine 322: 161–165

Pifer L L, Hughes W T, Stagno S et al 1978 *Pneumocystis carinii* infection: Evidence for high prevalence in normal and immunocompromised children. Pediatrics 61: 35–41

Pitchenik A E, Robinson H A 1985 The radiographic appearance of tuberculosis in patients with the acquired immunodeficiency syndrome (AIDS) and pre-AIDs. American Review of Respiratory Disease 131: 393–396

Pitchenik A E, Rubinstein H A 1985 A radiographic appearance of tuberculosis in patients with the acquired immunodeficiency syndrome (AIDS) and pre-AIDS. American Review of Respiratory Disease 131: 393–396

Pitchenik A E, Cole C, Russel B W et al 1984 Tuberculosis, atypical mycobacteriosis and the acquired immunodeficiency syndrome among Haitian and non-Haitian patients in South Florida. Annals of Internal Medicine 101: 641–645

Pitchenik A E, Gangei R, Torres A et al 1986 Sputum examination for the diagnosis of *Pneumocystis carinii* pneumonia in the acquired immunodeficiency syndrome. American Review of Respiratory Disease 133: 226–229

Polsky B, Gold J W M, Whimbey E et al 1986 Bacterial pneumonia in patients with the acquired immunodeficiency syndrome. Annals of Internal Medicine 104: 38–41

Rankin J A, Collman R, Danide R P 1988 Acquired immune deficiency syndrome and the lung. Chest 94: 155–164

Rosen M J, Cueco R A, Tierstein A S 1986 Outcome of intensive care in patients with the acquired immunodeficiency syndrome. Journal of Intensive Care Medicine 1: 55–60

Rosen P P, Martini N, Armstrong D 1975 *Pneumocystis carinii* pneumonia: Diagnosis by lung biopsy. American Journal of Medicine 58: 795–802

Sattersfield J R, McLauglin J S 1979 Open lung biopsy in diagnosing pulmonary infiltrates in immunosuppressed patients. Annals of Thoracic Surgery 28: 359–362

Sattler F R, Cowan R, Nielsen D M et al 1988 Trimethoprim–sulfamethoxazole compared with pentamidine for treatment of *Pneumocystis carinii* pneumonia in the acquired immunodeficiency syndrome. Annals of Internal Medicine 109: 280–281

Schein R M H, Fischl M A, Pitchenik A E et al 1986 ICU survival of patients with the acquired immunodeficiency syndrome. Critical Care Medicine 14: 1026–1027

Selwin P A, Feingold A R, Hertel D et al 1988 Increased risk of bacterial pneumonia in HIV-infected intravenous drug users without AIDS. AIDS 2: 267–272

Selwin P A, Hartel D, Lewis J A et al 1989 A prospective study of the risk of tuberculosis among intravenous drug users with human immunodeficiency virus infection. New England Journal of Medicine 320: 545–550

Shaw R J, Roussak C, Forster S M et al 1988 Lung function abnormalities in patients infected with the human immunodeficiency virus with and without overt pneumonitis. Thorax 43: 436–440

Shelhamer J H, Ognibene F P, Macher A M et al 1984 Persistence of *Pneumocystis carinii* in lung tissue of acquired immunodeficiency syndrome patients treated for pneumocystis pneumonia. American Review of Respiratory Disease 130: 1161–1165

Simberkoff M S, El-Sadr W, Schiffman G et al 1984 *Streptococcus pneumoniae* infections and bacteremia in patients with acquired immune deficiency syndrome with a report of a pneumococcal vaccine failure. American Review of Respiratory Disease 130: 1174–1176

Simmonds A K, Johnson M A, Clarke S W et al 1989 Simple nebuliser modification to enhance alveolar deposition of pentamidine. Lancet ii: 953

Smith D E, McLuckie A, Wyatt J et al 1988 Severe exercise hypoxaemia with normal or near normal x-rays: A feature of Pneumocystis carinii infection. Lancet ii: 1049–1051

Smith R L, Ripps C S, Lewis M L 1988 Elevated lactate dehydrogenase values in patients with Pneumocystic carinii pneumonia. Chest 93: 987–929

Solal-Celigny D, Coudere L J, Herman D et al 1985 Lymphoid interstitial pneumonitis in the acquired immunodeficiency syndrome-related complex. American Review of Respiratory Disease 131: 956–960

Steinbrook R, Lo B, Tirpack J, Dilley J W et al 1985 Ethical dilemmas in caring for patients with the acquired immunodeficiency syndrome. Annals of Internal Medicine 103: 787–790

Stover D E, White D A, Romano P A et al 1984 Diagnosis of pulmonary disease in the acquired immune deficiency syndrome: Roles of bronchoscopy and bronchoalveolar lavage. American Review of Respiratory Disease 130: 659–662

Stover D E, White D A, Romano P A et al 1985 Spectrum of pulmonary disease associated with the acquired immunodeficiency syndrome. American Journal of Medicine 78: 429–437

Suffredini A F, Ognibene F P, Lack E E et al 1987 Non-specific interstitial pneumonitis: A common cause of pulmonary disease in the acquired immunodeficiency syndrome. Annals of Internal Medicine 107: 7–13

Sunderam G, McDonald R J, Maniatis T et al 1986 Tuberculosis as a manifestation of the acquired immunodeficiency syndrome (AIDS). Journal of the American Medical Association 256: 362–366

Sunderam G, Mangura B T, Lombardo J M et al 1987 Failure of optimal four drug short course tuberculosis chemotherapy in a compliant patient with human immunodeficiency virus. American Review of Respiratory Disease 136: 1475–1478

Suster B, Ackerman M, Orenstein M et al 1986 Pulmonary manifestation of AIDS: Review of 106 episodes. Radiology 161: 87–93

Tanabe K, Fuchimoto M, Egawa K et al 1988 Use of Pneumocystis carinii genomic DNA clones for DNA hybridization analysis of infected human lungs. Journal of Infectious Diseases 3: 593–596

Toma E, Fournier S, Poisson M et al 1989 Clindamycin with primaquine for Pneumocystis carinii pneumonia. Lancet i: 1046–1048

Venn G E, Kay P H, Midwood C J et al 1985 Open lung biopsy in patients with diffuse pulmonary shadowing. Thorax 40: 931–935

Wachter R M, Luce J M, Turner J et al 1986 Intensive care of patients with the acquired immunodeficiency syndrome: Outcome and changing patterns of utilisation. American Review of Respiratory Disease 134: 891–896

Wachter R M, Cooke M, Hopewell P C et al 1988 Attitudes of medical residents regarding intensive care for patients with the acquired immunodeficiency syndrome. Archives of Internal Medicine 148: 149–152

Wachter R M, Russi M B, Hopewell P C et al 1989 The improving survival rate after intensive care for Pneumocystis carinii pneumonia and respiratory failure [abstract]. Fifth International Conference on AIDS, Montreal, p 127

Wakefield A E, Pixley F J, Banerji S et al 1990 Detection of Pneumocystis carinii with DNA amplification. Lancet 336: 451–453

Walzer P D 1988 Diagnosis of Pneumocystis carinii pneumonia. Journal of Infectious Diseases 157: 629–632

Wharton J M, Coleman D L, Wofsy C B 1986 Trimethoprim–sulfamethoxazole or pentamidine for Pneumocystis carinii pneumonia in the acquired immunodeficiency syndrome: A prospective randomised trial. Annals of Internal Medicine 105: 37–44

Wong B, Edwards F F, Kiehn T E et al 1985 Continuous high grade Mycobacterium avium intracellulare bacteraemia in patients with the acquired immunodeficiency syndrome. American Journal of Medicine 78: 35–40

Young L S 1987 Antigen detection in Pneumocystis carinii infection. Serodiagnosis and Immunotherapy 1: 163–167

Young L S, Berlin O G W, Inderlied C B 1987 Activity of ciprofloxacin and other fluorinated quinolones against mycobacteria. American Journal of Medicine 82: 23–26

Zaman M K, White D A 1988 Serum lactate dehydrogenase levels and Pneumocystis carinii pneumonia: Diagnostic and prognostic significance. American Review of Respiratory Disease 137: 796–800

Zaman M K, Wooken O J, Supramanya B et al 1988 Rapid non-invasive diagnosis of *Pneumocystis carinii* from induced liquified sputum. Annals of Internal Medicine 109: 7–10

Ziza J M, Brun-Vezinet F, Venet A et al 1985 Lymphadenopathy-associated virus isolated from bronchoalveolar lavage fluid in AIDS-related complex with lymphoid interstitial pneumonitis (letter). New England Journal of Medicine 313: 183

9

The impact of infection with human immunodeficiency virus on tuberculosis

K. Styblo   D. A. Enarson

Infection with human immunodeficiency virus (HIV) is now the greatest risk factor for tuberculosis, having caused the greatest deterioration in the epidemiological situation in the last 100 years. Its impact upon the incidence of tuberculosis is so great that it has disrupted the balance between the tubercle bacillus and man, which in the absence of interventions (i.e. case-finding and chemotherapy) had existed in the 'pre-HIV' era. Consequently, the tools currently available for tuberculosis control in countries where both tuberculous and HIV infections are prevalent will fail to restrain the increase in the incidence of tuberculosis caused by HIV infection.

The progressive immunodeficiency caused by HIV infection may lead to an increase in tuberculosis incidence in three ways: firstly, by the multiplication of tubercle bacilli in quiescent foci after a *remote* tuberculous infection; secondly, through progression of a *recent* tuberculous infection to the disease among HIV-positive subjects whose progressive immuno-deficiency substantially increases the breakdown rate to tuberculosis disease; thirdly, through *superinfection* with tubercle bacilli in HIV-positive individuals who had been previously infected with tubercle bacilli. This is less likely than the first two.

Unlike the situation in developed countries, in developing countries the last two causes for the excess incidence of tuberculosis may result in a considerable number of tuberculosis cases among HIV-positive subjects. Even so, in such countries, most of the tuberculosis cases in HIV-infected individuals are attributable to endogenous reactivation of a remote tuberculous infection.

The impact of HIV infection on the epidemiology of tuberculosis depends mainly on the prevalence of, and trend in, HIV infection in the community, and the prevalence of tuberculous infection, particularly in the 15–49-year age group. It also depends on the breakdown rate from tuberculous infection to the disease in those dually infected, the level and trend in the risk of tuberculous infection in the community, and the efficacy and efficiency of case-finding and chemotherapy in the area under study (Styblo 1989, 1990a).

Finally, the impact of HIV infection on the tuberculosis problem depends on the pattern of HIV transmission (Mann 1988). Mann's pattern II, including large parts of Africa — mainly central and southern but increasingly also western — and parts of the Caribbean, is of greater consequence to tuberculosis than pattern I. In pattern II, transmission is predominantly heterosexual and therefore the ratio for AIDS cases (and most probably also for HIV infection) is approximately equal between the sexes. Very high-risk groups in the second pattern are prostitutes (50–80% infected), individuals receiving blood and blood products (at least before the introduction of effective screening), and those receiving injections or other skin-piercing procedures where adequate sterilization is not practised. Also, transplacental transmission is an increasing problem in such areas.

As already mentioned, the occurrence of tuberculosis in HIV-infected subjects depends mainly on the prevalence of tuberculous infection in those aged 15–49 years, and the level of, and trend in, the risk of tuberculous infection. The present prevalence of tuberculous infection in the 15–49-year age group is the result of the risk of infection in the community many years ago and the magnitude of the decrease in the risk of infection during the subsequent period. In many developing countries (especially the countries of sub-Saharan Africa), the prevalence of tuberculous infection does not appear to have ever reached the very high levels observed at the beginning of the present century in the countries of Europe. Nevertheless, the very slow (or lack of any) decline in the risk of infection has meant that the present prevalence and risk of infection have remained relatively high. It is evident that the situation is very different in developed countries where, in the last 40 years, the risk of infection has decreased by about 10–14% annually, with the consequence that the current prevalence and risk of infection in these countries are very low indeed. Consequently, the impact of HIV infection on the tuberculosis problem will differ greatly in developed and developing countries, and we will therefore deal with them separately.

PREVALENCE OF HIV INFECTION AND ITS TREND

Reliable information on the level of and the trend in HIV infection among the general population in countries where HIV infection is prevalent is not readily available. This lack of information severely hampers our ability to determine the extent and impact of HIV infection on tuberculosis. There is an urgent need for careful, prospective investigation of the prevalence and natural history of HIV infection.

On the other hand, information on AIDS worldwide is more complete and we will therefore deal first with AIDS.

AIDS

The best available information on the number of AIDS cases is based on data reported by countries to the WHO Global Programme on AIDS (WHO 1990a). However, reporting from certain countries (in particular those in sub-Saharan Africa, some in Latin America and some in Asia) is incomplete and irregular.

Table 9.1 shows cumulative AIDS cases reported to the WHO as of September 30, 1990. In analysing these data, it is useful to calculate the rate of increase to determine the trend of the epidemic. This is particularly important where the changes may be non-linear and where a 'zenith' or 'saturation point' might be postulated. Thus, the time required to double the cumulative number of cases (the doubling time) may be utilized to determine the trend.

In the last 4 years, the doubling time has increased: doubling time was slightly more than 12 months for AIDS cases between 1985 and 1986, about 13 months between 1986 and 1987, and 18 months between 1987 and 1988. It is probable that it will be nearly 2 years between 1988 and 1989 (the figures for 1989 in Table 9.1 are incomplete). Estimation of this increase in the doubling time is relatively reliable for the USA and European countries, where the notification of AIDS cases is comparatively complete. Although the figures for Africa are incomplete, an increase in the doubling time appears to be occurring there as well.

Table 9.2 shows the incidence of AIDS cases in 1987, 1988 and 1989. Again, the incompleteness of the reported cases suggests that we must view comparisons with caution. Since 1987 the incidence of AIDS cases in Africa has been the second highest among the regions of the world. The estimated numbers for 1989 suggest that Africa may have the highest number (and probably the highest rate) in the world by the early 1990s. Table 9.3 shows the seven countries in Africa, in the Americas and in Europe with the highest rates of reported AIDS cases in 1989.

In some African countries, the rates for AIDS cases will be higher than 100 per 100 000 general population in the early 1990s (and more than 200 per 100 000 in those aged 15–49 years). In the Americas, the absolute number of AIDS cases continues to be highest in USA, namely 33 183 in 1989 (13.3 per 100 000) compared with 31 377 cases in 1988 (an increase

Table 9.1 Cumulative AIDS cases reported to WHO from 1985 to 1989 as of 30 September 1990, and percentage increase from one year to the next

Year	Africa No.	%	Americas No.	%	Europe No.	%	Total No.	%
1985	382		23 761		2 843		27 218	
1986	3 743		44 386	87	6 408	125	55 069	102
1987	15 707	320	76 469	72	13 035	103	106 268	93
1988	36 632	133	116 111	52	22 792	75	177 298	67
1989	67 461 .	84	158 509	37	34 384	51	262 942	48

Total includes a further 642 cases in Asia and 1946 cases reported in Oceania.
% is percentage increase in cumulative reported AIDS cases compared with those reported in the previous year.

Table 9.2   Number of AIDS cases reported to the WHO for 1987, 1988 and 1989 (as of 30 September 1990)

| | No. of reported cases | | | Increase From '87 to '88 | | From '88 to '89 | |
Continent	1987	1988	1989	No.	%	No.	%
Africa	11 964	20 925[a]	30 829[a]	8 961	75	9 904	47
Americas	32 083	39 642	42 398	7 559	24	2 756	7
Asia	122	156	254	34	28	98	63
Europe	6 627	9 757	11 592	3 130	47	1 835	19
Oceania	403	550	571	147	36	21	4
Total	51 199	71 030	85 644	19 831	39	14 614	21

[a]   Incomplete data.

Table 9.3   The seven countries in Africa, in the Americas and in Europe with the highest rates (per 100 000 general population) of AIDS[a] reported to the WHO in 1989 as of 30 September 1990

Africa Country	No.	Rate	Americas Country	No.	Rate	Europe Country	No.	Rate
Malawi	3 124	37.1	Bahamas	168	68.6	Switzerland	413	6.3
Uganda	5 225	28.3	Bermuda	35	61.4	Spain	2 162	5.5
Burundi[b]	1 054	19.3	Fr. Guiana	54	61.4	France	2 828	5.0
Kenya	4 825	19.2	St. Chr. Nevis[b]	17	37.0	Italy	2 335	4.1
Congo[b]	346	17.4	Guadeloupe	54	15.9	Denmark	168	3.3
Zaire	6 188	17.2	Martinique	50	15.1	Luxemburg	11	3.0
Ivory Coast	1 930	15.3	USA	33 183	13.3	Netherlands	365	2.5

[a]   More than 10 cases; [b]   1988.

of 1806 or 5.8%). In certain small countries in the American region, the rate of AIDS cases was high (Bahamas, Bermuda and French Guiana: more than 60 per 100 000) but the absolute number was relatively small. In Europe the highest rate was in Switzerland (5.8 per 100 000 in 1988 and 6.3 in 1989), followed by Spain (4.6 and 5.5 per 100 000 in 1988 and 1989 respectively).

HIV infection

Even today, very little is known about the natural history of HIV infection. As already mentioned, transmission of HIV infection in Mann's first pattern is predominantly through male homosexual contact and through sharing inadequately sterilized needles and syringes by i.v. drug abusers. In Africa and other countries, where Mann's second pattern prevails, seroprevalence studies of HIV infection show the infection predominantly in young adults (the peak frequency in women is between 20 and 24 years and in men between 30 and 34 years). A second peak is observed in small children, aged up to 2 years, due to transplacental transmission from HIV-infected mothers (Rwandan 1989). Blood transfusion and infections from inadequately sterilized needles and syringes are the main contributors to HIV infections in children aged 2–14 years (Mann et al 1986).

Although in certain HIV pattern II countries HIV infection is rather high in young adults (in some areas up to 25%: Mann 1988), the *overall* proportion of those infected with HIV rarely exceeds 2–3% at present in those aged 15–49 years.

There is considerable uncertainty in estimates of the current and future prevalence of HIV infection worldwide, arising both from limited knowledge of key factors that determine transmission and disease progression, and from limitations in the surveillance data. The WHO Global AIDS Programme estimated the prevalence of HIV infection, worldwide, at 5 million as of mid-1988. However, the WHO recently revised the global estimates for HIV infection to 8–10 million. The new estimate was based on a detailed review and analysis of the global status of infection with HIV and of AIDS disease. It is apparent that the incidence of HIV infection is accelerating dramatically in some parts of the world (WHO 1990b). The new figures reflect a continued worsening of the epidemic of HIV/AIDS in developing countries, especially in sub-Saharan Africa and Asia. WHO estimates for persons infected with HIV in sub-Saharan Africa have increased from 2.5 million in 1987 to about 5 million at present (1990b). Thus about one in 40 adult men and women in sub-Saharan Africa are infected with HIV. Another important development is the spread in most sub-Saharan African countries of HIV infection from large cities to rural areas which contain the majority of the population. This is an unfavourable development for tuberculosis control, since excess incidence of tuberculosis caused by HIV infection will affect (and already has affected) rural areas where case-finding and treatment of tuberculosis are very difficult.

From the point of view of worldwide tuberculosis control, the most serious aspect of the new estimates of HIV infection is the rapid increase in HIV-infected persons in Asia. The estimated total number of HIV-infected persons may be currently as high as 500 000, from a small number of infected individuals 2 or 3 years ago. It is extremely important to know to what extent HIV infection will spread in Asia, since the global epidemiological situation for tuberculosis will depend to a great extent on excess tuberculosis cases caused by HIV infection in Asia. This continent contains most of the adults infected with tubercle bacilli, and a high prevalence of HIV infection would dramatically increase the number of tuberculosis cases, thus increasing the total cases around the world.

In contrast to the situation in many developing countries, the rate of HIV infection has been slowing in the developed world during the last few years, which may continue to limit the impact of HIV infection on tuberculosis.

TUBERCULOUS INFECTION

The incidence of tuberculosis in patients with HIV infection depends on the overlap between the population infected with HIV and the population previously (and recently) infected with tubercle bacilli. It is relatively easy to establish the prevalence of tuberculous infection in age groups in which AIDS cases are most commonly reported. As already mentioned, it is also important to know the present risk of tuberculous infection in the studied population particularly in developing countries where it is still high and its decrease is very slow.

It is obvious that the present prevalence of tuberculous infection in individuals aged 15–49 years (in whom most HIV infections occur) depends on the level of the risk of tuberculous infection 50 years ago, and the average annual decrease in the risk of infection during those 50 years up to the present day.

The transmission of tubercle bacilli

Several studies (Shaw & Wynn-Williams 1954, Hertzberg 1957, Geuns van et al 1975, Grzybowski et al 1975, Rouillon et al 1976) among close contacts of tuberculosis patients demonstrate that smear-positive patients play the greatest role in the spread of infection. Patients whose sputum is culture positive only, or who are culture negative, are much less important in the transmission of infection.

The risk of being infected with tubercle bacilli is related to the number of sources of infection existing in a community. It is estimated that one undiagnosed smear-positive case infects 10 persons during one year of contact (Styblo 1980). Since the patient's and doctor's delay in diagnosing smear-positive cases in the Netherlands is about 2.5 months (Baas et al 1982), one open case may infect 2–3 persons before being discovered. In America, it is estimated that an open case infects, on average, 2–3 persons (Johnston & Wildrik 1974).

The annual risk of tuberculous infection and its trend

The average annual risk of infection indicates what proportion of the population will be infected, and is usually expressed as a percentage or a rate. It is derived from the results of tuberculin testing. Techniques for converting information on prevalence of infection into a smooth series of annual incidence rates of infection are described by Styblo et al (1969) and Sutherland (1976). To obtain a reliable estimate of the risk of infection and its change over a given period of time, several tuberculin surveys are required at intervals, each survey taking a representative sample of non-BCG-vaccinated subjects of the same age tested by the same technique.

As already mentioned, the level of, and the trend in, the risk of infection markedly differ in developed and developing countries. Fig. 9.1 shows the risks of infection in several developed countries covering the period 1950–1975 (Styblo & Meijer 1978). It is seen that the risk of infection was low in 1975, ranging between 20 and 200 per 100 000 population, and was decreasing by more than 10% each year. Between 1975 and the present (1990), it has halved itself twice.

In most developing countries the rate of decrease in the risk of tuberculous infection has been very slow during the last four decades — in some countries as low as 1%. Estimates for Uganda, Lesotho and Mozambique are shown in Fig. 9.2. A similar decrease has been observed in Tanzania, where the first round of the National Tuberculin Survey was carried out between 1983 and 1987 and covered a representative sample of nearly 80 000 children (TSRU Progress Report 1989). The estimated risk of tuberculous infection in more than 34 000 non-BCG-vaccinated schoolchildren aged 10 years was between 1.1% and 1.2%. Comparing the prevalences of tuberculous infection for the same age, it is estimated that

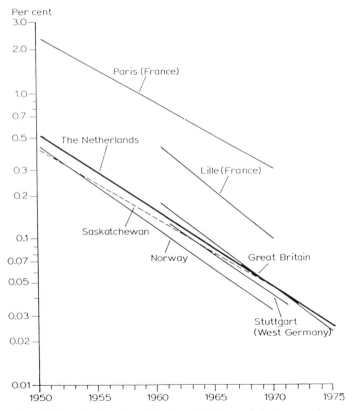

Fig. 9.1 Annual risks of tuberculous infection and their trends in low-prevalence countries 1950–1975. Reproduced from Styblo & Meijer 1978.

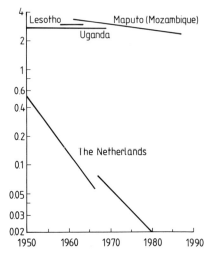

Fig. 9.2   Annual risks of tuberculous infection and their trends in high-prevalence countries, 1950–1987.

there has been an annual decrease in the risk of infection of between 1% and 2% between the first study, in 1957, and the most recent one, carried out from 1983 to 1987.

Prevalence of tuberculous infection

It is obvious that the rapid decline in the risk of tuberculous infection in developed countries and the very slow decrease in many developing countries during the last 40 years has resulted in very different prevalence rates in those aged 15–49 years (Styblo 1986).

In the Netherlands, the prevalence of tuberculous infection in 1985 was 0.8% in subjects aged 20 years and 24.2% in those aged 50 years (Table 9.4) (Styblo 1990b). The corresponding figures in 1995 will be 0.3% and 7.6%, respectively. In other developed countries prevalence rates of tuberculous infection may be slightly higher than in the Netherlands but the downward trend is similar.

In many developing countries 40–50% of persons aged 15–49 years have been infected with tubercle bacilli. Because of the slow decrease in the risk of tuberculous infection the prevalence of infection has also been decreasing slowly.

THE RELATION BETWEEN HIV AND TUBERCULOUS INFECTION AND THE IMPACT OF HIV INFECTION UPON TUBERCULOSIS INCIDENCE

In order for HIV infection to increase the incidence of tuberculosis within a community, it must occur along with tuberculous infection. That this is

Table 9.4   Estimated prevalence of tuberculous infection by age groups, Netherlands, 1945, 1975, 1985 and 1995

Age group (years)	Estimated prevalence of tuberculous infection (%) in			
	1945	1975	1985	1995
0–14	11.0	0.3	0.1	< 0.1
15–24	44.7	2.2	0.8	0.3
25–34	72.1	7.4	2.4	0.9
35–44	90.8	24.0	7.5	2.5
45–54	97.2	48.8	24.2	7.6
55–64	99.2	74.0	48.9	24.2
65–74	99.5	91.5	74.1	48.9
75 or more	99.8	97.4	91.5	74.1
Total	59.7	26.4	18.3	11.3

true was shown in a prospective study of drug addicts in New York City (Selwyn et al 1989). HIV-infected individuals who subsequently developed clinical tuberculosis were those who were already infected with tuberculosis (positive tuberculin test) at the outset and subsequently reactivated.

The role of primary infection (or reinfection) resulting in clinical tuberculosis in countries with a high prevalence is definitely greater than that reflected in the study from New York City, but is still unlikely to be as important as reactivation in increasing the incidence of tuberculosis cases.

The impact of HIV infection on tuberculosis incidence depends not only upon the prevalence of the two infections and the time interval between them but also upon the natural history of HIV infection and the pathogenesis of tuberculosis caused by HIV infection.

The natural history of HIV infection

Two types of virus (termed HIV-1 and HIV-2) have been identified as causing AIDS. The latter is found primarily in West Africa. Most information pertains to HIV-1. The presence of HIV infection can be determined in its asymptomatic phase by screening tests. This allows the study of its natural history.

Infection with HIV is usually followed by a long latent period prior to the development of AIDS (Lui et al 1988). Only 21 of 318 newly infected men had developed AIDS by 54 months of follow-up and the median period following infection, free of AIDS, was computed from mathematical modelling to be 11 years. Factors influencing progression to disease have not been fully determined. It is likely that opportunistic infections may hasten disease (Phair et al 1989). It is also likely that medical treatment may prolong the course of the disease and the period of infectiousness.

Information concerning HIV infection in pattern II countries is less readily available. The IUATLD-assisted National Tuberculosis Programmes in a number of African countries initiated during the period 1978–1984 will enable the study of the interactions between HIV and tuberculosis. In sub-Saharan Africa, more than 10 000 cases of smear-positive tuberculosis have been enrolled annually and followed during treatment (8 months of medication) for the past 5 years. There has been a striking rise in fatality rates during therapy, in some regions as high as 16–24%. This 'excess' of deaths is largely related to HIV infection as most die late in the course of treatment, after sputum conversion, and many are young (Mohamed et al 1990). These observations suggest an adverse effect of active tuberculosis on the course of HIV infection, as noted in countries with pattern I transmission.

Pathogenesis of tuberculosis in the presence of HIV infection

The development of tuberculosis in HIV-infected persons has been studied mainly in pattern I countries. Tuberculosis develops at an earlier stage in HIV disease than other opportunist infections. Retrospective studies have suggested that at least one-half of patients have no other indication of HIV infection at the time of diagnosis of tuberculosis (Chaisson et al 1987). Such patients usually demonstrate a significant reaction on tuberculin testing (MMWR 1989); only those who have tuberculosis after the onset of AIDS are likely to have no reaction to tuberculin and, even in this group, a minority (25%) have a tuberculin reaction.

The influence of HIV infection on tuberculosis relates to the extent of immunodeficiency due to HIV. In cases which are markedly immunocompromised, haematogenous dissemination or progressive primary tuberculosis appears to be more common. Pulmonary cavities are uncommon and granulomas in lung tissue are poorly developed (Chaisson et al 1987). In those HIV-infected tuberculosis patients without AIDS, the clinical appearance does not differ from other tuberculosis patients (Chaisson & Slutkin 1989).

The incidence of tuberculosis in those dually infected, with or without AIDS, has not been studied extensively. In one detailed prospective study of drug abusers in New York City, it was determined that approximately one-third of dually infected individuals would develop active tuberculosis (Selwyn et al 1989). In British Columbia, Canada, we have observed that approximately one-half of AIDS patients who are infected with tuberculosis develop clinical tuberculosis.

It is unknown, in pattern II countries, whether a similar series of events occurs in the development of tuberculosis in HIV-infected persons. The high risk of tuberculous infection in such countries results in a higher proportion of cases of tuberculosis resulting from recent infection. The pathogenesis (as well as the resulting clinical appearance) of tuberculosis is quite different, depending upon the time that has elapsed since the tuberculosis patient was infected. Studies of the clinical appearance of tuberculosis in children in Europe, prior to the introduction of chemotherapy, when the disease was very common (Legrand 1933), indicate disease with wide dissemination throughout the body, with large bacterial populations, even when bacilli were difficult to isolate from the sputum. Moreover, even when the disease was relatively isolated, the appearance was 'bizarre', with large pleural and pericardial effusions and pulmonary infiltrations affecting mid and lower zones. When evaluating the pathogenesis and clinical appearance of tuberculosis in pattern II countries, it must be remembered that these so-called 'atypical' appearances may be expected in young people recently infected with both *M. tuberculosis* and HIV.

Implications of the level of dual infection for tuberculosis incidence

In developed countries the impact of HIV infection on tuberculosis incidence will remain relatively small, since the prevalence of tuberculous infection in subjects aged 15–49 years is low and rapidly decreasing (Table 9.4). In the USA the impact is detectable (Murray 1989). On the other hand, in most other Western countries, the overall impact of HIV infection on the trend in tuberculosis incidence is virtually undetectable (Ferlinz 1990).

In developing countries, most notably those in sub-Saharan Africa where the prevalence of tuberculous infection is relatively high (40–50%) and the prevalence of HIV infection is also relatively high (at least 2%), the excess incidence of tuberculosis resulting from HIV infection is evident and continuously increasing (Slutkin et al 1988, Chum 1989, Murray 1989, Styblo 1990). The increase in the incidence of tuberculosis in some large cities of Tanzania and Malawi is placing an unbearable strain on already overstretched human and technical resources. This increase has been observed for all newly reported cases (pulmonary smear-positive and smear-negative as well as extrapulmonary), without an appreciable increase in the number of smear-positive pulmonary relapse cases (Fig. 9.3).

HIV INFECTION AND THE CLINICAL PICTURE OF TUBERCULOSIS

The effects of HIV infection upon the human host are wide ranging and severe. Tuberculosis is only one of the opportunistic infections which causes disease and death in the HIV-infected individual, as a result of the severe immunodeficiency induced by the virus.

Diagnosis of tuberculosis in HIV-infected subjects

The principal presenting features of patients with AIDS are relatively non-

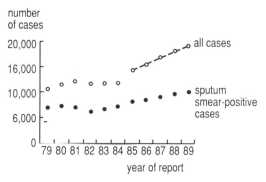

Fig. 9.3   Reported tuberculosis cases, Tanzania, 1979–1989.

specific. In a study of 1378 consecutive cases in Zambia there were four common groups of symptoms: loss of weight or malnutrition, generalized lymphadenopathy, chronic diarrhoea, and chronic chest infection (Fleming 1990). The relative frequency of the presenting features differed according to age, with loss of weight being most prominent in young children and adults, and chest infection being more common among older children and adolescents. Two of these presentations are similar to the presentation of tuberculosis. Part of the reason for the similarity between patients with AIDS and those with tuberculosis may be that, in developing countries, a high proportion of patients with AIDS coincidentally have tuberculosis: in Malawi, 115 of 352 HIV-1-seropositive patients admitted to hospital had concurrent tuberculosis (Reeve 1989). Where tuberculosis is common, the diagnosis of the disease in patients with HIV infection is more likely to be considered. Where tuberculosis is uncommon, it might not be considered. The likelihood of imputing symptoms of tuberculosis to other illnesses, which it may resemble, is great, and can have fatal consequences (Enarson et al 1978).

Even when tuberculosis is considered, the diagnosis may still be difficult because of haematogenous spread or non-pulmonary involvement (Fleming 1988, Reeve 1989). These forms of tuberculosis can be difficult to diagnose because the presenting symptoms are frequently non-specific, and isolation of tubercle bacilli from such cases is difficult. The occurrence of rare forms of tuberculosis, for example tuberculous pericarditis and serous cavity involvement, are being seen in countries where HIV infection is frequent.

However, in the majority of cases there is pulmonary involvement, and in a high proportion of cases this is infectious (sputum smear positive). Such cases can be diagnosed, by smear microscopy, and form the most important group of tuberculosis patients resulting from HIV infection, because of their infectious potential. Among smear-negative cases, some studies from developed countries have indicated that atypical radiographic appearances are more frequent. A review of radiographs from a low-prevalence country (Canada) with a series from a high-prevalence country for tuberculosis but with a low prevalence for HIV infection with another country with a high prevalence for tuberculosis and HIV infection indicated that patients from the country with a high prevalence for tuberculosis were most likely to have disease extending beyond the apex of the lung, regardless of whether HIV infection was common. However, patients from the area with a high prevalence for HIV infection were less likely to have cavities than were patients from either of the two other countries (unpublished data). These results are similar to those from the USA (Chaisson & Slutkin 1989). Nevertheless, all patients were more likely to have disease in the upper zones of the lungs on the chest radiographs and very unlikely to have isolated lower zone disease, regardless of which group they came from.

Treatment of tuberculosis in the presence of HIV infection

Patients with HIV infection who have tuberculosis are more likely to die while on treatment for tuberculosis than patients without HIV (Kibuga et al 1989). Thus, in countries with a relatively high prevalence of HIV infection, the fatality rate for tuberculosis is rising. In reviewing patients with both HIV infection and tuberculosis, it is frequently observed that those who die while on treatment do so after sputum conversion and their tuberculosis has improved clinically (Mohamed et al 1990). Death is more likely to be due to causes other than tuberculosis. Indeed, such patients often develop severe diarrhoea or overwhelming bacterial infection, to which they succumb.

Of patients who survive treatment, response to therapy does not appear to differ whether the patient is infected with HIV or not (Chaisson et al 1987). In IUATLD-assisted national tuberculosis programmes where HIV prevalence has been rapidly rising, rates of sputum conversion have not changed and appear to be the same in districts with a known high prevalence of HIV infection as compared with districts where HIV infection is uncommon. It is not yet known whether relapse after cure is the same, or higher, in HIV-infected patients as compared with HIV-negative patients. Since the life expectancy after completion of treatment of patients with HIV infection is relatively short, the likelihood of relapse is necessarily reduced.

While on treatment for tuberculosis, adverse reactions to medications have been noted to be more common among those who are HIV positive (Chaisson et al 1987). This is especially true in developing countries where resources are limited and programmes must use thiacetazone. The occurrence of Stevens–Johnson syndrome appears to be significantly increased among those patients who are HIV positive (Kibuga et al 1989). These reactions may be severe enough, and frequent enough, to limit the use of thiacetazone where HIV infection is common.

The safety of staff and of other patients is a matter for consideration where HIV infection is common. It is clear that tuberculosis patients are a group with a high prevalence of HIV infection. It is extremely important that when injections (for example, streptomycin) are given, or when blood from such patients is handled, proper sterilization and disposal procedures for hazardous materials be strictly practised.

CURTAILING THE IMPACT OF HIV INFECTION ON TRANSMISSION OF TUBERCULOSIS

Prevention of tuberculosis in HIV-infected persons

Because HIV infection is the greatest risk factor for the development of tuberculosis, this group should benefit from preventive chemotherapy. Although the efficacy of preventive chemotherapy with isoniazid has been well established in non-HIV-infected subjects in numerous control trials in a wide variety of populations and in many different countries, there is virtually no evidence on the efficacy of preventive chemotherapy for tuberculous infection in dually infected subjects. An informal consultation on preventive tuberculosis chemotherapy among HIV-infected persons was held by the WHO in Geneva in early 1990 and guidelines for efficacy study protocols were elaborated.

However, even if preventive chemotherapy can be shown to be efficacious in preventing tuberculosis in HIV-infected individuals, the likelihood that it could be implemented efficiently in the poorest developing countries, where HIV infection is common, is questionable. The increasing burden of patients with active tuberculosis caused by HIV infection, who require treatment, are beginning to stress the limited capacity of even well-organized treatment programmes. It is likely that the number of patients will further increase and further resources will be required to treat such patients. Moreover, the screening of the population for HIV infection is likely to be prohibitive in cost, manpower and logistics.

Preventing transmission of tuberculous infection in the community

The key to containing the adverse effects of HIV infection on transmission of tuberculosis in the community in pattern II countries must be by effective treatment of known cases and extension of case-finding throughout the community (the basic elements of a National Tuberculosis Programme). It is possible that these activities might be sufficient to prevent an increase in the risk of tuberculous infection in the community. An evaluation of this possibility is currently underway in the National Tuberculosis Programme in Tanzania. The level and trend of the risk of infection were known prior to the advent of AIDS in the community. The trend is being systematically evaluated by tuberculin surveys of a representative sample of children throughout the country, repeated every 5 years. Within several years, the evaluation will be sufficiently complete to determine the answer to this question.

REFERENCES

Baas M A, Geuns H A van, Hellinga H S, Meijer J, Styblo K 1982 Surveillance of diagnostic and treatment measures of bacillary pulmonary tuberculosis reported in the Netherlands from 1973 to 1976. Selected Papers 21: 41–80

Chaisson R E, Slutkin G 1989 Tuberculosis and human immunodeficiency virus infection. Journal of Infectious Diseases 159: 96–100

Chaisson R E, Schecter G F, Theuer C P et al 1987 Tuberculosis in patients with the acquired immunodeficiency syndrome. American Review of Respiratory Disease 136: 570–574

Chum H J 1989 Ten years of the National Tuberculosis and Leprosy Programme in Tanzania. Bulletin of the International Union against Tuberculosis 64: 34–36

Enarson D A, Gryzbowski S, Dorken E 1978 Failure of diagnosis as a factor in tuberculous mortality. Canadian Medical Association Journal 118: 1520–1522

Ferlinz R 1990 Deutsches Zentralkomitee zur Bekämpfung der Tuberkulose (p 14). Informationsbericht, Mainz

Fleming A F 1988 AIDS in Africa: An update. AIDS Forschung 3: 116–138

Fleming A F 1990 Opportunistic infections in AIDS in developed and developing countries. Transactions of the Royal Society of Tropical Medicine and Hygiene 84 (suppl 1): 1–6

Geuns H A van, Meijer J, Styblo K 1975 Results of contact examination in Rotterdam 1967–1969. Bulletin of the International Union against Tuberculosis 50: 107–121

Grzybowski S, Barnett G D, Styblo K 1975 Contacts of cases of active pulmonary tuberculosis. Bulletin of the International Union against Tuberculosis 50: 90–106

Hertzberg G 1957 The infectiousness of human tuberculosis. Munksgaard, Copenhagen

Johnston R F, Wildrik H K 1974 'State of art' review: The impact of chemotherapy on the care of patients with tuberculosis. American Review of Respiratory Disease 109: 636–664

Kibuga D K, Gathu S, Nunn P 1989 A study of HIV infection in association with tuberculosis seen in Infectious Diseases Hospital, Nairobi. Fifth International Conference on AIDS, Montreal, Th G 0.5, p 989

Legrand A (ed) 1933 La tuberculose pulmonaire et les maladies de l'appareil respiratoire de l'enfant et de l'adolescent. Kapp, Paris, p 499

Lui K J, Darrow W W, Rutherford G W 1988 A model-based estimate of the mean incubation period for AIDS in homosexual men. Science 240: 1333–1335

Mann J 1988 Global AIDS: Epidemiology, impact, projections, global strategy. In: AIDS prevention and control. Pergamon Press, Oxford, pp 3–13

Mann J M, Francis H, Davachi F et al 1986 Human immunodeficiency virus seroprevalence in pediatric patients 2 to 14 years at Mama Yemo Hospital, Kinshasa. Pediatrics 78: 673–677

Mohamed A, Lwechunguru S, Chum H J, Styblo K, Broekmans J 1990 Excess fatality, caused — to a great extent — by HIV infection, in smear-positive patients enrolled on short-course chemotherapy, after sputum conversion. American Review of Respiratory Disease 141: A267

Mortality and Morbidity Weekly Report 1989 Tuberculosis and human immunodeficiency virus infection: Recommendations of the Advisory Committee for the elimination of tuberculosis (ACET). Mortality and Morbidity Weekly Report 38: 236–250

Murray J F 1989 The white plague: Down and out, or up and coming? J Burns Amberson Lecture. American Review of Respiratory Disease 140: 1788–1795

Phair J P, Munoz A, Detels R et al 1989 Incidence of Pneumocystis carinii pneumonia in men infected with human immunodeficiency virus type 1 (HIV-1). Fifth International Conference on AIDS, Montreal

Reeve P A 1989 HIV infection in patients admitted to a general hospital in Malawi. British Medical Journal 298: 1567–1568

Rouillon A, Perdrizet S, Parrot R 1976 Transmission of tubercle bacilli: The effects of chemotherapy. Tubercle 57: 275–299

Rwandan HIV Seroprevalence Study Group 1989 Nationwide community-based serological survey of HIV-1 and other human retrovirus infections in a Central African country. Lancet i: 941–943

Selwyn P A, Hartel D, Lewis V A et al 1989 A prospective study of the risk of tuberculosis among intravenous drug users with human immunodeficiency virus infection. New England Journal of Medicine 320: 545–550

Shaw J B, Wynn-Williams N 1954 Infectivity of pulmonary tuberculosis in relation to sputum status. American Review of Tuberculosis 69: 724–732

Slutkin G, Leowski J, Mann J 1988 Tuberculosis and AIDS: The effects of the AIDS epidemic on the tuberculosis problem and tuberculosis programmes. Bulletin of the International Union against Tuberculosis 67: 21–24

Styblo K 1980 Recent advances in epidemiological research in tuberculosis. Advances in Tuberculosis Research 20: 1–63

Styblo K 1986 Tuberculosis control and surveillance. In: Flenley D S, Petty T L (eds) Recent advances in respiratory medicine, vol 4. Churchill Livingstone, Edinburgh

Styblo K 1989 Overview and epidemiologic assessment of the current global tuberculosis situation with an emphasis on control in developing countries. Review of Infectious Diseases 2 (suppl 2): S339–346

Styblo K 1990a Impact of HIV infection on the tuberculosis problem worldwide. Kekkaku 65: 429–438

Styblo K 1990b The elimination of tuberculosis in the Netherlands. Bulletin of the International Union against Tuberculosis 65: 49–55

Styblo K, Meijer J 1978 Recent advances in tuberculosis epidemiology with regard to formulation or re-adjustment of control programmes. Bulletin of the International Union against Tuberculosis 53: 283–294

Styblo K, Meijer J, Sutherland I 1969 The transmission of tubercle bacilli: Its trend in a human population. Tuberculosis Surveillance Research Unit Report No. 1. Bulletin of the International Union against Tuberculosis 42: 5 104

Sutherland I 1976 Recent studies in the epidemiology of tuberculosis, based on the risk of being infected with tubercle bacilli. Advances in Tuberculosis Research 19: 1–63

TSRU Progress Report 1989 The first round of the National Tuberculin Survey in Tanzania, 1983–1987, vol 2, pp 101–116

World Health Organization 1990a Global Programme on AIDS. Surveillance, Forecasting and Impact Assessment Unit. AIDS cases reported as of 1 October 1990

World Health Organization 1990b Press release WHO/38 of 31 July 1990

10

Interstitial lung diseases

R. L. Mortenson   R. M. Bogin   T. E. King Jr

The interstitial lung diseases are a heterogeneous group of lung parenchymal disorders which are classified together because of common clinical, radiological, physiological and pathological features. The term interstitial is somewhat misleading in that most of these disorders have extensive alteration of alveolar architecture as well. While there continues to be progress in understanding, the aetiology for approximately two-thirds of these diseases remains unknown and these diseases are, therefore, classified by their clinical and/or pathological features (Crystal et al 1984). The most common known causes of the interstitial lung diseases are related to occupational and environmental exposures, especially to inorganic dust (Table 10.1).

Table 10.1 Aetiological classification of interstitial lung disease

I. *Occupational and environmental exposures*
    Inorganic dust
      Silica
      Silicates (i.e. asbestos, talc, kaolin or 'china clay')
      Aluminium
      Carbon (i.e. coal dust, graphite)
      Hard metal dusts (i.e. cadmium, titanium oxide)
      Beryllium
    Organic dusts[a]
      Thermophilic bacteria (i.e. *Micropolyspora faeni*,
        Thermactinomyces vulgaris, *T. sacchari*)
        Farmer's lung
        Grain-handler's lung
        Humidifier or air conditioner lung
        Bagassosis[b]
        Mushroom-worker's lung
      Other bacteria (i.e. Bacillus subtilis, B. sereus)
        Humidifier lung
      True fungi (i.e. *Aspergillus, Cryptostroma corticale, Aureobasidium pullulans,*
        Penicillin spp.)
      Animal proteins (e.g. bird-fancier's disease)
      Bacterial products
        Byssinosis
    Chemical sources
      Synthetic-fibre lung
      Bakelite-worker's lung
    Gases
      Oxygen, sulphur dioxide, chlorine gas

Table 10.1 continued:

Fumes
  Oxides of zinc, copper, manganese, cadmium, iron, magnesium, nickel, brass, selenium, tin and antimony
Vapours
  Thermosetting resins (rubber tyre workers)
  Toluene diisocyanate (TDI, asthmatic reactions prominent)
  Trimellitic anhydride toxicity
  Mercury
Aerosols
  Fats, pyrethrum, 'Bordeau mixture'
Paraquat
Radiation

II. *Drugs and Poisons (partial list)*
  Chemotherapeutic agents
    Busulfan
    Bleomycin
    Methotrexate
  Antibiotics
    Nitrofurantoin
    Sulfasalazine
  Drug-induced lupus
    Diphenylhydantoin
    Procainamide
  Miscellaneous
    Gold salts
    Amiodarone
    Radiation

III. *Connective tissue disease*
  Systemic lupus erythematosus
  Rheumatoid arthritis
  Progressive systemic sclerosis
  Sjogren's syndrome
  Polymyositis and dermatomyositis
  Mixed connective tissue disease
  Ankylosing spondylitis

IV. *Other systemic diseases*
  Sarcoidosis
  Vasculitides
    Wegener's granulomatosis
    Churg–Strauss syndrome
  Haemorrhagic syndromes
    Goodpasture's syndrome
    Idiopathic pulmonary haemosiderosis
  Histiocytosis X (eosinophilic granuloma)
  Chronic gastric aspiration
  Lymphangitic carcinomatosis
  Chronic pulmonary oedema
  Chronic uraemia
  Alveolar proteinosis

V. *Idiopathic pulmonary fibrosis*

VI. *Infections* (residue of active infection of any type)

[a] Hypersensitivity pneumonitis or extrinsic allergic alveolitis.
[b] Primarily of historical interest only.

Sarcoidosis and idiopathic pulmonary fibrosis (cryptogenic fibrosing alveolitis), with or without an associated connective tissue disease, are the most common interstitial lung diseases of unknown aetiology.

A common pathogenetic sequence underlies most interstitial lung diseases regardless of aetiology. The development of pulmonary fibrosis is thought to follow injury to the alveolar wall via either the vasculature or the airways. Following this injury, there is an influx of inflammatory and immune effector cells, i.e. an 'alveolitis'. The precise pathway leading from injury to fibrosis is not known. The major mechanism may involve either continued exposure to the inciting agent or aberrant perpetuation of the lung injury process after an initial insult. In the presence of this ongoing alveolitis, derangement of alveolar and interstitial architecture occurs. The ensuing fibrosis and honeycombing result in loss of alveolar gas-exchanging units. With some exceptions, this process is typically chronic in nature.

Because these conditions are uncommon and their aetiologies often obscure, patients with interstitial lung disease may present a diagnostic and therapeutic challenge. The goal of this chapter is to review the current understanding of these diseases and to present a guide to the work-up and management of the patient presenting with one of these disorders.

EVALUATION OF PATIENT WITH SUSPECTED INTERSTITIAL LUNG DISEASE

History and physical examination

The evaluation of a patient with suspected interstitial lung disease begins with an in-depth history. Common presenting symptoms are those of progressive breathlessness with exertion and/or persistent cough which is typically non-productive. Frequently the patient will have attributed the insidious onset of these symptoms to ageing, deconditioning, obesity, or a recent flu-like illness. In addition to defining the duration and extent of dyspnoea, cough and sputum production (if any), symptoms of the connective tissue diseases should be carefully sought. This group of disorders may be difficult to rule out since the pulmonary manifestations occasionally precede the more typical systemic manifestations by months or even years. Occupational, environmental and medication history are also important. Review of the environment (home and work), especially as it relates to pets, air conditioners, humidifiers, hot tubs, evaporative cooling systems (e.g. swamp coolers), etc., is valuable as well.

Physical examination commonly reveals tachypnoea, reduced chest expansion and bibasilar end-inspiratory dry ('Velcro') crackles. Clubbing of the digits is common in some patients (idiopathic pulmonary fibrosis) and rare in others (sarcoidosis). Signs of pulmonary hypertension and cor pulmonale are generally secondary manifestations of advanced interstitial lung disease, although they may be primary manifestations of a connective tissue disorder (progressive systemic sclerosis/CREST).

Laboratory findings

The routine laboratory evaluation of a patient suspected of having interstitial lung disease is often not helpful but should include biochemical tests to evaluate liver and renal function, and haematological tests to check for evidence of polycythaemia and leucocytosis.

An elevated erythrocyte sedimentation rate and hypergammaglobulinaemia are commonly observed but are non-diagnostic. Antinuclear antibodies, anti-immunoglobulin antibodies (rheumatoid factors) and circulating immune complexes are identified in many of these patients even in the absence of a defined connective tissue disorder. Elevation of serum lactate dehydrogenase may be noted but is a non-specific finding common to other pulmonary disorders (e.g. alveolar proteinosis). An increase in the angiotensin-converting enzyme (ACE) level may be observed in sarcoidosis but is non-specific, as elevated ACE levels have been reported in several other interstitial diseases including hypersensitivity pneumonitis. Antibodies to organic antigens may be helpful when hypersensitivity pneumonitis is suspected, although non-diagnostic. The electrocardiogram is usually normal in the absence of pulmonary hypertension or concurrent cardiac disease.

Radiological studies

Chest radiograph

The diagnosis of interstitial lung disease will often be suspected initially on the basis of a chest radiograph (Fig. 10.1A). The most common radiographic abnormality is a reticular or reticulonodular pattern, although mixed patterns of alveolar filling and increased interstitial markings are not unusual (Felson 1979). Although the chest radiograph is useful in suggesting the presence of interstitial lung disease, the correlation between the radiographic pattern and the stage of disease (clinical or histopathological) is generally poor. Only the radiographic finding of honeycombing (small cystic spaces) correlates with pathological findings and when present portends a poor prognosis.

There are additional radiographic features that when present may assist in the diagnosis of interstitial diseases (Table 10.2) (Schwarz & King 1988). Radiographic findings of increased interstitial markings in association with increased lung volumes, upper zone predominant radiographic findings, pneumothorax, pleural disease, Kerley B lines, hilar or mediastinal lymphadenopathy, a miliary pattern, or the presence of subcutaneous calcinosis, may be useful in narrowing the differential diagnosis and directing appropriate diagnostic studies. Of importance, the chest radiograph may be normal in as many as 10% of patients with interstitial lung disease (Table 10.2) (Epler et al 1978). A frequent mistake is for the physician to fail to evaluate a symptomatic patient because of a normal chest X-ray. Equally troubling is the incomplete evaluation of the asymptomatic patient with radiographic evidence of interstitial lung disease, as this often leads to

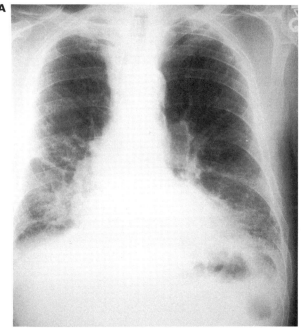

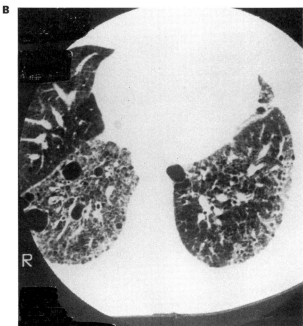

Fig. 10.1 **A** Chest radiograph showing diffuse reticular interstitial infiltrates most prominent at the lung bases. Open lung biopsy revealed moderately severe usual interstitial pneumonitis. **B** High-resolution, thin-section CT scan. The CT scan shows extensive parenchymal involvement, especially in the lower lobes. The right lower lobe is essentially a destroyed honeycombed lung. The left lower lobe reveals the characteristic subpleural reticular pattern seen in idiopathic pulmonary fibrosis.

Table 10.2   Helpful radiographic patterns in interstitial lung disease

Upper zone predominance
Granulomatous disease
    Sarcoidosis
    Histiocytosis X (eosinophilic granuloma)
    Chronic hypersensitivity pneumonitis
    Chronic infectious diseases (e.g. tuberculosis, histoplasmosis)

Pneumoconiosis
    Silicosis
    Berylliosis
    Coal-miner's pneumoconiosis
    Hard metal disease

Miscellaneous
    Rheumatoid arthritis
    Ankylosing spondylitis
    Radiation fibrosis
    Drug-induced (amiodarone, gold)

Associated with pneumothorax
Histiocytosis X (eosinophilic granuloma)
Lymphangioleiomyomatosis
Tuberous sclerosis

Increased lung volumes
Lymphangioleiomyomatosis
Tuberous sclerosis
Sarcoidosis (stage 3)
Eosinophilic granuloma (chronic with cyst formation)
Neurofibromatosis
Chronic hypersensitivity pneumonitis

Pleural involvement
Asbestosis
Connective tissue disorders
    1.   Systemic lupus erythematosus
    2.   Rheumatoid arthritis
    3.   Scleroderma
    4.   Mixed connective tissue disease
Lymphangitic carcinomatosis
Lymphangioleiomyomatosis (chylous effusion)
Drug induced
    Nitrofurantoin
Sarcoidosis (lymphocytic effusion)
Radiation pneumonitis (chronic with mediastinal lymphatic obstruction)

Hilar or mediastinal lymphadenopathy
Sarcoidosis
Lymphoma
Lymphangitic carcinomatosis
Berylliosis

Associated with Kerley B lines
Chronic left ventricular failure
Mitral valve disease
Lymphangitic carcinomatosis
Lymphoma
Lymphangioleiomyomatosis

Table 10.2 continued

Subcutaneous calcinosis
Scleroderma (CREST)
Dermatopolymyositis

Miliary pattern
Infectious granulomatous disease (tuberculosis, histoplasmosis, coccidioidomycosis)
Metastatic malignant disease
  Hypernephroma
  Adenocarcinoma of breast
  Malignant melanoma
Miscellaneous
  Sarcoidosis
  Silicosis
  Hypersensitivity pneumonitis
  Bronchiolitis obliterans

Normal
Hypersensitivity pneumonitis
Sarcoidosis
Bronchiolitis obliterans
Idiopathic pulmonary fibrosis (especially early 'cellular' stage)
Asbestosis
Lymphangioleiomyomatosis

After Schwarz M I, Radiologic recognition of chronic diffuse lung disease. In: Schwarz M I, King T E Jr (eds) Interstitial lung disease. Decker, Toronto, 1988, pp 27–36.

---

progressive disease which may be irreversible by the time significant symptoms develop.

High-resolution computed tomography

High-resolution computed tomography (HRCT) is particularly well suited for evaluation of diffuse pulmonary parenchymal disease (Fig. 10.1B) (Aberle et al 1988a, b, Mueller et al 1986, 1987, 1989, Staples et al 1987). Pattern recognition in diffuse lung disease is enhanced because HRCT avoids the problem of superimposition of structures and is exposure independent (Swensen et al 1989). While still in the midst of extensive research, HRCT is likely to offer (1) more accuracy than conventional radiographic studies in the distinction of air space from interstitial lung disease; (2) earlier detection and confirmation of suspected diffuse lung disease; (3) better assessment of the extent and distribution of disease; (4) the ability to discern occult mediastinal adenopathy; and (5) possible utility in more specifically selecting appropriate biopsy sites.

Gallium-67 scan

Gallium-67 lung scanning has been tried as a means of evaluating the inflammatory component of interstitial lung disease, as gallium is not taken up by normal lung parenchyma. Uptake may be diffuse or patchy and is felt to reflect an increased accumulation of inflammatory cells in the lung (Line et al 1978). To date, gallium scans have not been proven useful in staging or follow-up of interstitial lung disease.

Pulmonary function testing

Pulmonary function tests are an important aspect of the evaluation of any patient with suspected interstitial lung disease. The finding of an obstructive or restrictive pattern is important in narrowing the number of possible diagnoses (Cherniack 1988). There are few disorders that produce interstitial infiltrates and an obstructive ventilatory defect (e.g., sarcoidosis, lymphangioleiomyomatosis, hypersensitivity pneumonitis, tuberous sclerosis, and chronic obstructive pulmonary disease with superimposed interstitial lung disease. Most of the interstitial disorders have a restrictive defect with reduced total lung capacity (TLC), functional residual capacity (FRC) and residual volume (RV). Flow rates are decreased (forced expiratory volume in 1 second) (FEV_1) and functional vital capacity (FVC) but this is related to the decreased lung volumes. The FEV_1/FVC ratio is usually normal or increased (Fig. 10.2A). Smoking history must be considered when interpreting the functional studies. Reduction in lung compliance is also common. It is important to realize that, in symptomatic patients with a normal chest radiograph and minimal or no restrictive disease, the measurement of elastic recoil (pressure–volume curve) may be helpful by identifying lung stiffness (decreased compliance) (Fig. 10.2B).

The measurement of gas transfer as measured by the diffusing capacity for carbon monoxide (DLCO) may also be useful. The decrease in DLCO is due in part to effacement of the alveolar capillary units but more important to the extent of mismatching of ventilation and perfusion in the alveoli. Lung regions with reduced compliance due either to fibrosis or excessive cellularity may be poorly ventilated, but still be well perfused. A frequent mistake is to equate the severity of reduction in DLCO with disease stage. In some interstitial lung disease there can be considerable reduction in lung volumes and/or severe hypoxaemia but normal or only slight reduction in DLCO.

The resting arterial blood gases may be normal or reveal hypoxaemia (secondary to a mismatching of ventilation to perfusion) and respiratory alkalosis (Austrian et al 1951). Carbon dioxide retention is rare and usually a manifestation of far-advanced endstage disease. Importantly, a normal resting arterial oxygen tension (PaO_2) does not rule out significant hypoxaemia during exercise or sleep (Fulmer et al 1979). Furthermore, although hypoxaemia with exercise and sleep is very common, secondary erythrocytosis is rarely observed in uncomplicated interstitial lung disease. Because resting hypoxaemia is not always evident and because severe exercise-induced hypoxaemia may go undetected, it is important to perform exercise testing with arterial blood gases (Kelley & Daniele 1984, Risk et al

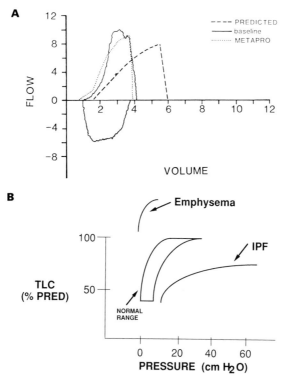

Fig. 10.2 A The pattern of ventilatory dysfunction in a patient with interstitial lung disease is usually restrictive. Lung volume is reduced and flow rates are higher than expected for a given lung volume because of the elevated driving pressure due to increased elastic recoil. There is no improvement after bronchodilator (metapro–metaproterenol). **B** The pressure–volume relationship in a patient with idiopathic pulmonary fibrosis reveals a shift down and to the right and a decreased slope consistent with a restrictive disorder and decreased lung compliance. The maximal transpulmonary pressure is increased, reflecting the very high negative pressure required to open the fibrotic alveoli present in this patient. The boxed area is the predicted normal range for this patient. The typical curve for a patient with pulmonary emphysema is shown for comparison.

1984). Arterial oxygen desaturation, a failure to decrease dead space appropriately with exercise (i.e. a high dead space/tidal volume (VD/VT) ratio), and an excessive increase in respiratory rate with a lower than expected recruitment of tidal volume provide useful information regarding physiological abnormalities and extent of disease (Austrian et al 1951, Cherniack 1988, Fulmer et al 1979).

Bronchoalveolar lavage

Subsegmental lavage through the wedged bronchoscope has been used to retrieve and examine cells and soluble constituents of the lower respiratory air spaces (Cherniack et al 1990, Haslam et al 1980, Hunninghake et al 1979, 1981, Reynolds et al 1977, Reynolds 1987). Bronchoalveolar lavage

(BAL) studies have been performed on patients with many types of interstitial lung disease (Table 10.3). As a result of these studies, numerous hypotheses have been advanced regarding the pathogenesis of the interstitial diseases. Differences in the quantity and distribution of BAL cells and other components in the interstitial disorders have been the basis for hypotheses suggesting that BAL constituents can (1) narrow the differential diagnostic possibilities between various types of interstitial lung disease, (2) define the stage of disease, and (3) assess the progression of disease or response to therapy. However, the utility of BAL in the clinical assessment and management of interstitial lung disease patients remains to be established.

Lung biopsy

Following the initial evaluation, it is important to confirm the diagnosis and establish the stage of disease. Lung biopsy is usually indicated because (1) it provides a more accurate diagnosis, (2) it will exclude neoplastic and infectious processes that occasionally mimic chronic, progressive interstitial disease, (3) it will occasionally identify a more treatable process than originally suspected (for example, extrinsic allergic alveolitis), and (4) it will provide a better assessment of disease activity. Often fibreoptic bronchoscopy with transbronchial lung biopsy is the initial procedure of choice, especially when sarcoidosis, lymphangitic carcinomatosis, eosinophilic pneumonia, Goodpasture's syndrome or infection is suspected. If a specific diagnosis is not made by transbronchial biopsy then an open lung biopsy is indicated (Fortoul 1988). A frequent mistake is to fail to obtain a definitive diagnosis and to fail to determine the stage of disease prior to the initiation of treatment. Open lung biopsy is the definitive method for diagnosis and staging of disease allowing appropriate prognostic and therapeutic decisions to be made (Gaensler & Carrington 1980). It is a relatively safe procedure with low morbidity and less than 1% mortality (Ray et al 1976). Relative contraindications to open lung biopsy include serious cardiovascular disease, radiographic evidence of diffuse 'honeycombing', severe pulmonary dysfunction or other major operative risks (especially in the elderly population).

Table 10.3 Bronchoalveolar lavage: common cellular patterns in common interstitial lung diseases

	Lymphocytes	Neutrophils	Eosinophils	Mast cells
Asbestosis[a]	N[b]	++	+	N
Idiopathic pulmonary fibrosis	+	+++	+	N
Sarcoidosis	++	N or +	N	N
Hypersensitivity pneumonitis	+++	N or +	N	+

[a] Ferruginous bodies may be identified.
[b] +, increase; N, normal values.

The remainder of this chapter will give a concise review of the major categories of disease which can produce the clinical, radiological and physiological features characterizing the interstitial disorders (Table 10.1).

COMMON CAUSES OF INTERSTITIAL LUNG DISEASE

Occupational and environmental causes of interstitial lung disease (see also Chapter 13)

By far the most important step in considering occupational or environmental exposures as a cause of disease is the taking of the history (Fink 1982). In order to establish a potential link to environmental causes of disease, it is insufficient to merely record the title of the occupation of the patient; the physician should have a clear understanding of exactly what tasks the patient performed in each job throughout his life. A chronological listing of the patient's employment, including specific duties and known exposures to dust, gases and chemicals, is important. The degree of exposure, duration, latency of exposure and the use of protective devices in the workplace should be elicited. Since certain diseases are not related to the duration of exposure, all occupations, regardless of duration, must be considered important. Specific enquiries should also be made regarding the patient's perception of dust or fume exposure and illnesses of coworkers.

Coal-worker's pneumoconiosis, silicosis and asbestosis are the most common inhalation exposures that result in pulmonary fibrosis. These processes usually occur in individuals with an exposure history in excess of 10 years to the offending agent.

Coal-worker's pneumoconiosis

Coal-worker's pneumoconiosis is a rare cause of significant pulmonary fibrosis. A small percentage of coal-workers, particularly those who work underground as opposed to strip mining, may develop coal-worker's pneumoconiosis. Even among underground workers there are substantive differences in exposure to coal dust depending upon the specific job site, with those in close proximity to the coal face (where excavation of the coal seam occurs) at highest risk. Two forms of disease predominate: (1) simple pneumoconiosis, represented by small opacities (less than 1 cm in diameter) predominantly in the upper lung zones; and (b) complicated pneumoconiosis or progressive massive fibrosis (opacity 1 cm or more in diameter) (Parkes 1982). Simple pneumoconiosis is not associated with increased incidence of dyspnoea while progressive massive fibrosis is characterized by marked dyspnoea. The prevalence rate among coal-miners is approximately 10%, of which 0.4% develop progressive massive fibrosis. Pulmonary function abnormalities in simple coal-worker's pneumoconiosis generally occur only in the presence of a history of cigarette smoking despite the presence of radiographic involvement.

Silicosis

Silicosis is found in miners, sandblasters, glass manufacturers, quarry workers, stone dressers, foundry workers and boiler scalers (Silicosis and Silicate Disease Committee 1988, Ziskind et al 1976). Radiographically, silicosis appears as bilateral multinodular rounded densities predominantly in the upper lung zones. The radiographic changes usually occur before the clinical and functional abnormalities. Progression from simple to progressive massive fibrosis occurs in a minority of patients. Patients with silicosis are susceptible to infection by *Mycobacterium tuberculosis* and other atypical mycobacteria (Snider 1978). Also, scleroderma and rheumatoid arthritis are unusually prevalent in silicotics. Laboratory findings in simple silicosis may include an increased sedimentation rate, immunoglobulins, immune complexes, antinuclear antibodies and anti-immunoglobulin antibodies (rheumatoid factors). There is no known effective treatment at present for silicosis.

Asbestosis

Asbestos exposure is widespread because it is used extensively as an insulation material, fire retardant and noise reduction agent in many public facilities. Workers employed in the shipyard, automotive, insulation, cement, textile and asbestos mining industries are at greatest risk. There is a long latent period between exposure and the development of lung diseases. Smoking appears to facilitate the damaging effects of asbestos inhalation. It is important to distinguish evidence of asbestos exposure from asbestosis (Mossman & Gee 1989). Asbestosis is characterized by a history of exposure to asbestos and the presence of interstitial pulmonary fibrosis manifested by dyspnoea, cough, and bibasilar inspiratory crackles with or without digital clubbing on examination. Bilateral pleural thickening along the lower or mid-thoracic walls, calcified pleural plaques and hazy infiltrates composed of irregular or linear small opacities especially in the lower lung zones are the most common radiological changes (Friedman et al 1988). Pulmonary function studies may reveal a restrictive pattern, and the DLCO is often reduced. The clinical course is usually one of slow but progressive deterioration, and death is often a result of either respiratory compromise or cancer. Pleural and peritoneal mesotheliomas and bronchogenic carcinoma are established complications of asbestos exposure. The synergistic effect of cigarette smoking and asbestos exposure on the development of lung cancer is well established.

Hypersensitivity pneumonitis (extrinsic allergic alveolitis)

This group of diseases is associated with repeated inhalation of finely dispersed organic dusts. This produces diffuse patchy interstitial and/or alveolar infiltrates in the lung following the formation of antigen–antibody complexes (Arthus reaction). Farmer's lung (exposure to mouldy hay containing fungal spores) is the prototype. In urban areas, air conditioner or humidifier lung disease (due to fungal overgrowth and aerosolization) and bird fancier's lung are more common.

The disease can present in two forms (Reynolds 1982). The first form is an acute reaction following heavy exposure, which is characterized by the abrupt onset (4–6 hours later) of fever, chills, malaise, nausea, cough, chest tightness and dyspnoea without wheezing. These symptoms subside over hours or days. Diffuse fine crackles throughout the chest, mild hypoxaemia and a restrictive ventilatory defect accompany these symptomatic episodes. A fleeting, micronodular, interstitial pattern in the lower and mid-lower zone may be identified on chest radiograph. Removal from exposure usually results in complete resolution. Pathologically, this stage is characterized by bronchiolocentric non-caseating interstitial granulomatous pneumonitis. The second form of the disease is an insidious form which results if repeated acute episodes or continued antigen exposure occurs.

A patient with chronic hypersensitivity pneumonitis may not have any acute episodes. Disabling and frequently irreversible respiratory findings, i.e. pulmonary fibrosis, are characteristic. Mixed obstructive and restrictive physiology is often present on pulmonary function testing, as well as reduced diffusing capacity, and hypoxaemia. The chest radiograph shows progressive fibrotic changes with fewer nodular densities and loss of lung volume, particularly of the upper lobes. Diagnosis of the chronic form of hypersensitivity pneumonitis usually requires open lung biopsy. Besides the granulomatous pneumonitis, biopsy specimens at this stage reveal bronchiolitis obliterans with distal destruction of alveoli (honeycombing) in association with densely fibrotic zones.

The diagnosis of hypersensitivity pneumonitis is important since it is a reversible disease when diagnosed early. It often requires intensive detective work to uncover the source of the antigen. The serum can be tested against common antigens (the thermophilic actinomycetes, especially *Micropolyspora faeni* and *Theramoactinomyces vulgaris*). However, the presence of serum precipitins does not make a definite diagnosis. For example, 30–40% of farmers will have positive serum precipitins without clinical disease. Furthermore, the absence of serum precipitins does not rule out this disease. Inhalation challenge may very occasionally be required, although it should generally be avoided as it may exacerbate disease. Bronchoalveolar lavage with the measurement of antibodies, IgG and IgM, and examination of immunoreactive cells for specific immune responses may eventually become a useful diagnostic procedure (Reynolds et al 1977).

Drug-induced interstitial lung disease

Many drugs are known to have the potential to induce diffuse interstitial infiltrates with associated symptoms of dyspnoea and non-productive cough. In most cases, the pathogenesis of this aberrant pulmonary response to a given drug is unknown, although a combination of direct toxic effects of the drug (or its metabolite) and indirect inflammatory and immunological events is probable (Rosenow 1980). Although too extensive a topic to discuss in detail here, several generalizations can be made: (1) the extent of disease is usually dose related; (2) many classes of drugs may cause disease; (3) the onset of illness may be insidious over weeks or months, or may be abrupt and fulminant; (4) treatment always includes discontinuation of any possible offending drug and supportive care; and (5) since the addition of corticosteroids is often ineffective, the decision to use steroids must be based on the available data for a given drug. Table 10.1 lists the drugs most commonly associated with interstitial lung disease.

Connective tissue disorders

Interstitial lung disease associated with connective tissue disorders usually occurs after the connective tissue disorder has been recognized, although occasionally interstitial lung disease does precede the development of the characteristic systemic signs and symptoms of the particular disease. The most common form of pulmonary involvement is a chronic interstitial pattern indistinguishable from idiopathic pulmonary fibrosis (Hunninghake & Fauci 1979, King & Dunn 1988). However, determining the precise nature of lung involvement in most of the connective tissue diseases is difficult, due to the high incidence of lung disease caused by the disease-associated complications of oesophageal dysfunction (predisposing to aspiration and secondary infections), respiratory muscle weakness (atelectasis and secondary infections), complications due to therapy (opportunistic infections) and associated malignancies.

Rheumatoid arthritis

Although rheumatoid arthritis has a female predominance, pulmonary disease associated with rheumatoid disease is more common in men. Manifestations of rheumatoid disease in the lung include pleurisy with or without effusion, interstitial lung disease, necrobiotic nodules (non-pneumoconiotic intrapulmonary rheumatoid nodules) with or without cavities, Caplan's syndrome (rheumatoid pneumoconiosis), pulmonary hypertension secondary to rheumatoid pulmonary vasculitis, bronchiolitis obliterans, and upper airway obstruction due to arytenoid arthritis. Interstitial lung disease in association with rheumatoid disease occurs in up to 20% of cases and is similar clinically, physiologically and pathologically to idiopathic pulmonary fibrosis (Walker & Wright 1968). The course of the disease is usually a slowly progressive one, but rapid deterioration can occur. If therapy is required, the approach is similar to that described for idiopathic pulmonary fibrosis below.

Progressive systemic sclerosis (scleroderma)

Progressive systemic sclerosis is a systemic disease characterized by dermatological changes (skin thickening, ulcerations), visceral microvascular abnormalities and oesophageal dysfunction. The incidence of interstitial lung disease associated with it ranges from 14% to 90% in clinical studies and from 60% to 100% in autopsy studies (Rodnan 1963, Weaver et al 1968, Young & Mark 1978). Pulmonary function tests usually reveal a restrictive pattern with reduced lung compliance and impaired diffusing capacity, often before any clinical or radiographic evidence of lung disease appears. Pulmonary vascular disease alone or in association with pulmonary fibrosis, pleuritis, recurrent aspiration pneumonitis and carcinoma also occur. The interstitial lung disease and pulmonary hypertension associated with scleroderma are strikingly resistant to current modes of therapy.

Systemic lupus erythematosus (SLE)

SLE is a systemic disorder of unknown aetiology characterized by immunologically mediated tissue damage, with a variable presentation and multiple organ system involvement. Pleuritis with or without effusion is the most common pulmonary manifestation of SLE. Other lung manifestations include atelectasis, diaphragmatic dysfunction with loss of lung volumes, pulmonary vascular disease, pulmonary haemorrhage, uraemic pulmonary oedema, infectious pneumonia, bronchiolitis obliterans, and interstitial lung disease. The latter is uncommon (less than 5% of patients) and may present in two forms, i.e. acute interstitial pneumonitis (tachypnoea, dyspnoea, high fever, cyanosis and pulmonary haemorrhage that can be fatal) and chronic interstitial pneumonia (dyspnoea, non-productive cough, pleuritic chest pain, hypocapnia, impaired diffusing capacity and a restrictive ventilatory defect). Chest radiographs may reveal diffuse or patchy infiltrates, located primarily (though not exclusively) in the lower zones. Corticosteroids, cyclophosphamide, azathioprine and plasmapheresis have been employed in treatment with variable clinical responses.

Sjogren's syndrome

Sjogren's syndrome manifested by keratoconjunctivitis sicca, xerostomia and recurrent swelling of the parotid gland may be associated with interstitial lung disease. Although the most common interstitial process is indistinguishable from idiopathic pulmonary fibrosis, lymphocytic interstitial pneumonitis, lymphoma, pseudolymphoma, bronchiolitis and bronchiolitis obliterans can also be associated with Sjogren's syndrome (Fairfax et al 1981, Strimlan et al 1976). Thus, open lung biopsy is frequently required to make a precise diagnosis. Biopsy tissue can be frozen for immune marker studies to help differentiate malignant from benign lymphoproliferation. In the absence of controlled trials, corticosteroids have been used in the management of Sjogren's syndrome associated interstitial lung disease with some degree of clinical success.

Polymyositis/dermatomyositis

Interstitial lung disease occurs in approximately 10% of patients with polymyositis or dermatomyositis, and the clinical features are similar to idiopathic pulmonary fibrosis. Less commonly, a rapidly progressive Hamman–Rich type syndrome may occur with respiratory failure. Diffuse reticular or reticular–nodular infiltrates with or without an alveolar component occur radiographically, with a predilection for the lung bases. The response rate to corticosteroid therapy has been reported to be somewhat higher than interstitial lung disease associated with other connective tissue disorders (Dickey & Myers 1984, Schwarz et al 1976).

Idiopathic pulmonary fibrosis

Idiopathic pulmonary fibrosis (cryptogenic fibrosing alveolitis) is one of the more commonly occurring interstitial lung diseases of unknown aetiology. It has specific clinical–pathological manifestations and so it is important to reserve this diagnosis for this particular disease entity, and not to assume that increased interstitial markings on a chest radiograph necessarily represent idiopathic pulmonary fibrosis.

The clinical manifestations of idiopathic pulmonary fibrosis include dyspnoea on exertion, non-productive cough, and 'Velcro'-type inspiratory crackles with or without digital clubbing. The chest radiograph typically reveals diffuse interstitial infiltrates, although as many as 10% of patients with idiopathic pulmonary fibrosis have a normal radiograph. Pulmonary function tests often reveal restrictive impairment with decreased static lung volumes, reduced diffusing capacity for carbon monoxide and arterial hypoxaemia exaggerated or elicited by exercise. The pathogenesis of idiopathic pulmonary fibrosis is unknown, although genetic, viral and immunological aberrations are hypothesized. The diagnosis of idiopathic pulmonary fibrosis generally requires open lung biopsy since tissue obtained by transbronchial biopsy is usually insufficient. Pathologically, idiopathic pulmonary fibrosis is characterized by variable degrees of cellular infiltration of alveolar walls, fibroblast proliferation, collagen deposition and cystic spaces in areas of advanced disease (honeycomb lung). The clinical course is variable, with a mean survival of 4–6 years from diagnosis. Response to treatment is variable, but patients with a more cellular biopsy are more likely to improve with corticosteroid and/or cytotoxic therapy (Panos et al 1990).

Sarcoidosis

Sarcoidosis is a multisystem disease of unknown aetiology manifested by granulomatous infiltration in a perivascular pattern. The granulomas are non-caseating and may occur in any organ, although the lung, peripheral lymph nodes, skin, eyes and liver are most commonly affected. The clinical presentation of sarcoidosis is quite variable. Classically, the patient presents asymptomatically with an abnormal chest radiograph discovered incidentally. Dyspnoea, with or without exertion, and non-productive cough are the most common respiratory system complaints. Laboratory evaluation may reveal abnormal liver function tests, hypercalcaemia and hypergamma-globulinaemia. Serum ACE levels, formerly thought to reflect the activity of the disease, are of limited value in management. Pulmonary function tests may reveal normal function, a restrictive pattern or an obstructive defect, the latter inferring endobronchial sarcoid involvement. The DLCO may be reduced.

The 'classic' chest radiograph in sarcoidosis reveals bilateral hilar adenopathy, but this may be absent or occur in combination with parenchymal infiltrates depending on the stage of disease. Parenchymal infiltrates may be interstitial, alveolar or both. Nodular lesions also occur. An upper zone predominant distribution of disease is typical.

The diagnosis of sarcoidosis is made histologically, by demonstrating non-caseating granulomas in tissue. The frequent involvement of the lung makes this organ the most accessible tissue for biopsy. Even if an interstitial infiltrate is not present radiographically, the diagnosis may be made by transbronchial biopsy in over 90% of cases if a sufficient number of biopsies are obtained.

Treatment of the disease with corticosteroids is indicated for symptomatic patients, patients with declining lung function and for those who have significant involvement of the eye, heart, central nervous system or hypercalcaemia. Sarcoidosis is generally very responsive to corticosteroids although long-term outcome is probably not affected. For patients with sarcoidosis found to be unresponsive to steroids, alternative strategies include chloroquine, and high-dose i.v. pulsed methyl prednisolone, although data from clinical trials are sparse (see Chapter 11).

MANAGEMENT OF INTERSTITIAL LUNG DISEASE

Many interstitial lung diseases are not responsive to therapy. Therefore, it is extremely important that all treatable possibilities be carefully considered. Since therapy will not reverse fibrosis, the major goals are: (1) early identification and aggressive treatment directed at suppressing the acute and chronic inflammatory process, thereby, preventing further lung damage; (2) permanent removal of the offending agent when known; and (3) palliation of complications. While the course of interstitial lung disease is variable, progression of disease is common and often insidious. Careful monitoring with 6 or 12-month clinical evaluations and pulmonary function testing (especially exercise testing) is essential. Hypoxaemia (PaO_2 less than 7.3 kPa, 55 mmHg) at rest and/or with exercise should be managed by supplemental oxygen. Not providing supplemental oxygen to the patient with exercise-induced hypoxaemia is a frequent error. This often leads to progressive reduction in the patient's level of activity and earlier onset of right heart failure. With the appearance of cor pulmonale, diuretic therapy and phlebotomy may occasionally be required.

Drug therapy

Corticosteroids remain the mainstay of therapy for suppression of the 'alveolitis' present in these processes but the success rate is low. In idiopathic pulmonary fibrosis, 40–50% of patients experience subjective improvement but only 20–30% have objective improvement. Besides the immediate removal of the aetiological agent in occupational and environmental diseases, corticosteroid therapy is recommended for symptomatic patients with acute inorganic dust exposure, acute radiation pneumonitis and drug-induced disease. In organic dust disease, corticosteroids are recommended for both the acute and chronic stages.

Cyclophosphamide (1–2 mg/kg ideal body weight per day), with or without corticosteroids, has been tried with variable success in idiopathic pulmonary fibrosis and some other interstitial lung diseases. An objective response commonly will take at least 12 weeks to occur (and often longer) in most forms of interstitial lung disease. A treatment trial should therefore not be for less than this period unless complications or side effects occur. If the patient shows clinical and physiological improvement and medication is discontinued, careful monitoring on a 6 or 12-month basis is essential to identify relapses. Further clinical investigation is needed to establish the efficacy of cyclophosphamide in the interstitial lung disorders. Other agents have been used for the treatment of interstitial lung diseases, for example, azothiaprine, methotrexate, colchicine and cyclosporin (Schwarz & King 1988), but further clinical evaluation and controlled trials are needed.

In general, the 'responsive' patient will: (1) report a decrease in symptoms; (2) show radiographic improvement; (3) demonstrate physiological improvement, i.e. increased TLC, DLCO or have an improvement in the exercise-induced oxygen desaturation; or (4) show no further decline in lung function or other parameter of disease activity. Patients who fail to respond to medical management should now be considered for heart–lung or single lung transplantation (see chapters 14–17 on heart–lung transplantation.)

Problems in management (Panos et al 1990)

Clinical deterioration may occur due to disease or therapy-associated complications (Table 10.4). The cause of the decline obviously determines therapy and influences prognosis. Because the manifestations of interstitial lung disease are multiple, non-specific, and often similar to the disease-associated complications, careful assessment of deterioration is required, and includes chest radiology and pulmonary function tests (including lung volumes, DLCO, resting and exercise gas exchange), in addition to a thorough history and physical examination. Other specialized diagnostic studies may be indicated based on the clinical suspicion of complicating problems such as cardiovascular disease, pulmonary infection, pulmonary embolism, bronchogenic carcinoma, pneumothorax or complications of therapy (see Table 10.4).

Table 10.4 Key points for clinical practice

ASSESSMENT IN SUSPECTED INTERSTITIAL LUNG DISEASE

History and physical examination

Laboratory findings: Generally non-specific

Chest X-ray: Useful to narrow differential diagnosis, insufficient for diagnosis; insensitive indicator of physiological function, insufficient to follow efficacy of therapy; useful in assessment of deterioration to rule out new masses/infiltrates

High-resolution computed tomography: Distinguishes air space from interstitial lung disease; earlier detection of suspected interstitial lung disease; better assessment of extent and severity of disease; may discern occult mediastinal lymphadenopathy

Gallium scan: Has not been proven useful in staging or follow-up of interstitial lung disease

Pulmonary function tests: Spirometric measures of lung function do not correlate well with lung histopathology changes in interstitial lung disease; resting and exercise gas exchange is most useful in establishing degree of physiological impairment at presentation and to monitor disease course and response to therapy

Bronchoalveolar lavage: May be useful in narrowing differential diagnosis. In idiopathic pulmonary fibrosis lymphocytosis tends to correlate with increased responsiveness to corticosteroids, while neutrophilia and eosinophilia without lymphocytosis predict lack of steroid sensitivity

Transbronchial biopsy: Useful in diagnosis of some interstitial lung diseases e.g. sarcoidosis, infections, lymphangitic carcinomatosis; insufficient tissue to diagnose many of the interstitial lung diseases such as idiopathic pulmonary fibrosis

Open lung biopsy: Most sensitive and specific test to determine both diagnosis and stage of disease in idiopathic pulmonary fibrosis and some other interstitial lung diseases; the extent and severity of the fibrotic component corresponds best with stage and prognosis

DISEASE PROGRESSION

Clinical manifestations: multiple, non-specific

Symptoms: Increased dyspnoea or cough, reduced exercise capacity

Physical examination: Progression of crackles from bibasilar region to throughout the lung fields; worsening right heart failure

Table 10.4 continued

Pulmonary function: Worsening hypoxaemia; increased supplemental oxygen requirement; progressive restrictive disease; reduced DLCO; increased alveolar–arterial oxygen gradient at rest or with exercise

Chest X-ray: Progression of interstitial infiltrates and volume loss; honeycombing; pulmonary hypertension; enlarging heart

COMPLICATIONS OF INTERSTITIAL LUNG DISEASE OR THERAPY

Cardiovascular disease: Right ventricular hypertrophy and cor pulmonale due to progressive pulmonary hypertension; left ventricular failure is also frequent and is generally due to concurrent ischaemic heart disease

Pulmonary infections: Increased incidence in many of the interstitial lung disorders; risk may be heightened by corticosteroid and cytotoxic therapy

Acute pulmonary embolism: Occasional cause of clinical deterioration in interstitial lung disease; sudden worsening of dyspnoea, with unexplained deterioration in arterial blood gases, and without evidence of superimposed infection should prompt the clinician to consider lung ventilation–perfusion scan or pulmonary angiography

Malignancy (particularly adenocarcinoma): can develop in idiopathic pulmonary fibrosis and perhaps in some other types of interstitial lung disease with increased frequency

Pneumothorax: Characteristic of eosinophilic granuloma, but also occurs in other interstitial lung diseases

Complications of therapy

Prolonged high-dose corticosteroids: Myopathy; peptic ulcer; cataracts; osteoporosis; fluid/ electrolyte abnormalities; increased susceptibility to infection

Cytotoxic agents: Increased susceptibility to infection; bone marrow supression; hepatitis; haemorrhagic cystitis

REFERENCES

Aberle D, Gamsu G, Ray C et al 1988a Asbestos-related pleural and parenchymal fibrosis: Detection with high-resolution CT. Radiology 166: 729–734
Aberle D R, Gamsu G, Ray C S 1988b High-resolution CT of benign asbestos-related diseases: Clinical and radiographic correlation. American Journal of Roentgenology 151: 883–891
Austrian R, McClement J H, Renzetti A D J et al 1951 Clinical and physiologic features of some types of pulmonary disease with impairment of alveolar–capillary diffusion. American Journal of Medicine 11: 667–685
Cherniack R M 1988 Physiologic disturbances in interstitial lung disease. In: Schwarz M I, King T E Jr (eds) Interstitial lung disease. Decker, Philadelphia, pp 37–44
Cherniack R M, Banks D E, Bell D Y et al and the BAL Cooperative Group Steering Committee 1990 Bronchoalveolar lavage constituents in healthy individuals, idiopathic pulmonary fibrosis, and selected comparison groups. American Review of Respiratory Disease 141: S169–S202
Crystal R G, Bitterman P B, Rennard S I et al 1984 Interstitial lung diseases of unknown cause: Disorders characterized by chronic inflammation of the lower respiratory tract. New England Journal of Medicine 310: 154–166
Dickey B F, Myers A R 1984 Pulmonary disease in polymyositis/dermatomyositis. Seminars in Arthritis and Rheumatism 14: 60–76
Epler G R, McLoud T C, Gaensler E A et al 1978 Normal chest roentgenograms in chronic diffuse infiltrative lung disease. New England Journal of Medicine 298: 934–939
Fairfax A J, Haslam P L, Paria D et al 1981 Pulmonary disorders associated with Sjogren's syndrome. Quarterly Journal of Medicine 50: 279–295

Felson B 1979 A new look at pattern recognition of diffuse pulmonary disease. American Journal of Roentgenology 133: 183–189

Fink J N 1982 Evaluation of the patient for occupational immunologic lung disease. Journal of Allergy and Clinical Immunology 70: 11–14

Fortoul T 1988 Comparison of transbronchial and open lung biopsies in interstitial lung diseases. Archivos de Investigacion Medica 19: 7–11

Friedman A C, Fiel S B, Fisher M S et al 1988 Asbestos-related pleural disease and asbestosis: A comparison of CT and chest radiography. American Journal of Roentgenology 150: 269–275

Fulmer J D, Roberts W C, von Gal E R et al 1979 Morphologic–physiologic correlates of the severity of fibrosis and degree of cellularity in idiopathic pulmonary fibrosis. Journal of Clinical Investigation 63: 665–676

Gaensler E A, Carrington C B 1980 Open biopsy for chronic diffuse infiltrative lung disease: Clinical, roentgenographic, and physiological correlations in 502 patients. Annals of Thoracic Surgery 30: 411–426

Haslam P L, Turton C W G, Heard B et al 1980 Bronchoalveolar lavage in pulmonary fibrosis: Comparison of cells obtained with lung biopsy and clinical features. Thorax 35: 9–18

Hunninghake G W, Fauci A S 1979 Pulmonary involvement in the collagen vascular diseases. American Review of Respiratory Disease 119: 471

Hunninghake G W, Gadek J E, Kawanami O et al 1979 Inflammatory and immune processes in the human lung in health and disease: Evaluation by bronchoalveolar lavage. American Journal of Pathology 97: 149–206

Hunninghake G W, Kawanami O, Ferrans V J et al 1981 Characterization of the inflammatory and immune effector cells in the lung parenchyma of patients with interstitial lung disease. American Review of Respiratory Disease 123: 407–412

Kelley M A, Daniele R P 1984 Exercise testing in interstitial lung disease. Clinics in Chest Medicine 5: 145–156

King T E Jr, Dunn T L 1988 Connective tissue disease. In: Schwarz M I, King T E Jr (eds) Interstitial lung diseases. Decker, Toronto, pp 171–210

Line B R, Fulmer J D, Reynolds H Y et al 1978 Gallium-67 citrate scanning in the staging of idiopathic pulmonary fibrosis correlation with physiologic and morphologic features and bronchoalveolar lavage. American Review of Respiratory Disease 118: 355–365

Mossman B T, Gee J B L 1989 Asbestos-related diseases. New England Journal of Medicine 320: 1721–1730

Mueller N L, Miller R R, Webb W R et al 1986 Fibrosing alveolitis CT: Pathologic correlation. Radiology 160: 585–588

Mueller N, Staples C, Miller R et al 1987 Disease activity in idiopathic pulmonary fibrosis: CT and pathologic correlation. Radiology 165: 731–734

Mueller N, Kullnig P, Miller R 1989 The CT findings of pulmonary sarcoidosis: Analysis of 25 patients. American Journal of Roentgenology 152: 1179–1182

Panos R J, Mortenson R, Niccoli S A et al 1990 Clinical deterioration in patients with idiopathic pulmonary fibrosis: Causes and assessment. American Journal of Medicine 88: 396–404

Parkes W R 1982 Pneumoconiosis due to coal and carbon. In: Parkes W R (ed) Occupational lung disorders. Butterworths, Boston, p 175

Ray J F III, Lawton B R, Myers W O et al 1976 Open pulmonary biopsy: Nineteen-year experience with 416 consecutive operations. Chest 69: 43–47

Reynolds H Y 1982 Hypersensitivity pneumonitis. Clinics in Chest Medicine 3: 503–519

Reynolds H Y 1987 Bronchoalveolar lavage. American Review of Respiratory Disease 135: 250–263

Reynolds H Y, Fulmer J D, Kazmierowski J A et al 1977 Analysis of cellular and protein content of bronchoalveolar lavage fluid from patients with idiopathic pulmonary fibrosis and chronic hypersensitivity pneumonitis. Journal of Clinical Investigation 59: 165–175

Risk C, Epler G R, Gaensler E A 1984 Exercise alveolar–arterial oxygen pressure difference in interstitial lung disease. Chest 85: 69–74

Rodnan G P 1963 The natural history of progressive systemic sclerosis (diffuse scleroderma). Bulletin on the Rheumatic Disease 13: 301–304

Rosenow E C III (ed) 1980 Drug-induced lung diseases. Seminars in Respiratory Medicine 2: 45–96

Schwarz M I, King T E Jr (eds) 1988 Interstitial lung disease. Decker, Toronto

Schwarz M I, Matthay R A, Sahn S A et al 1976 Interstitial lung disease in polymyositis and dermatomyositis. Medicine 55: 89–104

Silicosis and Silicate Disease Committee 1988 Diseases associated with exposure to silica and nonfibrous silicate minerals. Archives of Pathology and Laboratory Medicine 112: 673–720

Snider D E 1978 The relationship between tuberculosis and silicosis. American Review of Respiratory Disease 118: 455–460

Staples C, Mueller N, Vedal S et al 1987 Usual interstitial pneumonia: Correlation of CT with clinical, functional, and radiographic findings. Radiology 162: 377–381

Strimlan V C, Rosenow E C III, Divertie M B et al 1976 Pulmonary manifestations of Sjogren's syndrome. Chest 70: 354–361

Swensen S J, Aughenbaugh G L, Brown L R 1989 High-resolution computed tomography of the lung. Mayo Clinic Proceedings 64: 1284–1294

Walker W C, Wright V 1968 Pulmonary lesions and rheumatoid arthritis. Medicine 48: 501–520

Weaver A L, Divertie M B, Titus J L 1968 Pulmonary scleroderma. Diseases of the Chest 54: 490–498

Young R H, Mark G J 1978 Pulmonary vascular changes in scleroderma. American Journal of Medicine 64: 998–1003

Ziskind M, Jones R N, Weill H 1976 Silicosis. American Journal of Respiratory Disease 113: 643–665

11

Sarcoidosis

D. N. Mitchell

The purpose of this chapter is to evaluate the fruits of recent research and the use of modern clinical techniques in the investigation of patients presenting with probable sarcoidosis and in the management of this disorder.

EPIDEMIOLOGY

Sarcoidosis may affect subjects of any nationality or ethnic group of either sex at any age. In Great Britain it is more frequent among the Irish, British and West Indian than among the Asian population. Thus, Mikhail et al (1980) found that of 401 consecutive patients with sarcoidosis referred from all departments of a district general hospital in London, 135 (33.7%) were British, 101 (25.2%) Irish, 112 (27.9%) West Indian and 16 (4%) were Asian. In view of earlier reports emphasizing the rarity of the disease among the Chinese it is relevant that in a study of the prevalence of sarcoidosis amongst the patients attending the National Tuberculosis Centre, Kuala Lumpur, Ampikaipakan et al (1983) reported the finding of intrathoracic and/or extrathoracic sarcoidosis in 17 patients (6 Malays, 9 Chinese and 2 Indians).

A comparative study of four contrasted areas of Great Britain was undertaken by the British Thoracic and Tuberculosis Association (1969) during the 5-year period 1961–1966. The annual incidence increased from north to south, from 2.1 per 100 000 in the most northerly area to 4.1 in the most southerly; the female/male ratio of annual incidence was 1.1 in the south and increased to 1.72 in the north. The peak incidence in all areas and both sexes was in the age group 25–34 years. Because of the protean nature of many of the manifestations of sarcoidosis — the few studies of incidence to which uniform standards have been applied — and because of the rapid changes in population trends in recent years, we can have no true appreciation of the incidence of sarcoidosis in Great Britain at the present time. In this context it is relevant that in the city of Malmo in Sweden (population 230 000) where autopsies were conducted during the years 1957–1962 on 6707 individuals comprising approximately 60% of all deaths, evidence for sarcoidosis founded on critical criteria was found in 43 individuals, only 3 of whom were known to have sarcoidosis during life, giving a prevalence of 641 per 100 000, some ten times higher than that detected by mass screening (Hägerstrand & Linell 1963). Similarly, Parkes et al (1985), in a 7-year study in the Isle of Man in which a special effort was made to identify all cases, found a mean incidence of 14.7 per 100 000 per annum in the years 1977–1983 compared with an annual incidence of 3.5 per 100 000 in the preceding 15 years, when no specific attempts were made to identify cases of sarcoidosis. Although the peak incidence is in the age group 20–45 years, there are many reports of sarcoidosis among children and adolescents (Mandi 1964, Siltzbach & Greenberg 1968, Hosoda 1974, Kendig & Brummer 1976, Hetherington 1982). From these and other reports it seems probable that even considering the absence of routine radiography the relative frequency of sarcoidosis in children has not been underestimated. The majority of cases reported in children are symptomatic; moreover, although rare, sarcoidosis in the very young tends to present in bizarre forms which may carry a worse prognosis. In late childhood the frequency of sarcoidosis increases and it assumes clinical features and a prognosis which is at least as good and possibly more favourable than that for adults. There have been many reports of sarcoidosis presenting among patients over the age of 60 years (Cowdell 1954, Maycock et al 1963). Beyond awareness of the possibility of this diagnosis in the elderly, there are no special features.

CLINICAL PRESENTATIONS

There are many detailed accounts of the clinical presentation and natural history of sarcoidosis (Fanburg 1983, Scadding & Mitchell 1985, James & Jones-Williams 1985, Lieberman 1986). This chapter will highlight points of interest arising from clinical practice and, where relevant, will discuss their investigation and management.

'Lone' erythema nodosum

In the absence of any other clinical or radiographic evidence of sarcoidosis and in the knowledge that the lesions are likely to resolve spontaneously, there is usually no indication to proceed to more detailed investigations or biopsy procedures. Bradstreet et al (1980) found that of 278 such patients presenting in London, 56 (21%) gave granulomatous 'positive' and 13 (5%) partly granulomatous 'equivocal' Kveim test responses. On the not unreasonable assumption that these findings reflect the presence of a generalized granulomatosis (and since a negative Kveim test response mitigates little, if at all, against a diagnosis of sarcoidosis) it seems probable that in some 50% of these patients the presence of 'lone' erythema nodosum (EN) may be a manifestation of sarcoidosis. A further difficulty arises because these patients are usually followed up for a period of 3–6 months only; thus, although it is known that a few subsequently develop other clinical features of sarcoidosis, there is no real measure of the rate or extent of any subsequent clinical progression.

The 'normal' chest radiograph

The number of patients who present with a normal chest radiograph is of course related to the nature of the principal sources of their referral and is of the order of 5–10% (Dunbar 1978). Computed tomography (CT) may in some cases show quite marked mediastinal nodal involvement and/or unexpected parenchymal disease even in the presence of a virtually normal chest radiograph (Fig. 11.1). Moreover, CT changes may match pulmonary function abnormalities more closely than the chest radiograph (Putman et al 1977). Accordingly, if a patient with extrathoracic manifestations of sarcoidosis but with a normal or near normal PA chest radiograph shows significant impairment of standard lung function tests, it may well be profitable to proceed to CT, which may assist in a more critical assessment of subsequent progress.

Hilar lymphadenopathy

In the majority of patients (> 90%) hilar node enlargement is bilateral, but apparently unilateral and usually right-sided hilar adenopathy and/or unilateral paratracheal adenopathy is present in some 4% of patients (Kirks & Greenspan 1973, Kent 1965, Mikhail et al 1980). It is important that this possibility be appreciated because of the increasing recognition of the prevalence of sarcoidosis among the Asian population of Great Britain, in whom it is especially important to exclude the possibility that mediastinal lymphadenopathy may be attributable to tuberculosis. Bilateral hilar enlargement is characterized by a relatively translucent space between the nodes and the cardiovascular margin (Frazer & Paré 1978) but CT has shown that the subcarinal, posterior mediastinal and aorticopulmonary nodes may also be enlarged. Evidence to support the possibility that mediastinal lymphadenopathy is due to sarcoidosis may be ascertained from the presence of other affected organs or tissues which may provide a convenient source of biopsy material. Transbronchial biopsy of the radiologically normal lung will yield the presence of epithelioid and giant cell granulomas in some 60% of such patients (Mitchell et al 1981).

Alternatively, and provided the diagnosis of sarcoidosis remains highly probable on clinical grounds so as to justify the delay of 4–6 weeks incurred between its insertion and biopsy of the resultant test site, a Kveim test will provide histological support for the diagnosis in a substantial proportion (50–60%) of such cases, although rates of Kveim reactivity fall off with increasing duration of disease (Munro & Mitchell 1987). If, however, there is suspicion on clinical or radiological grounds that mediastinal lymphadenopathy may be attributable to a more sinister cause, such as

A

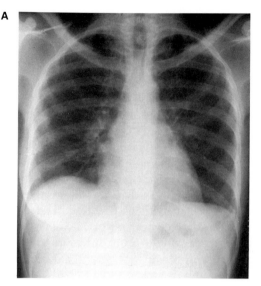

B

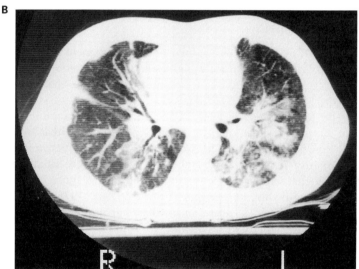

Fig. 11.1 **A** Chest radiograph of patient with severe extrathoracic sarcoidosis showing minimal abnormalities. **B** CT scan of the same patient and at the same date, showing much greater extent of intrathoracic involvement.

tuberculosis or lymphoma, recourse should be made to mediastinal lymph node biopsy via mediastinoscopy or mediastinotomy. In the latter context it is relevant that Brinker & Wilbek (1974) reported a high incidence of malignant lymphoma in their survey of 2544 patients with sarcoidosis which, even after a review by Rømer (1980) had removed dubious diagnoses, was six times that expected for the general population; the actual number of cases of lymphoma, however, was only three. Accordingly, if there is clinical doubt sufficient to warrant mediastinal lymph node biopsy it is important to obtain biopsies from sites which are fully representative of the mediastinal lymph node enlargement so as to exclude the possibility of lymphoma or of a lymphoma coexisting with sarcoidosis (Brinker 1972). It is important that biopsy tissue is sent not only for histology and culture for acid-fast bacilli but is also preserved at −70°C in case immunocytochemistry is required.

It is also important to bear in mind that sarcoid granulomas may be found in association with Hodgkin's disease and other lymphomas, both in lymph nodes and other tissues affected by lymphoma, and also in unaffected tissues. Thus, Kadin et al (1970) performed multiple biopsies at staging laparotomy in 185 patients with Hodgkin's disease, and found granulomatous reactions in 31 of them; of these, 8 were in tissues overtly affected by Hodgkin's disease and 23 in tissues not so affected. Moreover, the histology of local sarcoid reactions may be indistinguishable from that of generalized sarcoidosis, and may be so extensive within one or more affected lymph nodes as to be confused with it. All these problems are compounded by the fact that there is a small but significant group of patients in whom sarcoidosis is clinically manifest only by the presence of mediastinal and/or paratracheal lymph nodes, which persist often with little or no change in size over many years. In such cases the nodal enlargement may indent major bronchi as seen on tomography but does not give rise to superior vena caval obstruction.

UPPER RESPIRATORY TRACT

Although upper respiratory involvement by sarcoidosis is often associated with long-standing pulmonary and other chronic extrathoracic sarcoid lesions, it may be asymptomatic, so that it is only detected by routine examination (Di Benedetto & Lefrak 1970, Neville et al 1976). Nasal stuffiness or blockage and crusting are common and when a discharge is present it is often purulent or bloodstained. Changes in the nasal mucosa are most frequently seen over the septum and inferior turbinates. Pale yellow excrescences are seen projecting from the mucosa, are firm on touch and occasionally form plaques. The mucosa is often hypertrophied, causing airway obstruction, and surface erosion with crust formation are commonly seen. Septal perforation may be present. There may be collapse of the bridge of the nose from destruction of septal cartilage, and involvement of the nasal bones may be demonstrable radiographically. Indirect laryngoscopy may reveal granularity of the inferior surface of the epiglottis, and asymptomatic inflammation and oedema of the vocal cords. In more severe cases grossly inflamed and granular arytenoid folds may give rise to stridor or the whole larynx may be inflamed and scarred, with distortion of the normal architecture (Wilson et al 1988). These authors found that the use of an alkaline nasal douche was helpful in relieving crusting of the nose prior to the application of corticosteroid drops. However, the majority of their patients required treatment with oral corticosteroids to control either nasal symptoms or some other aspect of their disease. In 3 of their 27 patients with nasal involvement, the brain was also involved by sarcoidosis (Table 11.1 and Fig. 11.2).

CARDIAC SARCOIDOSIS

In 1962 Forbes & Usher reported a single case of cardiac sarcoidosis and this was followed by six further cases (Ghosh et al 1972). Subsequently, Fleming (1980, 1986, 1988) collected the records of patients throughout the UK in whom the diagnosis was reached during life or at autopsy. This collection of cases has provided further information regarding the epidemiology, natural history and effects of treatment of this condition. It appears probable that cardiac sarcoidosis is underdiagnosed even at autopsy in cases of sudden death. Fleming (1988) reported a series of 138 fatal cases in 300 patients with sarcoid heart disease, nearly all of whom were white. At presentation 73% had ventricular or supraventricular arrhythmias, 26% had complete heart block and 24% had 'cardiomyopathy'. A further 61% had right or left bundle branch block or partial heart block. Only 5% had a presentation that simulated myocardial infarction. Sudden death occurred

Table 11.1 Other organs affected and clinical symptoms present in 27 patients with nasal sarcoidosis

	No. of patients	Percentage
Organ		
Lung	18	67
Skin	15	56
Lupus pernio	7	26
Peripheral lymph nodes	8	30
Lacrimal glands	4	15
Bone	5	19
Eyes	6	22
Conjunctiva	3	11
Uveitis	3	11
Brain	3	11
Joints	3	11
Spleen	1	4
Symptom		
Stuffiness or blockage	24	89
Crusting	17	63
Bloodstained discharge	10	37
Purulent discharge	8	30
Facial pain	6	22
Mucoid discharge	4	15
Stridor	3	11
Anosmia	1	4

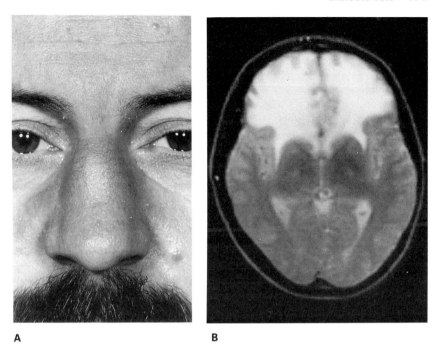

A   B

Fig. 11.2 **A** Front facial view of patient presenting with nasal sarcoidosis. **B** Extension of sarcoid infiltration to involve most of the frontal lobe of the brain via cribriform plate.

in 77 cases, and in 49 of these cardiac sarcoidosis had not been previously diagnosed.

Oakley (1989) reviewed these findings and compared them with a series of black American patients with cardiac sarcoidosis (Wait & Movahed 1989). The latter authors suggest that anginal chest pain is common in black male patients with sarcoidosis and that it may indicate sarcoid infiltration of the myocardium, whereas anginal pain is not mentioned in the series reported by Fleming (1988), even though the average age at presentation was 50 years and more than half the patients were male. It has become clear that the heart may be extensively involved, with inconspicuous evidence of sarcoidosis in other organs, and that sudden death is the most common manifestation of cardiac sarcoidosis although there may be antecedent arrhythmias or atrioventricular block. Subclinical cardiac involvement is probably common; thus Silverman et al (1978) in a clinicopathological study found cardiac granulomas in 27% of 84 unselected patients with generalized sarcoidosis; Fleming (1988) suggests that suspected cases should be investigated by 24-hour ECG tape monitoring, echocardiography, exercise testing and radionuclide imaging. Endo-myocardial biopsy will occasionally yield sarcoid granulomas, but because of the patchy distribution of the disease in the myocardium a negative result is of no importance. Oakley (1989) considers that sarcoid infiltration is one of the few causes of focal left ventricular abnormality in the absence of disease of the major coronary arteries. The distribution is typically in the proximal part of the left ventricle and upper septum, where it produces akinesia of the affected region; with healing the previously akinetic wall becomes thin or aneurysmal. Reidy et al (1988) discussed the role of magnetic resonance imaging in the investigation of myocardial sarcoidosis. They report a patient in whom the magnetic resonance image identified discrete myocardial abnormalities that changed the initial diagnosis from asymmetric septal hypertrophy to a multifocal myocardial disease and directed the biopsy that established the definitive diagnosis. Their magnetic resonance study characterized the patchy distribution of the cardiac granulomas and their predilection for involvement of the left ventricle and basal portion of the septum.

The treatment of arrhythmias, conduction defects and heart failure due to sarcoidosis do not differ from established cardiological practice. The effects of corticosteroid treatment on the lesions of cardiac sarcoidosis are probably similar to those on sarcoidosis involving other organs or tissues, with suppression of active granulomas but with little effect on established fibrosis. Published reports suggest that reduction in numbers of premature beats and episodes of tachycardia with easier control of arrhythmias follows corticosteroid treatment in many cases, and improvement in conduction defects may occur, although less frequently (Stein et al 1976, Lash et al 1979, Yamamato et al 1980). The danger of sudden death may also be diminished, yet it remains.

MAGNETIC RESONANCE IN CENTRAL NERVOUS SYSTEM SARCOIDOSIS

In reported series the proportion of patients with sarcoidosis found to have nervous system involvement has been approximately 5% (Siltzbach et al 1974, Delaney, 1977). In order to obtain some idea of the relative frequency of the various clinical features of intracranial sarcoidosis Scadding & Mitchell (1985) reviewed the literature over a 20-year period, which yielded information on 102 cases. Two-thirds of these cases presented with neurological or neuro-endocrinological problems without current or past clinical evidence of sarcoidosis, the histological diagnosis being made from tissue removed at craniotomy or, in a minority of cases, at necropsy. Two major pathological changes account for the central nervous system features: firstly, the presence of sarcoid tissue in the meninges and brain parenchyma, and, secondly, areas of infarction as a result of occlusion of small blood vessels by granulomas (Matthews 1986, Herring & Urich 1969). For example, Zollinger (1941) reported a case who presented with a syndrome resembling atypical multiple sclerosis. At necropsy one year later multiple sarcoid granulomas were found in the leptomeninges and scattered through the brain, as well as in the hilar and paratracheal lymph nodes. Association of central nervous system sarcoidosis with peripheral neuropathy may further complicate the clinical presentation. Miller et al (1988) reported the results of magnetic resonance scans on 21 patients with central nervous system sarcoidosis. Parenchymal lesions were seen in 17 of 21 with magnetic resonance, compared to 9 of 18 with CT. The most frequent magnetic resonance findings were periventricular abnormalities, which were seen in 14 of 21 patients. These authors point out that such abnormalities are non-specific and that their differential diagnosis includes multiple sclerosis (Young et al 1981), inflammatory and non-inflammatory cerebral vascular disease (Miller et al 1988), cranial irradiation (Bradley et al 1984), head injury (Zimmerman et al 1986) and periventricular oedema secondary to hydrocephalus (Bydder et al 1982). Six patients had multiple white matter lesions indistinguishable from those of multiple sclerosis. Measurements of T_1 and T_2 in the regions of abnormal signal were similar in both conditions.

Clinically, the two conditions may be confused, especially when the presentation of sarcoidosis is with an optic neuropathy or spinal cord or brain stem disturbance. Moreover, oligoclonal bands may be present in central nervous system sarcoid, and the visually evoked responses may be prolonged. Miller et al (1988) concluded that magnetic resonance and CT have complementary roles in the investigation of neurosarcoidosis. Magnetic resonance was found to be the best means of detecting parenchymal lesions and lesions in the posterior fossa, whereas contrast-enhanced CT proved useful in detecting diffuse meningeal involvement. Magnetic resonance can prove useful in following response to treatment (Fig. 11.3), with the further advantage over CT of no cumulative radiation dosage. Smith et al (1989) have stated that neurosarcoidosis should be considered in the differential diagnosis of isolated periventricular lesions in patients less than 50 years of age. They reported five sarcoidosis patients with central nervous system symptoms in whom isolated periventricular with occasional subcortical lesions were the only findings noted on magnetic resonance, again indicating the difficulties of distinguishing between neurosarcoidosis and multiple sclerosis in some cases.

CLINICAL VALUE OF MEASUREMENTS OF DISEASE 'ACTIVITY'

Bronchoalveolar lavage

Lavage cell counts in active pulmonary sarcoidosis are characterized by an increase in the proportion of lymphocytes, many of which are activated T-cells. The total number of cells obtained at lavage is increased so that although the proportion of macrophages is less than that in normal subjects their absolute numbers are increased. It is probable that the proportion of T-lymphocytes in the lavage is an index of their contribution to new granuloma formation, more than 28% indicating a high level of activity

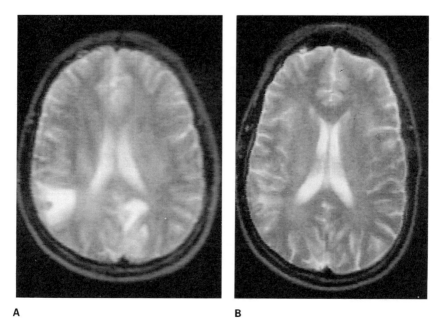

A   B

Fig. 11.3 A Magnetic resonance scan of a patient presenting with convulsions and found to have brain infiltration due to sarcoidosis. **B** Magnetic resonance scan of brain of the same patient showing regression of brain infiltration following 3 months' treatment with i.v. methylprednisolone and oral prednisolone.

(Keogh et al 1983, Crystal et al 1983). A similar increase in lavage lymphocytes is observed in patients with extrinsic allergic alveolitis, whereas in patients with cryptogenic fibrosing alveolitis the neutrophil count may be increased. However, in non-smoking patients with pulmonary sarcoidosis there may be an increase in the percentage of neutrophils in the lavage if the pulmonary infiltrates are of long standing. Thus, although the percentage of lymphocytes in the lavage of patients presenting with sarcoidosis provides an index as to disease activity, lavage is not helpful in the differential diagnosis of patients presenting with pulmonary infiltration of long standing.

Serum angiotensin I-converting enzyme (ACE)

Serum ACE levels are significantly elevated (2 SD > mean of values in a control group) in about half of patients presenting with untreated sarcoidosis. Levels tend to be higher in black than in white patients and in children than in adults. Elevated levels are also found in about 5% of patients with miscellaneous pulmonary diseases. Turton et al (1979) found that ACE levels fell rapidly toward normal following treatment with corticosteroids, but noted similar falls from initially normal levels among patients given corticosteroids for other diseases. Elevated and rising levels in patients with sarcoidosis usually indicate increasing disease activity, but the value of ACE levels in deciding about the need for treatment and in assessing the response to it is limited.

Gallium citrate scanning

[67Ga]Gallium citrate is taken up at sites of active sarcoidosis and also by inflammatory and malignant diseases, including tuberculosis and lymphomas. Heshiki et al (1974) found that radiographically normal lungs showed no abnormal uptake and that uptake in lungs and hila correlated poorly with clinical activity, although uptake diminished after corticosteroid treatment. Israel et al (1976) confirmed the avidity of mediastinal and pulmonary sarcoidosis for gallium, but found that gallium scanning did not reveal clinically evident extrapulmonary sarcoidosis in several cases. The pattern of gallium uptake may change rapidly, with different regions of the lung being involved with varying intensity patterns. Hunninghake & Crystal (1981) performed lavage in sarcoidosis patients who had just had gallium scans. Ninety-five per cent of the radioactivity was associated with macrophages and 5% with lymphocytes. In vitro, gallium was taken up by macrophages from sarcoidosis patients but not by those from normal subjects. Beaumont et al (1982) performed gallium scans in 54 patients with intrathoracic sarcoidosis, repeated in 23. These scans distinguished fibrotic from active lung changes and also demonstrated some previously undetected localizations in mediastinum, spleen and salivary glands.

With these reservations, serum ACE measurements, bronchoalveolar lavage and gallium scanning can assist in the diagnosis of sarcoidosis and in determining its extent and activity. In the majority of patients, however, the combination of the clinical, radiological and laboratory findings including ACE measurement are sufficient to reach a definite or highly probable diagnosis of sarcoidosis. Histological support for the diagnosis can usually be obtained from biopsy of an accessible tissue, by bronchial and/or transbronchial biopsy or by Kveim test. In all doubtful cases and in cases where treatment is likely to be needed, support for the diagnosis from biopsy or by Kveim testing is, wherever possible, essential. Finally, it should be noted that serial lavage lymphocyte counts, serum ACE measurements and gallium scans are not more sensitive methods for monitoring patients during treatment than are serial radiographs and the results of lung function tests (Turner-Warwick et al 1986).

TREATMENT

The management of sarcoidosis, including the assessment of disease activity, indications for treatment, results of controlled studies of corticosteroid therapy, policies of long-term management and the use of antimalarial, immunosuppressive and cytotoxic drugs, have been discussed previously (Scadding & Mitchell 1985). More recent developments in therapy will be discussed here.

Intravenous 'pulse' methylprednisolone

Prolonged treatment with high doses of oral prednisolone is usually required for the treatment of severe neurological sarcoidosis, with the consequent risk of serious side effects (Delaney 1977). Concomitant anticonvulsant therapy (inducers of hepatic microsomal enzymes) will reduce the plasma prednisolone concentration and hence the efficacy of steroids when given orally (McAllister et al 1982).

Prompted by unpublished reports of the successful use of i.v. 'pulse' methylprednisolone in pulmonary sarcoidosis from the National Institutes of Health, Bethesda, Maryland, USA, Allen & Merory (1985) successfully treated a 26-year-old man with severe widespread sarcoid polyneuropathy with associated pulmonary involvement using 'pulse' methylprednisolone. He had failed to respond clinically to high-dose oral prednisolone after 2 months' treatment. He received i.v. methylprednisolone 1 g once a week for 8 weeks, in addition to 10 mg of daily oral prednisolone. Neurological improvement began after the third 'pulse' dose, with complete remission after the eighth week. More than 12 months after cessation of treatment he remained in good health, with no clinical or laboratory evidence of sarcoidosis.

Warrens et al (1986) treated eight patients with difficult histologically confirmed sarcoidosis with a course of eight weekly 'pulses' of i.v. methylprednisolone 1 g per week. Simultaneously the oral dose of 20 mg prednisolone daily was reduced during the first week, to 20 mg on alternate days by the end of the eighth week. Seven of these eight patients showed considerable regression of their sarcoidosis after 8 weeks. In one, this represented an increase in visual acuity and improvement in peripheral neuropathy. A second patient lost radiological evidence of an intracerebral granuloma which had been associated with convulsions. Very few adverse effects were experienced and only one patient showed significant increase in weight.

More recently, Landh & Wikkelsö (1987) reported the case of a patient presenting with sarcoidosis with hydrocephalus who was successfully treated with a ventriculoperitoneal shunt and methylprednisolone 'pulse' therapy. We have also found i.v. pulsed methylprednisolone therapy successful in the treatment of two patients with sarcoidosis and hydrocephalus and in the treatment of several other patients with severe central nervous system sarcoidosis. The long-term follow-up of these patients remains to be assessed, and a prospective study to assess the role of i.v. 'pulsed' methylprednisolone in the treatment of sarcoidosis would appear to be justified.

Cyclosporin

There have been conflicting reports as to the value of cyclosporin in the treatment of sarcoidosis. Three patients with pulmonary disease were reported to have responded well to cyclosporin after steroid therapy had failed to secure a remission (Rebuck et al 1984), whilst a further six patients whose sarcoidosis had not responded to high-dose steroids and who had developed serious steroid side effects showed less encouraging results (Rebuck et al 1987). Against this background, we treated a patient with cyclosporin who had severe pulmonary and cutaneous sarcoidosis. Following treatment with oral prednisolone he had developed bilateral necrosis of the femoral heads, requiring hip replacements. His extensive pulmonary involvement and disease progression were such that he was likely to come to transplant unless his disease could be controlled. He was treated with cyclosporin (9 mg/kg daily) and after subsequent reduction of the dose to 225 mg twice daily his blood levels were maintained between 150 and 200 mg/l. After two months of treatment he was much improved, with almost complete clearing of his skin lesions and with some improvement of his extensive and predominantly fibrotic pulmonary sarcoidosis, as judged by CT scans (Fig. 11.4) and by improvements in his lung function tests and arterial blood gases.

Patients with progressive central nervous system sarcoidosis have been treated with cyclosporin with mixed results. Kavanaugh et al (1987) in a single case report suggested a beneficial effect, whilst Cunnah et al (1988) reported relentless progression of disease in a case of neurosarcoidosis using a similar dosage regimen.

It should be emphasized that the use of cyclosporin and the mixed responses reported both in pulmonary and in neurosarcoidosis have been largely restricted to patients who had already failed to respond to high doses of oral prednisolone. Our own findings support the suggestion of Cunnah et al (1988) that a formal trial is required in order to evaluate the results of treatment with cyclosporin in these poor prognostic groups.

Transplantation

Valentine et al (1987) reported the results of heart transplantation in three patients with cardiac sarcoidosis who had failed to respond to conventional steroid therapy. Their subsequent successful course suggested that heart transplantation could improve prognosis and quality of life.

We have performed lung transplantation on a 26-year-old man with end-stage pulmonary sarcoidosis (Fig. 11.5). Postoperatively he has done very well and has returned to full-time work, leading a normal life.

Waltzer et al (1984) have reported the successful results of kidney transplantation for sarcoidosis.

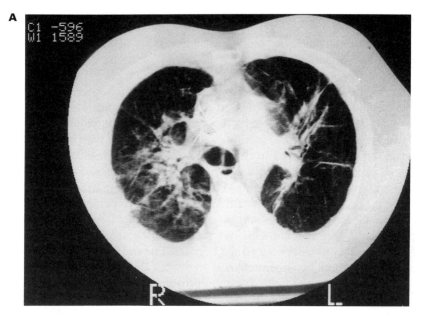

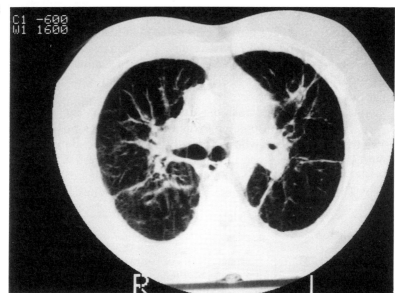

Fig. 11.4 A CT scan showing intrathoracic changes at inception of treatment with cyclosporin. **B** Comparable CT scan showing resolution of intrathoracic changes after 2 months' treatment with cyclosporin.

The lack of recurrence of sarcoidosis in the transplanted organs (heart, lung and kidney) cited above may be related to the use of steroids and potent immunosuppressive agents in the routine management of transplant recipients, yet close attention to the possibility of recurrence of sarcoidosis

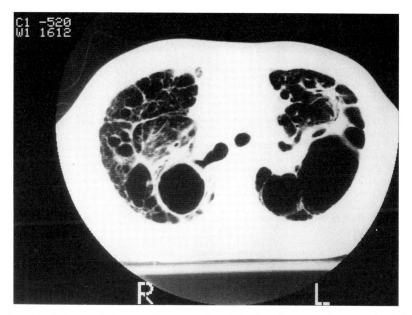

Fig. 11.5 CT scan of thorax: patient treated by single (left) lung transplantation despite previous left talc pleurodesis (pre-transplant).

in the transplanted organ must be borne in mind (see also chapters 14–17 on lung transplantation).

Radiotherapy

Although radiotherapy has been used for various manifestations of sarcoidosis (Florange 1910, Jackson 1925) there was no evidence that it had any beneficial effect (Donlan 1938). Recently, there had been reports of possible beneficial effects from radiotherapy used in the treatment of central nervous system sarcoidosis (Bejar et al 1985, Cunnah et al 1988, Martin et al 1989). It is possible that a trial of fractionated low-dose external beam radiotherapy to the whole brain or spinal cord may be justified where conventional measures have failed.

REFERENCES

Allen R K A, Merory J 1985 Intravenous pulse methyl prednisolone in the successful treatment of severe sarcoid polyneuropathy with pulmonary involvement. Australian and New Zealand Journal of Medicine 15: 45–46

Ampikaipakan K, Prathap G, Mitchell D N 1983 Sarcoidosis in Malaysia. In: Chrétien J, Marsac J, Saltiel J (eds) Proceedings of the 9th International Conference on Sarcoidosis, Paris. Pergamon Press, Oxford, p 626

Beaumont D, Herry J Y, Sapene M et al 1982 Gallium 67 in the evaluation of sarcoidosis: Correlation with serum angiotensin converting enzyme and bronchoalveolar lavage. Thorax 37: 11–18

Bejar J M, Kirby G R, Ziegler D K et al 1985 Treatment of central nervous system sarcoidosis with radiotherapy. Annals of Neurology 15: 258–260

Bradley W G, Waluch V, Yadley R A et al 1984 Comparison of CT and MRI in 460 patients with suspected disease of the brain and cervical spinal cord. Radiology 152: 695–702

Bradstreet C M P, Dighero M W, Mitchell D N 1980 The Kveim test: analysis of results of test using K19 materials. In: Jones-Williams W, Davies B H (eds) Proceedings of the 8th International Conference on Sarcoidosis, Cardiff. Alpha Omega Publishing Ltd, Cardiff, pp 674–677

Brinker H 1972 Sarcoid reactions and sarcoidosis in Hodgkin's disease and other malignant lymphomata. British Journal of Cancer 26: 120–128

Brinker II, Wilbek E 1974 The incidence of malignant tumours in patients with respiratory sarcoidosis. British Journal of Cancer 29: 247–251

British Thoracic and Tuberculosis Association 1969 Geographic variations in the incidence of sarcoidosis in Great Britain: A comparative study of four areas. Tubercle 50: 211–232

Bydder G M, Steiner R E, Young I R et al 1982 Clinical NMR imaging of the brain: 140 cases. American Journal of Radiology 139: 215–236

Cowdell R H 1954 Sarcoidosis with special reference to diagnosis and prognosis. Quarterly Journal of Medicine 23: 29–55

Crystal R G, Hunninghake G W, Gadek J E et al 1983 State of the art: The pathogenesis of sarcoidosis. In: Chrétien J, Marsac J, Saltiel J C (eds) Proceedings of the 9th International Conference on Sarcoidosis, Paris. Pergamon Press, Oxford, p 13

Cunnah D, Chew S, Wass J 1988 Cyclosporin for central nervous system sarcoidosis. American Journal of Medicine 85: 580–581

Delaney, P 1977 Neurologic manifestations of sarcoidosis: Review of the literature, with a report of 23 cases. Annals of Internal Medicine 87: 336–345

Di Benedetto R, Lefrak S 1970 Systemic sarcoidosis with severe involvement of the upper respiratory tract. American Review of Respiratory Disease 102: 801–807

Donlan C P 1938 X-ray therapy of Boeck's sarcoid. Radiology 51: 237–240

Dunbar R D 1978 Sarcoidosis and its radiologic manifestations. CRC Critical Review in Diagnostic Imaging, December: 185–221

Fanburg B L 1983 Sarcoidosis and other granulomatous diseases of the lung. Marcel Deckker Inc, New York, Basel

Forbes G, Usher A 1962 Fatal mycocardial sarcoidosis. British Medical Journal 2: 771–778

Fleming H A 1980 Sarcoid heart disease: A review and an appeal. Thorax 35: 641–643

Fleming H A 1986 Cardiac sarcoidosis. Seminars in Respiratory Medicine 8: 65–71

Fleming H A 1988 Death from sarcoid heart disease. United Kingdom series 1871 to 1986. 300 cases with 138 deaths. In: Grassi C, Rizzato G, Pozzi E (eds) Sarcoidosis and other granulomatous disorders. 11th world congress, Milan, 1987. Elsevier, Amsterdam, p 19

Florange A 1910 Uber einem Fall von Lupus Pernio und Seine Reaktion auf Rötgenbestrahlung. Dermatologica 17: 558–564

Frazer R G, Paré J A P 1978 Diagnosis of diseases of the chest. Saunders, Philadelphia, p 1665

Ghosh P, Fleming H A, Gresham G A et al 1972 Myocardial sarcoidosis. British Heart Journal 34: 769–773

Hägerstrand I, Linell F 1963 The prevalence of sarcoidosis in the autopsy material from a Swedish town. In: Löfgren S (ed) Proceedings of the IIIrd International Conference on Sarcoidosis. Acta Medica Scandinavica (suppl 425, 1964): p 171

Herring A B, Urich H 1969 Sarcoidosis of the central nervous system. Journal of Neurological Science 9: 405–422

Heshiki A, Schatz S L, McKusick K A et al 1974 Gallium 67 citrate scanning in patients with pulmonary sarcoidosis. American Journal of Roentgenology 122: 744–749

Hetherington S 1982 Sarcoidosis in young children. American Journal of Diseases of Children 136: 13–15

Hosoda Y 1974 Epidemiology of sarcoidosis in Japan. In: Iwai K, Hosoda Y (eds) Proceedings of the 6th International Conference on Sarcoidosis. University of Tokyo Press, Tokyo p 297

Hunninghake G W, Crystal R G 1981 Pulmonary sarcoidosis: A disorder mediated by excess helper T lymphocyte activity at sites of disease activity. New England Journal of Medicine 305: 429–434

Israel H L, Park C H, Mansfield C M 1976 Gallium scanning in sarcoidosis. Annals of the New York Academy of Sciences 278: 514–516

Jackson B H 1925 Use of X-ray in uveoparotitis. American Journal of Opthalmology 8: 361

James D G, Jones-Williams W 1985 Sarcoidosis. Major problems in internal medicine series. Saunders, London

Kadin M E, Donaldson S S, Dorfman R F 1970 Isolated granulomas in Hodgkin's disease. New England Journal of Medicine 283: 859–861

Kavanaugh A F, Andrew S L, Cooper B et al 1987 Cyclosporin therapy of central nervous system sarcoidosis. American Journal of Medicine 82: 387

Kendig E L, Brummer D L 1976 The prognosis of sarcoidosis in children. Chest 70: 351–353

Kent D C 1965 Recurrent unilateral hilar adenopathy in sarcoidosis. American Review of Respiratory Disease 91: 272–276

Keogh B A, Hunninghake G W, Line B R et al 1983 The alveolitis of pulmonary sarcoidosis: Evaluation of natural history and alveolitis dependent changes of lung function. American Review of Respiratory Disease 128: 256–265

Kirks D R, McCormick V D, Greenspan R H 1973 Pulmonary sarcoidosis: roentgenologic analysis of 150 patients. American Journal of Roentgenology 117: 777–786

Landh T, Wikkelsö C 1987 Sarcoidosis with hydrocephalus: Report of a case successfully treated with a ventriculo-peritoneal shunt and methylprednisolone pulse therapy. Acta Neurologica Scandinavica 76: 365–368

Lash R, Coker J, Wong B Y S 1979 Treatment of heart block due to sarcoid heart disease. Journal of Electrocardiology (San Diego) 12: 325–329

Lieberman J (ed) 1986 Sarcoidosis. Grune & Stratton (Harcourt Brace Jonanovich), Orlando

Mandi L 1964 Thoracic sarcoidosis in childhood. Acta Thuberculosis Scandinavica 45: 256–270

Martin N, Debroucker T, Mompoint D et al 1989 Sarcoidosis of the pineal region: CT and MR studies. Journal of Computer Assisted Tomography 13: 110–112

Matthews W B 1986 Neurologic manifestations of sarcoidosis. In: Asbury A K, McKhaun G M, McDonald W I (eds) Diseases of the nervous system: Clinical neurobiology (1st edn). Heinemann, London, pp 1563–1570

Maycock R L, Bertrand D, Morrison C E et al 1963 Manifestations of sarcoidosis: Analysis of 145 patients with a review of 9 series selected from literature. American Journal of Medicine 35: 67–89

McAllister W A C, Thompson P J, Al-Habet S et al 1982 Adverse effects of rifampicin on prednisolone disposition. Thorax 37: 792

Mikhail, J R, Mitchell D N, Sutherland I et al 1980 Sarcoidosis presenting in a district general hospital. In: Jones-Williams W, Davies B H (eds) Proceedings of the 8th International Conference on Sarcoidosis. Alpha Omega, Cardiff, p 532

Miller D H, Kendall B E, Barter G et al 1988 Magnetic resonance imaging in central nervous system sarcoidosis. Neurology 38: 378-383

Mitchell D M, Emerson C J, Collins J V et al 1981 Transbronchial lung biopsy (TBB) in 433 patients. In: Nakhosteen J A, Maassen W (eds) Bronchology. Martinus Nijhoff, The Hague p 333

Munro, C, Mitchell D N 1987 The Kveim test: Still useful, still a puzzle. Thorax 42: 321–331

Neville E, Mills R G S, Yash D G 1976 Sarcoidosis of the upper respiratory tract and its association with lupos pernio. Thorax 31: 660–664

Oakley C 1989 Cardiac sarcoidosis. Thorax 44: 371–372

Parkes S A, Baker S B de C, Bourdillon R E et al 1985 Incidence of sarcoidosis in the Isle of Man. Thorax 40: 284–287

Putman C E, Rothman S L, Littner M R et al 1977 Computerized tomography in pulmonary sarcoidosis. Computerized Tomography 1: 197–209

Rebuck A S, Stiller C R, Braude A C et al 1984 Cyclosporin for pulmonary sarcoidosis. Lancet i: 1174

Rebuck A S, Sanders B R, MacFadden D K et al 1987 Cyclosporin in pulmonary sarcoidosis. Lancet i: 1486

Reidy K, Fisher R, Belic N et al 1988 MR imaging in sarcoidosis. American Journal of Roentgenology 151: 915–917

Rømer F K 1980 Sarcoidosis and cancer — a critical view. In: Jones-Williams W, Davies B H (eds) Proceedings of the 8th International Conference on Sarcoidosis, Cardiff. Alpha Omega Publishing Ltd, Cardiff, pp 567–571

Scadding J G, Mitchell D N 1985 Sarcoidosis (2nd edn). Chapman & Hall, London

Siltzbach L E, Greenberg G M 1968 Childhood sarcoidosis: A study of 18 patients. New England Journal of Medicine 279: 1239–1245

Siltzbach L E, James D G, Neville E et al 1974 Course and prognosis of sarcoidosis around the world. Journal of the American Medical Association 147: 927–929

Silverman K J, Hutchins G M, Bulkley B H 1978 Cardiac sarcoid: A clinicopathological study of 84 unselected patients with systemic sarcoidosis. Circulation 58: 1204–1211

Smith A S, Meisler D M, Weinstein M A et al 1989 High signal periventricular lesions in patients with sarcoidosis: Neurosarcoidosis or multiple sclerosis? American Journal of Roentgenology 153: 147–181

Stein E, Stimmel B, Siltzbach L E 1976 Clinical course of cardiac sarcoidosis. Annals of the New York Academy of Sciences 278: 470–474

Turner-Warwick M, McAllister, W, Lawrence R et al 1986 Corticosteroid treatment in pulmonary sarcoidosis: Do serial lavage lymphocyte counts, serum angiotensin converting enzyme measurements, and gallium-67 scans help management? Thorax 41: 903–913

Turton C M G, Grundy E, Firth G et al 1979 Value of measuring serum angiotensin-I converting enzyme and serum lysozyme in the management of sarcoidosis. Thorax 34: 57–62

Valentine H A, Tagelaar H D, Macoviak J et al 1987 Cardiac sarcoidosis: Response to steroids and transplantation. Journal of Heart Transplantation 6: 245–250

Wait J L, Movahed A 1989 Anginal chest pain in sarcoidosis. Thorax 44: 391–395

Waltzer W, Anaise D, Friseher Z et al 1984 Renal transplantation and Boeck's sarcoidosis. Transplant Proceedings 14: 1359–1361

Warrens A N, Barnes P J, Cole P J et al 1986 'Pulsed' intravenous methylprednisolone therapy for refractory sarcoidosis. Thorax 41: 714–715

Wilson R, Lund V, Sweatman M et al 1988 Upper respiratory tract involvement in sarcoidosis and its management. European Respiration Journal 1: 269–272

Yamamato M, Muramatsu M, Suzuki T 1980 Successful corticosteroid treatment of 7 cases of probable myocardial sarcoidosis. In: Jones-Williams W (ed) Proceedings of the 8th International Conference on Sarcoidosis. Alpha Omega, Cardiff, p 615

Young R, Hall A S, Pallis C A et al 1981 Nuclear magnetic resonance imaging of the brain in multiple sclerosis. Lancet ii: 1063–1066

Zollinger H V 1941 Groszellig-granulomatöse lymphangitis cerebri (Morbus Boeck) unter dem Bilde einer multiplen sklerose verlaufeud. Virchows Archiv 307: 597–605

Zimmerman R D, Fleming C A, Lee B C P 1986 Periventricular hyperintensity as seen by magnetic resonance: Prevalence and significance. American Journal of Neuroradiology 7: 13–20

12

Cystic fibrosis

D. M. Geddes   A. Graham

BASIC RESEARCH

Advances in molecular biology have led to a most exciting and productive period in the history of cystic fibrosis (CF) research. The single most important discovery has without doubt been the identification and characterization of the CF gene, due to the combined efforts of many teams throughout the world. Most notable, however, has been the collaboration between the laboratories of L-C Tsui and JR Riordan, both at Toronto, and FS Collins at Michigan.

THE CYSTIC FIBROSIS GENE (Rommens et al 1989, Riorden et al 1989, Kerem et al 1989)

Before 1989 linkage analysis had assigned the cystic fibrosis locus to the long arm of chromosome 7, band q31 (Tsui et al 1985, Knowlton et al 1985, White et al 1985, Wainwright et al 1985). The finding of the closely linked flanking markers MET and D788 then allowed more precise localization to a region of $1–2 \times 10^6$ base pairs of DNA and this in turn made it possible to use various novel gene-cloning strategies to pinpoint the cystic fibrosis gene (Rommens et al 1989). The key approach used was a combination of chromosome walking and jumping. Walking consists of comparing known DNA with libraries derived from different tissues so that by matching segments along the gene a complete picture can be built up. Jumping involves circularizing a segment of DNA so that two distant parts can be brought together. Chromosome jumping (Collins et al 1987) proved to be powerful as it allows the production of a number of additional starting points for chromosome walks and also circumvents blocks caused by unclonable sequences.

About $2–3 \times 10^5$ base pairs were cloned before the end of the gene was found (Knowlton et al 1985). Thereafter sequences were accumulated and a picture of the gene was built up. Several transcribed and conserved sequences were identified, one of which, spanning about 250 000 base pairs, corresponded to the cystic fibrosis gene (Fig. 12.1).

Finally, 18 additional clones were isolated and although none corresponded

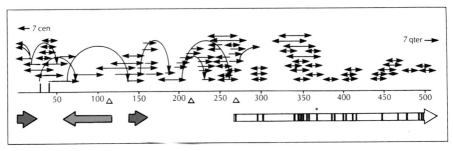

Fig. 12.1 The long march to the cystic fibrosis gene. The trek began at a site, shown here at the left of the diagram, that Tsui's group had identified as close to the cystic fibrosis gene on human chromosome 7. The 280 kb of DNA between the start site and the beginning of the gene was covered by a combination of chromosome 'walking' and 'jumping'. The straight arrows above the line represent the DNA segments cloned during the walk, and the curved arrows represent the jumps taken. The long arrow at the lower right depicts the cystic fibrosis gene, which spans about 250 kb. The dark bars are the 24 exons that specify the amino acid sequence of the protein encoded by the gene. These are separated by the non-coding sequences known as introns. The exon marked with the asterisk contains the mutation found in 70% of defective cystic fibrosis genes. The middle arrow at the lower left denotes the *IRP* gene that was identified by Robert Williamson's group during their search for the cystic fibrosis gene. The other two right arrows also mark sequences with protein-coding capabilities, and the three triangles point to sequences of a type frequently found near gene start sites. (From Marx 1989, Science 245: 925; with permission.)

to the length of the observed transcript a consensus sequence was derived from the overlapping regions. Together these clones span about 6.1 kilobases (kb) and contain an open reading frame for a protein of 1480 amino acids. The nucleotide sequence allowed deduction of the amino acid sequence and prediction of the protein structure.

Tissue distribution

In order to find out where the gene is expressed Riordan et al (1989) looked for the relevant mRNA in a range of different cells. RNA gel-blot hybridization with the first isolated complementary DNA (cDNA) clone (10-1) was used to assess the presence of the RNA transcript of the gene. A prominent band of about 6.5 kb was seen in T84 colonic carcinoma cells and similar strong signals were detected in pancreas and cell cultures from nasal polyps. The hybridization band intensity allows an estimate of the amount of RNA and suggests that the cystic fibrosis gene transcripts made up about 0.01% of total mRNA in the T84 cells. Similar mRNA was seen in lung, colon, sweat glands, placenta, liver and parotid glands, although the signal was weaker. Transcripts were not detectable in brain or adrenal gland nor in skin fibroblast or lymphocyte cell lines.

This suggested that the cystic fibrosis gene was expressed in tissues affected by cystic fibrosis and not in those such as brain and adrenal, which are spared by the disease. Furthermore, the amount and size of the transcripts were the same for cystic fibrosis and control tissues consistent with cystic fibrosis mutations being subtle changes at the nucleotide level.

Detection of mutation

This required detailed comparison of nucleotide sequences in cDNA from cystic fibrosis and unaffected individuals. A striking difference of a three-based deletion was found which would result in the loss of a phenylalanine residue at position 508. This mutation was present on 68% of chromosomes from cystic fibrosis and was not found in any of 198 normal chromosomes ($P < 10^{-57.5}$).

Haplotype analysis was carried out to explore the cystic fibrosis mutations further (Kerem et al 1989). There was a close association between the 508 deletion and the commonest haplotype and the existence of at least seven other less common haplotypes, suggesting that there may be as many (or more) further mutations. Subsequent analysis of different populations of cystic fibrosis patients has shown the frequency of this major mutation to be 75.8% in North America, 74.4% in the UK (McIntosh et al 1989), and lower in southern Europe; Spain 49%, Italy 43% (Estivill et al 1989) and in Ashkenazy families 30.3% (Lemne et al 1990). At least 50 different mutations have now been identified (Anon 1990).

Predicted protein structure

The 1480 amino acid predicted from the DNA sequence has a molecular mass of 168 138 and contains a number of repeated motifs. There are 12 hydrophobic helices capable of spanning the cell membrane and two nucleotide (ATP) binding folds likely to be situated in the cytoplasm. A further putative cytoplasmic domain (labelled the R domain) is in the centre of the polypeptide and contains sequences which could be phosphorylation sites for protein kinases A and C (Fig. 12.2). The 508 deletion occurs in one of the nucleotide binding folds and could interfere with ATP-mediated alterations in protein configuration.

This protein structure is similar to P-glycoprotein, which confers multiple drug resistance to some human cancer cells, perhaps by exporting the drug from the cell. It is also similar to a number of well-characterized bacterial membrane proteins (Higgins 1989) which have membrane transport functions dependent on ATP. Another similar protein is associated with chloroquine resistance in the malarial parasite and yet another is responsible for export of a mating pheromone in yeast. It is therefore likely that the CF gene-related protein resides in the cell membrane and is associated with transmembrane transport. While it is possible that the protein is an ion channel it seems more likely that it regulates a number of transmembrane functions and so has been labelled cystic fibrosis transmembrane regulator (CFTR).

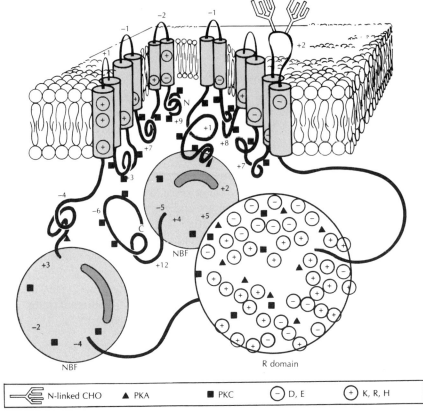

Fig. 12.2 Schematic model of the predicted cystic fibrosis transmembrane regulator protein. The six membrane-spanning helices in each half of the molecule are depicted as cylinders. The cytoplasmically oriented nucleotide binding folds are shown as hatched spheres with slots to indicate the means of entry by the nucleotide. The large polar R domain, which links the two halves, is represented by a stippled sphere. Charged individual amino acids are shown as small circles containing the charge sign. Net charges on the internal and external loops joining the membrane cylinders and on regions of the nucleotide binding folds are contained in open squares. Potential sites for phosphorylation by protein kinases A or C (PKA or PKC) and N-glycosylation (N-linked CHO) are as indicated. D, Asp; E, Glu; H, His; K, Lys; R, Arg. (From Riordan et al [2]; with permission.)

Implications

The identification of the gene and prediction of the protein are likely to have a major impact. The chief implications for cystic fibrosis research will be the rapid identification of the remaining mutations, the synthesis and cellular localization of the protein, the identification of the protein's function and its relationship to the ion transport defect in cystic fibrosis. The practical implications include carrier detection, population screening and accurate prenatal diagnosis. More visionary are the possibilities of gene therapy and new pharmacological approaches aimed at reversing the cystic fibrosis ion transport defect.

Carrier detection

The cloning of the cystic fibrosis gene and characterization of the most common mutation have immediate implications for the identification of carriers. A number of pilot projects are underway to assess the feasibility and benefits of population screening.

The results of screening programmes would depend upon the number of abnormal mutations and their frequency in the population studied. As the 508 mutation is present in about 75% of cases, screening for it would at best only detect 75% of carriers and therefore only 50% of couples at risk. Screening for all known mutations would increase the pick-up rate but this would be much more complex and expensive.

Screening could involve the whole population or selected groups such as those with a history of cystic fibrosis. There are strong arguments for restricting screening to such high-risk groups. Firstly, the tests will be more informative as the abnormal mutation in the family is usually known. Secondly, such families have knowledge of cystic fibrosis and so counselling is simpler and decisions about prenatal diagnosis and possible termination of pregnancy are better informed. Even in such families screening tests will not always give clear-cut results but only an estimate of probabilities (Welsh et al 1986).

The most important issue is the balance of benefit and loss to the community and to the carriers who are detected in a screening programme. In theory cystic fibrosis could be eliminated as a disease, but in practice this is most unlikely. The median survival for cystic fibrosis is already 25 years and rising, and many parents do not want to terminate an affected pregnancy under these circumstances. The issue of false-positive results and the stigma of being an identified carrier have also to be considered.

At present carrier detection should only be offered to those with a family history of CF. It is most unlikely that screening programmes will make a major impact on the incidence of new cases of CF, most of whom are born to parents with no such family history, for at least the next 10 years.

Ion transport

For many years abnormalities of ion concentration in body fluids have been reported in cystic fibrosis. The best known are the high levels of sodium and chloride in sweat but there have also been suggestions of a relative deficiency of water in some secretions. Abnormal ion transport has been found across epithelial cells in cystic fibrosis in sweat glands, airways, pancreas and gut, so uniting the clinically affected organs by a common defect. The ions studied have been predominantly sodium and chloride and research has focused on their passage through selective ion channels, the control of these channels by cyclic AMP and calcium and the overall effect of these ionic movements in terms of electrical current and potential differences as well as water flux. It is likely that the cystic fibrosis gene-associated protein in some way modifies the control of ion transport either directly or indirectly by facilitating the export of some controlling factor from the cell. Ion transport has recently been discussed in cystic fibrosis sweat duct (Reddy et al 1989) and secretory coil (Sato et al 1984), pancreatic ductal cells (Gray et al 1990) and gut (Hardcastle et al 1990).

The key findings in cystic fibrosis airway epithelia have been a raised transepithelial potential difference, an increase in sodium flux from the lumen across the apical cell membrane and a relative impermeability of this apical membrane to chloride ions. Since human airways normally absorb sodium from the lumen with little net chloride movement, it is likely that the increased sodium flux is the most important abnormality in cystic fibrosis and is responsible for the high negative charge. This is supported by the finding that amiloride, a specific blocker or apical sodium channels, lowers the potential difference by 80% and abolishes the difference in surface charge between normal and cystic fibrosis airways. In spite of the central importance of sodium transport, the chloride channel and its control have been more extensively studied.

The apical cell membrane in cystic fibrosis is almost completely impermeable to chloride ions, and manipulations which open chloride channels in normal airways, such as increases in cyclic AMP or activity of protein kinases A or C, have no effect in cystic fibrosis. In contrast, elevation of free intracellular calcium opens cystic fibrosis chloride channels but perhaps only at supraphysiological levels. Interestingly, when a patch of apical membrane is excised from the cell the cystic fibrosis and normal chloride channels are similar, so suggesting that there is a cytosolic inhibitor of chloride channel activation. In contrast, studies of the sodium channel and its control are few, although one preliminary report suggested that the cystic fibrosis sodium channel spends more time in an open state compared with normal. It is not yet clear whether the proposed cytosolic factor which affects chloride permeability is also modifying the function of apical sodium channels in cystic fibrosis. The most tempting speculation at present is that CFTR in its normal form removes an ion transport-modifying substance, perhaps a leukotriene, from the cell, while defective CFTR cannot. The substance may then accumulate and alter both chloride and sodium channel function (Ringe & Petski 1990). These changes and their net effect on the respiratory epithelium are illustrated schematically in Fig. 12.3.

Pathogenesis

The link between abnormal ion transport and bacterial infection has not yet been elucidated but there are at least three possible explanations (Geddes

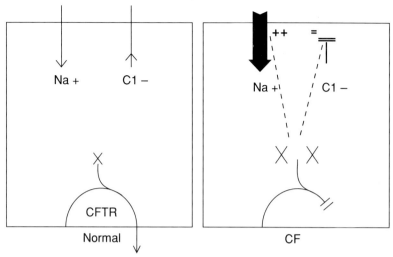

Fig. 12.3 CFTR normally exports an ion transport modifying factor (X). This function is deranged in cystic fibrosis.

1989). The first is that the increased sodium flux acts as an osmotic pump and removes excess water from the airway lumen. In support are the findings that airway surface liquid is relatively reduced in cystic fibrosis and amiloride increases airway liquid in sheep. In theory, such dehydration might reduce mucociliary clearance in cystic fibrosis, although clearance studies in vivo have given conflicting results. However, nebulized amiloride has been shown to improve clearance in cystic fibrosis. The second possibility is that the increased negative charge on the airway surface may modify mucus properties or bacterial adherence. There is as yet little supporting evidence, but amiloride has been shown to affect mucus rheology. Thirdly, other ions, and in particular sulphate, may be affected by the ion transport abnormality. Mucus and cell surface glycoproteins have been shown to have abnormally high sulphation levels in cystic fibrosis and in theory this might alter either bacterial adherence or mucociliary clearance.

CLINICAL ADVANCES

Diagnosis

Prenatal diagnosis

Prenatal diagnosis of cystic fibrosis by analysis of DNA obtained from chorionic villus sampling has been available since 1986 (Farrall et al 1986), based on comparing the fetal and parental pattern of markers around the cystic fibrosis locus. This approach requires DNA from a previously affected child and requires both parents to be fully informative (i.e. the cystic fibrosis bearing chromosome can be identified), conditions which are met in 85% of cases (Super et al 1987, Schwartz et al 1988). Identification of the ΔF 508 mutation, which is present in 78% of cystic fibrosis chromosomes in the UK (Watson et al 1990), now permits screening by direct gene analysis (Halley et al 1989, McIntosh et al 1989) and when both parents are heterozygous for ΔF 508 DNA from a previously affected child is not required. Studies of linked markers remain important in other families, and the number of non-informative families is decreasing with the increasing identification of new and more closely linked DNA markers such as KM 19 and XV2C (Kerem et al 1989, Estivill et al 1987).

The introduction of the polymerase chain reaction (PCR) (Saiki et al 1988) has enabled DNA for analysis to be obtained from buccal epithelial cells in mouth-wash samples (Williams et al 1988) and from old Guthrie cards of children who have died (Williams et al 1988, McIntosh et al 1988). Fibroblasts from previously affected children who have died have also been stored frozen for use in future prenatal diagnosis (Curtis et al 1988).

Partly informative couples who elect to have a further pregnancy may be faced with the decision as to whether to abort a fetus which has a 50% chance of being a normal carrier and 50% chance of having cystic fibrosis. Amniocentesis with microvillar enzyme assays enables further screening to be offered to such couples (Brock et al 1988). However, the optimal time of sampling for this measurement is at 17 weeks' gestation. Some couples may find a second-trimester abortion unacceptable. In addition, the technique carries a 2% false-positive and a 4% false-negative rate. This technique is a useful adjunct to genetic screening in appropriate cases but is no longer useful as a routine test.

Neonatal screening

Neonatal screening for cystic fibrosis is not widely practised at present, although a number of screening studies have now been carried out using the immunoreactive trypsin (IRT) assay on dried blood spots, since serum IRT levels are high in cystic fibrosis during the first year of life. This may be due to back-leakage of enzymes as the pancreatic ducts become blocked in the early stage of pancreatic damage (Durie & Forster 1989). The screening protocol involves an initial test at 5–8 days of age, followed by a further test at 3–7 weeks if the first is positive. If the second test is positive a sweat test is performed together with a full clinical assessment. Retesting rates in most studies are 0.37–0.8% (Adrianssens et al 1981, Wilken et al 1983, Ryley et al 1988, Bowling et al 1988) but have been as high as 5% (Roberts et al 1988). False-negative rates usually reported are 3–8% (Wilken et al 1983, Ryley et al 1988), but have been as high as 23% (Roberts et al 1988).

The potential advantages of neonatal screening for cystic fibrosis are that earlier diagnosis and institution of appropriate treatment may improve the prognosis of an affected child, and that genetic counselling can be offered to parents before a further pregnancy. The value of early diagnosis to an affected child is uncertain (Colten 1990), but two reports suggest that infants diagnosed on screening develop fewer chest infections and have better weight gain in the first 2 years of life (Bowling et al 1988, Wilken & Chalmers 1985). It is possible, however, that the groups of patients in these studies are not comparable, particularly as recent evidence suggests that screening is picking up considerable numbers of otherwise undiagnosed patients with milder disease (Ryley et al 1988). With regard to genetic counselling, neonatal screening will only identify one in four couples at risk of having an affected child in their next pregnancy, so the potential benefit compared with that of population screening of carriers is considerably less.

While IRT assays offer a simple and effective method of neonatal diagnosis of cystic fibrosis, genetic advances now mean that more than 50% of neonates (those homozygous for the F 508 mutation) can be reliably diagnosed by DNA analysis, specimens for which can also be obtained from dried blood spots (Williams et al 1988). Future neonatal screening programmes if considered justifiable may therefore use DNA studies instead of or in combination with IRT assays.

Routine diagnosis

The sweat test remains central to diagnosis (Littlewood 1986). When performed and repeated by experienced personnel, with fludrocortisone suppression where necessary, errors are few, yet a few false-positive and false-negative results still occur. Measurement of nasal potential difference has recently been introduced for equivocal cases (Knowles et al 1981, Hay & Geddes 1985, Alton et al 1987, Alton et al 1990). The technique is based on measurement of airway transepithelial potential difference, which is raised in patients with cystic fibrosis. The test is simple to do except in 2–5-year-olds. The sensitivity and specificity of this technique is comparable to the sweat test and it is a useful additional test, but is invalid during upper respiratory infection and in the presence of nasal polyps.

PULMONARY INFECTION

Microbiology

The main cause of morbidity and mortality in cystic fibrosis is bacterial lung infection, the bacteria most frequently involved being *Haemophilus influenzae, Staphylococcus aureus, Pseudomonas aeruginosa* and *Pseudomonas cepacia*. Infection with *H. influenzae* is often intermittent and, while it may produce acute exacerbations, its contribution to chronic lung damage is not as clearly defined as that of the other organisms (Hoiby 1988).

Staphylococcus aureus

Chronic colonization with *Staph. aureus* is common in children with cystic fibrosis, but intermittent infection also occurs. The reported prevalence of *Staph. aureus* varies between centres from 29% to 72% (Hoiby 1988, Penketh et al 1987, Bauernfeind et al 1988) and decreases with age. Advanced lung damage due to staphylococcal infection alone may occur before pseudomonal colonization, and in the past, before anti-staphylococcal antibiotics were available, was responsible for most of the morbidity and mortality (Hoiby 1988). Some centres use prophylactic anti-staphylococcal antibiotics either from the time of the initial diagnosis of cystic fibrosis or from the onset of bacteriologically proven staphylococcal infection (Govan & Glass 1990). While a lower incidence of staphylococcal colonization has been reported with prophylactic treatment (Neijens 1989), there may be a higher incidence of *Pseudomonas* colonization (Pedersen et al 1987). The restricted use of anti-staphylococcal antibiotics in some centres is claimed to have reduced the incidence of pseudomonal colonization (Govan & Glass 1990). These issues require further evaluation.

The presence of methicillin-resistant *Staph. aureus* in the sputum of patients with cystic fibrosis is increasing, but its prevalence is low at around 3% (Hoiby & Pedersen 1989) and causes little change in clinical condition.

Pseudomonas aeruginosa

Infection of the airways with *Ps. aeruginosa* is responsible for most of the pulmonary damage in cystic fibrosis. The incidence of pseudomonal colonization rises with age and is 70–90% in most adult patients (Neijens 1989). The source of initial colonization may be the environment or cross-infection from another cystic fibrosis patient. An increased rate of acquisition of *Ps. aeruginosa* in the sputum of Danish patients in whom hospital admissions resulted in increased patient contact raised initial concern (Pedersen et al 1987), and subsequent segregation of colonized and non-colonized patients reduced the rate at which colonization was acquired (Hoiby & Pedersen 1989). Studies suggesting that contamination of inanimate objects in hospital was important (Zimakoff et al 1983) have not been confirmed (Speert & Campbell 1987). Transient acquisition of new strains in patients sharing hospital rooms has been reported (Speert & Campbell 1987). Where pseudomonal strain types were studied by serological and more recently by genetic techniques, it was shown that siblings with cystic fibrosis usually share strain types (Kelly et al 1982, Grothues et al 1988, Speert et al 1989, Wolz et al 1989), but that this is uncommon for unrelated patients. It is prolonged, intimate contact that appears to be important. Segregation of colonized and non-colonized patients, although practised by some centres, is probably unnecessary.

Initial colonization is usually with non-mucoid strains. The emergence of mucoid strains, which genetic studies now suggest are derived from the existing non-mucoid strains (Govan & Glass 1990), and the development of the host immune response are factors correlated with a worsening prognosis (Van Bever et al 1988).

Bacterial production of toxins and proteases may be important in initial lung damage, but in later stages most lung damage results from neutrophil enzymes and oxidative processes (Doring et al 1988).

Pseudomonas cepacia

Ps. cepacia, a ubiquitous organism, is a relatively new pathogen in cystic fibrosis. Colonization is more common in those with poor pulmonary function (Isles et al 1984, Tablan et al 1985, Lewin et al 1990), but occurs with a worrying frequency in patients in whom pulmonary function remains good (Thomassen et al 1985). The observation of a greater prevalence of the organism and the association of initial colonization with a hospital admission led to concern about cross-infection, and precautions taken against this have reduced the incidence of colonization in some centres (Thomassen et al 1986). In the UK the incidence appears stable at present (Govan & Glass 1990). This organism was first reported to produce severe progressive respiratory failure associated with high fever, leucocytosis and a high erythrocyte sedimentation rate (Isles et al 1984). However, subsequent studies have shown that serious infection is rare and that colonization usually causes little change in clinical state or prognosis.

Other pulmonary infections

Viral infections

Patients with cystic fibrosis do not have an increased incidence of proven viral infections when compared to their normal siblings (Wang et al 1984). The frequency of viral infections in cystic fibrosis is, however, closely associated with pulmonary deterioration. Whether this is due directly to viral infection, to viral–bacterial interaction or a combination of the two remains to be clarified.

Mycobacterial infection

Mycobacterial infection in cystic fibrosis where routine sputum examination for acid-fast bacilli is performed has been reported as 3–11% (Wang et al 1984, Hjelle et al 1990). Organisms reported include *Mycobacterium tuberculosis* (in 17–43% of cases), and opportunistic mycobacteria in the remainder. The diagnosis is often not suspected clinically. Night sweats, which are unusual in patients with cystic fibrosis, may be a warning symptom. The majority of cases respond to appropriate chemotherapy, but occasional fatalities are reported (Efthimiou et al 1984).

Aspergillus fumigatus

The incidence of allergic bronchopulmonary aspergillosis is increased in cystic fibrosis. This is an allergic condition rather than an infection, and responds to treatment with steroids.

Treatment of pulmonary infection

The aim of treatment of pulmonary infection is to reduce the progression of lung damage. Physiotherapy is important but greater clinical improvement may be achieved with appropriate antibiotic therapy (Regelmann et al 1990). Antimicrobial therapy has a central role, but other drug treatments aimed at suppressing the host immune response may be beneficial, and clinical improvement has been reported following long-term alternate-day prednisolone therapy (Auerbach et al 1985). The value of inhaled steroids is being assessed.

There are many issues regarding antibiotic therapy. These include controversy about which antibiotics should be used, whether single or combined treatment is appropriate, what duration of therapy is best, which dosing schedules and means of delivery should be used and what is the significance of antibiotic sensitivity assays (Geddes 1988). A recent review concluded that placebo-controlled trials have failed to prove benefit for antibiotic therapy in acute exacerbations, suggesting that other treatment methods such as physiotherapy and improved nutritional care may be important. While treatment of infective exacerbations results in short-term improvement in terms of pulmonary function and weight gain, long-term benefit remains to be determined and there is no clear definition of what constitutes an infective exacerbation requiring antibiotic treatment (Govan & Glass 1990). Although trials have shown no advantage from combination antibiotic therapy, concern about later emergence of resistant strains persuade most clinicians to use two drugs. Acquired antibiotic resistance is often short term but becomes a greater problem in patients receiving frequent antibiotic courses (Geddes 1988). The need to prescribe antibiotic treatment according to in vitro bacterial sensitivities is not established, and clinical improvement often occurs when patients are treated with antibiotics to which their infecting organisms are resistant in vitro (Geddes 1988). This issue is the subject of further clinical trials. One reason may be that subinhibitory doses of many antibiotics can reduce the production of pseudomonal toxins and proteases (Grimwood et al 1989).

Home administration of i.v. antibiotics is increasing both in adults and children (David 1989, Kuzenko 1988). It reduces costs, is preferred by many patients, and the incidence of complications is extremely low. Use of long-term venous access devices has increased the availability of home treatment. Ciprofloxacin has enabled some infective exacerbations due to *Ps. aeruginosa* to be treated orally, but organisms frequently acquire resistance.

In addition to the short-term benefit of treating acute infectious exacerbations, long-term benefit may be achieved by regular or continuous antibiotic administration. An improved prognosis has been reported in patients treated with i.v. antibiotic courses at 3-monthly intervals regardless of the patient's condition (Pedersen et al 1987), and this policy is practised in some centres. Continuous aerosol antibiotic therapy, which is performed at home, is of clinical benefit in reducing the frequency of acute infective exacerbations and also improves lung function (Hodson et al 1981, Hodson 1988).

Haemoptysis and bronchial artery embolization

Minor episodes of haemoptysis are a common occurrence in cystic fibrosis, occurring in over 60% of patients (Penketh et al 1987). They usually settle with appropriate antibiotic therapy and correction of any clotting disorders. Bronchial artery embolization for life-threatening massive haemoptysis, which without intervention carries a high mortality (Holselaw et al 1970), is occasionally required. Results reported in two recent series (Cohen et al 1990, Sweezy & Fellows 1990) give immediate success rates of 55–84% with one embolization, increasing to 88–95% after a second embolization when required. Later severe recurrences which have been reported in more than 50% of patients have been treated by repeat embolization with a success rate of 89% (Sweezy & Fellows 1990). Side effects are usually limited to transient chest pain and pyrexia which can be treated symptomatically. Patients requiring bronchial artery embolization have a higher mortality than matched controls during the following 3 months, for which haemoptysis is a contributing cause in one-third (Sweezy & Fellows 1990).

HEART–LUNG TRANSPLANTATION (see also chapters 14–17 on heart–lung transplantation)

The first successful heart–lung transplant for cystic fibrosis was performed in 1985 (Jones et al 1988) and now more than 90 cystic fibrosis patients have received heart–lung transplants in the UK (including two heart–lung and liver transplants) (Scott et al 1988, Geddes & Hodson 1989, Yacoub & Bonner 1990, Hodson 1990). The first patient transplanted is alive and well more than 5 years after transplantation. The actuarial survival at 1 year is 63–69%. Most early deaths are due to bleeding, infection, adult respiratory distress syndrome (ARDS) and multisystem failure. Although the long-term prognosis of these patients is unknown, the results so far are encouraging and give new hope to cystic fibrosis patients with advanced pulmonary disease. Unfortunately, the number of donor lungs available will never satisfy demand, in spite of recent advances in lung preservation techniques providing an increase in the number of donors from more distant locations

(Yacoub & Bonner et al 1990), and patients accepted for heart–lung transplantation continue to die while on the waiting list. Careful selection of patients is therefore important (Table 12.1).

Assessment for transplantation

The major indication for heart–lung transplantation in cystic fibrosis is deteriorating chronic respiratory failure, which is assessed by lung function studies (usually forced expiratory volume at 1 second (FEV_1) and functional vital capacity (FVC) less than 40% predicted), blood gases, oxygen desaturation at rest and on exercise, the patient's level of exercise tolerance and frequency of admission for i.v. antibiotics. The optimum time for transplantation is when the prognosis is only a few months, but before the patient becomes moribund. This is, however, difficult to judge as the rate of clinical decline is very variable. Relative contraindications include major psychosocial problems usually associated with a history of poor compliance, poor nutritional state, pleural adhesions, renal failure, advanced liver disease and systemic corticosteroid therapy. Nutrition can be improved with dietary advice in some patients, while others require insertion of a feeding gastrostomy. Computed tomography scanning identifies pleural adhesions. As previous pleurectomy presents a major risk, the role of limited abrasion pleurodesis for patients with recurrent pneumothorax who may later be considered for transplantation is being assessed. Good renal function is necessary because of the use of cyclosporin for immunosuppression.

Table 12.1   Selection criteria for heart–lung transplant in cystic fibrosis

A Indications: Deteriorating chronic respiratory failure
B Contraindications:

	Major	*Minor*
Personal	Psychological disturbance Poor treatment compliance Age > 50 years	
Weight	50% predicted	75% predicted
Renal		Creatinine clearance < 70 ml/min
Hepatic	Cirrhosis[a] Portal hypertension[a]	
Endocrine		Diabetes
Pleural	Previous pleurectomy	Other pleural therapy
Microbiology	?Multiple resistant *Staph. aureus*	Mycobacterial *Aspergillus* infections

[a]Possible heart, lung and liver transplant.

Malabsorption needs to be assessed with faecal fat studies to help in appropriate dosing of oral cyclosporin postoperatively. Patients with severe liver disease or portal hypertension can only be considered for combined heart–lung and liver transplantation. Diabetes is not a contraindication. Cardiac assessment is needed as the recipient's heart is now frequently transplanted into another patient (domino procedure). Any steroid therapy must be withdrawn because of interference with healing of the tracheal anastomosis.

Full microbiological screening before surgery is important. Antibiotic sensitivities need to be known for postoperative treatment. Successful heart–lung transplantation has been performed in patients with methicillin-resistant *Staph. aureus* infection.

Management of terminal illness in patients awaiting heart–lung transplantation can be difficult as decisions have to be made regarding withdrawal of active treatment and whether ventilatory support should be considered. Most centres do not consider that intubation and formal ventilation is appropriate for these patients, but the value of non-invasive nasal ventilation for patients awaiting heart–lung transplantation is now being assessed.

The operation

The operation which has been preferred in the UK is heart and lung transplantation with retransplantation of the recipient's heart into another patient. Double lung transplantation is being assessed in North America.

Following transplantation lung function improves over a period of months towards normal values (Geddes & Hodson 1989), patients gain weight and finger clubbing resolves. Late complications, the frequency and prognosis of which are not yet known, include recolonization with *Pseudomonas*, malignancy secondary to immunosuppression and obliterative bronchiolitis. The latter is a serious clinical problem which is probably a manifestation of chronic rejection (Yacoub & Bonner 1990). It presents insidiously with cough and breathlessness associated with a decline in FEV_1/FVC, with the chest radiograph showing little change. Affected patients are treated with increased immunosuppression but this is usually of little benefit and lung function continues to decline, for which a further lung transplant is the only treatment. Lymphoproliferative disorders, which are most commonly of the B-cell type and are positive for Epstein–Barr virus nuclear antigen, respond to a reduction in immunosuppression combined with i.v. acyclovir. One T-cell lymphoma responded to a reduction in immunosuppression alone (Yacoub & Bonner 1990).

Physiotherapy

There have been no major changes in physiotherapy techniques for cystic fibrosis over the past few years and established treatment continues to be highly effective. Present treatment combines the forced expiration technique (Pryor et al 1979, Webber et al 1986, Sutton et al 1983), interspersed with controlled diaphragmatic breathing and thoracic expansion exercise, with gravity-assisted postural drainage and coughing. Interspersing the technique with pauses for controlled breathing and relaxation reduces fatigue and prevents hypoxias during therapy (Pryor et al 1990). During acute infective exacerbations patients often require assistance with postural drainage, but when well can achieve equally effective sputum clearances when performing postural drainage themselves (Pryor et al 1979). Chest percussion, which is frequently practised, is not an essential part of treatment if other techniques are performed effectively (Hofmeyr et al 1986).

Some centres advocate the use of periodic application of a face mask with positive expiratory pressure (PEP mask) during physiotherapy, with the proposed advantages that it can be performed in a sitting position, does not require an assistant and is associated with less oxygen desaturation (Falk et al 1984). Others have failed to show any advantage (Hofmeyr et al 1986).

The effect of exercise with standard physiotherapy has recently been evaluated and was found to have no effect on daily sputum production (Salh et al 1989). Whilst it has other benefits and should be encouraged, exercise is not a substitute for physiotherapy.

NUTRITIONAL CARE

Energy balance

Undernutrition is a common problem and is associated with a poor prognosis (Durie & Pencharz 1989). Its correction is central to management. It arises from inadequate energy intake, energy losses via the gastrointestinal tract and increased energy requirements.

Energy intake

Patients with cystic fibrosis require an energy intake 120–150% that of normal individuals to maintain their weight and need appropriate dietary advice on how to achieve this. A recent comparison of two patient populations in Boston and Toronto (Corey et al 1988) demonstrated that patients in Boston had lower body weights and a worse prognosis. The only difference in management was the fat content of the diet, which was high in the Toronto group. It is now recommended that patients with cystic fibrosis should have a full-fat diet, combined with adequate pancreatic enzyme supplementation to prevent steatorrhoea. Medical causes reduce food intake particularly during exacerbations when patients are anorexic and too breathless to eat.

Gastrointestinal energy loss

Losses due to malabsorption result from pancreatic enzyme deficiency, reduced pancreatic bicarbonate secretion allowing more acid duodenal contents to denature pancreatic lipase, thus encouraging precipitation of bile salts. Excessive abnormal intestinal mucus may further interfere with absorption (Corey et al 1988). Adequate pancreatic enzyme supplements control steatorrhoea in most patients and improved results have been obtained with the introduction of enteric-coated encapsulated microsphere preparations (Haymans 1989, Stead et al 1987).

New preparations containing more lipase activity have the advantage of reducing the number of capsules taken, but are otherwise no more effective than other enteric-coated microsphere preparations (Robinson et al 1989). In patients who continue to have steatorrhoea the addition of oral H2 receptor blockers such as cimetidine to reduce duodenal acid may be beneficial (Zentler-Munro et al 1985). Bile acid supplementation with taurine has also been used but with no confirmed benefit (Sinaasappel 1989).

Increased energy consumption

In patients with pulmonary infection increased energy requirements result from the increased work of breathing, but resting energy expenditure has also been shown to be elevated in patients with mild pulmonary disease (Durie & Pencharz 1989). In vitro studies have also shown increased oxygen consumption in cystic fibrosis tissues (Stutts et al 1986). It is possible that the basic defect in cystic fibrosis involves increased energy consumption, but this has yet to be shown.

Vitamin deficiencies

Although deficiencies of fat-soluble vitamins are often seen at diagnosis, supplementation is now standard and signs of deficiency of vitamins A, D and E are rare. A recent report describes asymptomatic conjunctival sclerosis associated with severe night blindness in three patients, suggesting that vitamin supplementation is not always adequate (Vernon et al 1989). Vitamin E deficiency occasionally manifests itself with evidence of haemolytic anaemia in newly diagnosed infants. In adults, in whom deficiency is rare with adequate supplementation, its manifestations are predominantly neurological and include diminished tendon reflexes, ataxia, muscle weakness and ophthalmoplegia (Cynamon et al 1988, Elias et al 1981, Sitrin et al 1987). This is often associated with the presence of advanced liver disease. Bile salt supplementation can improve vitamin E absorption in these patients (Sitrin et al 1987).

Essential fatty acid deficiency

Clinical features of essential fatty acid deficiency may be observed in undiagnosed infants but are rare in older patients (Durie & Pencharz 1989). Low plasma levels of essential fatty acids are usually, but not always, restricted to patients with pancreatic insufficiency (Standvik 1989). Recent interest has focused on the possible connection between increased fatty acid metabolism and the basic defect in cystic fibrosis (Standvik 1989). There is no evidence of clinical value in supplementation at the moment.

Nutritional management

Current nutritional strategy provides a full-fat, enzyme-rich diet with pancreatic enzymes and fat-soluble vitamins. Most problems arise later when chest infections become frequent and energy demands are increased. Short-term i.v. total parenteral nutrition may be beneficial during infective episodes but weight gain is usually not maintained (Durie & Pencharz 1989). Nasogastric feeding can have short-term benefits but few patients continue this because of problems with nasal irritation and keeping the tube in (Durie & Pencharz 1989). Recent approaches involving night-time feeds by gastrostomy (Levy et al 1985, Shepherd et al 1986) or jejunostomy (Boland et al 1986) have achieved better results in terms of nutritional gain. Gastrostomies can be inserted endoscopically under local anaesthetic and are generally well tolerated. Whether nutritional gains improve prognosis is yet to be clarified (Durie & Pencharz 1989).

OTHER ORGAN SYSTEMS

Liver

The incidence of liver disease in cystic fibrosis as defined by hepatomegaly, abnormal liver function tests or both has recently been reported as 24% (age range 16–45 years; Nagel et al 1989) and 40% (age range 4–19 years; Gaskin et al 1988). Splenomegaly in the latter series was 9%. The incidence of ascites and oesophageal varices varies, possibly because of differences in patient age groups, from one patient with ascites in a population of 153 to 2.6% with bleeding oesophageal varices in a population of 233 in the adult series. However, bleeding oesophageal varices have been reported in as many as 10% of one group of teenagers (Sinaasappel 1989). These complications are treated in the conventional way. Symptoms of upper abdominal pain are reported in up to 56% of patients with hepatosplenomegaly (Gaskin et al 1988), but liver disease is otherwise asymptomatic.

The variation in occurrence and severity of liver disease and the observation that cirrhosis may develop in patients with normal fat absorption indicates that factors additional to intrahepatic biliary obstruction are involved in its pathogenesis. One study (Gaskin et al 1988) reported a very high incidence (96%) of distal common bile duct obstruction in cystic fibrosis patients with liver disease, compared with zero in a control group without liver disease. However, another study reported an incidence of only 3.5% (Nagel et al 1989). A number of patients with distal biliary structures have been treated surgically, with relief of symptoms (Gaskin et al 1988).

Distal intestinal obstruction syndrome

Distal intestinal obstruction syndrome or meconium ileus equivalent occurs in 16% of patients (usually those with known pancreatic insufficiency) and may be recurrent (Penketh et al 1987). Conventional treatment has involved rehydration, oral and rectal N-acetylcysteine or gastrograffin, enzyme replacement and attention to diet. This is successful in most cases. A recent advance has been the use of a balanced intestinal lavage solution which contains polyethylene glycol to minimize transmucosal fluid flux (Cleghorn et al 1986). Following prophylactic antiemetics 5–6 litres of fluid is administered at a rate of 750–1000 ml per hour either orally or via a nasogastric tube. Reports of its use so far indicate that it is effective (Cleghorn et al 1986, Davidson et al 1986).

Joints

Joint symptoms are reported in 9% of patients (Penketh et al 1987). These are usually associated with exacerbations of chest disease, are not accompanied by abnormal physical signs and are treated symptomatically with minor analgesics and non-steroidal anti-inflammatory agents. Hypertrophic pulmonary osteoarthropathy has been reported.

Diabetes mellitus

The incidence of diabetes mellitus is 10%. The majority can be treated by diet or oral hypoglycaemics. One-third require insulin. Microvascular complications have now been reported (Penketh et al 1987).

Pregnancy and lactation

Improved survival in cystic fibrosis has resulted in increasing numbers of pregnancies. Spontaneous abortion in cystic fibrosis pregnancies is no higher than in the general population, but shortened gestation and increased perinatal mortality are more common. Maternal complications in pregnancy include poor weight gain, congestive heart failure and worsening of lung function, which does not always return to pregravid values. Intravenous antibiotics have been used during all stages of pregnancy and no cases of fetal congenital abnormalities have been reported. Successful breast feeding may be possible. In general the outcome of cystic fibrosis pregnancies has been excellent, although poor maternal lung function and nutrition increase the risks (Cohen et al 1980, Palmer et al 1983).

Psychological factors

As increasing numbers of cystic fibrosis patients survive into adult life, more interest is being focused on their social and psychological status. Many uncontrolled reports suggest few psychological problems in this patient group — an observation recently supported by a controlled study of the psychological status of adults with cystic fibrosis compared to their healthy peers (Shepherd et al 1990).

FUTURE TREATMENT APPROACHES

Amiloride

Recent advances in knowledge of the epithelial ion transport abnormalities in cystic fibrosis have led to interest in drugs which modify these more basic defects rather than treating the resulting disease. Amiloride, which selectively blocks sodium absorption across the epithelial cell apical membrane, is presently being evaluated as a treatment for cystic fibrosis. Oral administration does not achieve sufficiently high levels at the airway surfaces so interest has centred on its use as inhaled therapy. Studies of mucociliary clearance using radiolabelled inhaled particles in patients with cystic fibrosis have shown that a single dose of nebulized amiloride improves mucociliary clearance and cough clearance, presumably by increasing the depth of the periciliary fluid layer (Kohler et al 1986). The effect lasts for up to 80 minutes. Longer-term administration of twice-daily nebulized amiloride over a 3-week period increases the effect of a single dose (App et al 1990). In a recent pilot study of the overall clinical benefit of long-term nebulized amiloride in cystic fibrosis, it was administered four times daily for a 6-month period (Knowles et al 1990). Compared to a control period, the patients on treatment demonstrated a slower rate of decline in lung function and improvements in sputum viscosity and elasticity. No toxic effects were noted and further evaluation of the treatment has been recommended. One problem with this study is that in both the treated and untreated groups the rates of decline in lung function were higher than is usually observed. Two possible reasons for this are that the preceding treatment with i.v. antibiotics in all patients gave them an unrepresentatively high baseline or that withdrawal of all other respiratory treatment, including oral and inhaled antibiotics and bronchodilators, was responsible.

If amiloride is shown to be of value, then longer-acting preparations need to be developed or other drugs with similar effect but longer duration need to be evaluated. Therapeutic benefit with bradykinin may be useful, which induces chloride secretion in cystic fibrosis tissue via a receptor-mediated elevation of intracellular calcium (Boucher et al 1989).

Gene therapy

The normal gene has now been isolated and shown to correct the cystic fibrosis ion transport defect in in vitro systems. The possibility of treating cystic fibrosis by administering the normal gene to the respiratory tract is being pursued. The gene could be delivered via aerosol in a liposome or incorporated into the genome of a virus. Retroviruses are being investigated, as is an attenuated adenovirus. The preliminary results are encouraging. It will be important to know how well the gene can be incorporated and how long beneficial effects last. The safety of such novel treatment will need to be assessed. It will be necessary to establish that excessive expression of the normal cystic fibrosis gene has no undesirable effects, and that repeated administration is not damaging. There is still a long way to go.

REFERENCES

Adrianssens K, Janssens H and Van Soom H 1981 Two tier screen for cystic fibrosis. Lancet i: 833

Alton E W F W, Hay J G, Munro C et al 1987 Measurement of nasal potential difference in adult cystic fibrosis, Young's syndrome and bronchiectasis. Thorax 42: 815–817

Alton E W F W, Currie D, Logan-Sinclair R et al 1990 Nasal potential difference: A clinical diagnostic test for cystic fibrosis. European Respiratory Journal (in press)

App E M, King M, Helfesreider R et al 1990 Acute and long term amiloride inhalation in cystic fibrosis lung disease. American Review of Respiratory Disease 141: 605–612

Auerbach H S, Williams M, Kilpatrick J A et al 1985 Alternate day prednisolone reduces morbidity and improves pulmonary function in cystic fibrosis. Lancet ii: 686–688

Bauernfeind A, Horl G, Przyklenk B 1988 Microbiologic and therapeutic aspects of *Staphylococcus aureus* in cystic fibrosis patients. Scandinavian Journal of Gastroenterology 23 (suppl 143): 99–102

Boland M P, Stoski D S, MacDonald M E 1986 Chronic jejunostomy feeding with a non-elemental formula in undernourished patients with cystic fibrosis. Lancet i: 232–234

Boucher R C, Cheng E H C, Pardison A M et al 1989 Chloride secretory response of cystic fibrosis human airway epithelia: Preservation of calcium but not protein kinase C- and A-dependent mechanisms. Journal of Clinical Investigation 84: 1424–1431

Bowling F G, Cleghorn G, Chest A et al 1988 Neonatal screening for cystic fibrosis. Archives of Disease in Childhood 63: 726–729

Boxerbaum B, Jacobs M R, Cechner R 1988 Prevalence and significance of methicillin-resistant *Staphylococcus aureus* in patients with cystic fibrosis. Paediatric Pulmonology 4: 159–163

Brock E H, Clarke H A K, Barron L et al 1988 Prenatal diagnosis of cystic fibrosis by microvillar enzyme assay on a sequence of 258 pregnancies. Human Genetics 78: 271–275

Cleghorn G J, Stringer D A, Forstner et al 1986 Treatment of distal obstruction syndrome in cystic fibrosis with balanced intestinal lavage solution. Lancet i: 8–9

Cohen A M, Doershuk C F, Stern R C 1990 Bronchial artery embolisation to control haemoptysis in cystic fibrosis. Radiology 175: 401–405

Cohen L F, Sant'Agnese P A, Friedlander J 1980 Cystic fibrosis and pregnancy: A national survey. Lancet ii: 842–844

Collins F S, Drumon M L, Cole J L et al 1987 Construction of a general human chromosome jumping library, with application to cystic fibrosis. Science 235: 1046

Colten H R 1990. Screening for cystic fibrosis: Public policy and personal choices. New England Journal of Medicine 322: 328–329

Corey M, McLaoughlin F J, Williams M et al 1988 A comparison of survival, growth and pulmonary function in patients with cystic fibrosis in Boston and Toronto. Journal of Clinical Epidemiology 41: 583–591

Curtis A, Strain L, Mennie M et al 1988 First-trimester prenatal diagnosis of cystic fibrosis using fibroblasts from a deceased index child to establish haplotypes. Prenatal Diagnosis 8: 625–628

Cynamon H A, Milor D E, Valenstein E et al 1988 Effects of vitamin E deficiency on neurological function in patients with cystic fibrosis. Journal of Pediatrics 113: 637–640

David J T 1989 Intravenous antibiotics at home in children with cystic fibrosis. Journal of the Royal Society of Medicine 82: 130–131

Davidson A C et al 1986 Treatment of distal intestinal obstruction syndrome in patients with cystic fibrosis. Thorax 41: 732

Doring G, Albus A, Hoiby 1988 Immunologic aspects of cystic fibrosis. Chest 94 (suppl 2): 1095–1135

Durie P R, Forster G 1989 Pathophysiology of the exocrine pancreas in cystic fibrosis. Journal of the Royal Society of Medicine 2 (suppl 16): 2–10

Durie P R, Pencharz P B 1989 A rational approach to the nutritional care of patients with cystic fibrosis. Journal of the Royal Society of Medicine 82 (suppl 16): 11–20

Efthimiou J, Smith M J, Hodson M E et al 1984 Fatal pulmonary infection with *Mycobacterium fortuitum* in cystic fibrosis. British Journal of Diseases of the Chest 78: 299–302

Elias E, Muller D P R, Scott J 1981 Effects of vitamin E deficiency on neurological function in patients with cystic fibrosis. Journal of Pediatrics 113: 637–640

Estivill X, Farrall M, Scambler J 1987 A candidate for the cystic fibrosis locus isolated by selection for methylation-free islands. Nature 326: 257–263

Estivill X, Chillon M, Casals T et al 1989 508 gene deletion in cystic fibrosis in southern Europe. Lancet ii: 1404

Falk M, Kelstrup M, Andersen J R et al 1984 Improving the ketchup bottle method with positive expiratory pressure, PEP, in cystic fibrosis. European Journal of Respiratory Diseases 65: 423–432

Farrall M, Law H-Y, Rodech C H et al 1986 First trimester prenatal diagnosis of cystic fibrosis with linked DNA probes. Lancet i: 1402–1405

Gaskin K J, Waters D, Howman-Giles R et al 1988 Liver disease and common bile duct stenosis in cystic fibrosis. New England Journal of Medicine 318: 340–346

Geddes D M 1988 Antimicrobial therapy against *Staphylococcus aureus, Pseudomonas aeruginosa* and *Pseudomonas cepacia.* Chest 94: 1405–1435

Geddes D M, Slurier R 1989 Cystic fibrosis — from lung damage to symptoms. Acta Paediatrica Scandinavica (suppl 363): 52–57

Geddes D M, Hodson M E 1989 The role of heart and lung transplantation in the treatment of cystic fibrosis. Journal of the Royal Society of Medicine 82 (suppl 16): 49–53

Govan J R W, Glass S 1990 The microbiology and therapy of cystic fibrosis lung infections. Reviews in Medical Microbiology 1: 19–28

Gray M A, Pollard C E, Harris A et al 1990 Paediatric Pulmonology (suppl 5): 181–183

Grimwood K, To A, Rabin H R et al 1989 Inhibition of *Pseudomonas aeruginosa* exoenzyme expression by subinhibitory antibiotics concentrations. Antimicrobial Agents and Chemotherapy 33: 41–47

Grothues D, Koopman V, van der Haart H et al 1988 Genome finger printing of *Pseudomonas aeruginosa* indicates colonization of cystic fibrosis siblings with closely related strains. Journal of Clinical Microbiology 1973–1977

Halley D J J, Von Damme N H M, Deelan W H et al 1989 Prenatal detection of major cystic fibrosis mutation. Lancet ii: 972

Hardcastle J, Hardcastle P T, Taylor C J 1990 Paediatric Pulmonology (suppl 5): 181–183

Hay J G, Geddes D M 1985 Transepithelial potential difference in cystic fibrosis. Thorax 40: 493–396

Haymans H S A 1989 Gastrointestinal dysfunction and its effects on nutrition in cystic fibrosis. Acta Paediatrica Scandinavica (suppl 363): 74–79

Higgins C 1989 Protein joins transport family. Nature 301: 103

Hjelle L, Petrini B, Kallenius G et al 1990 Prospective study of mycobacterial infections in patients with cystic fibrosis. Thorax 45: 401–402

Hodson M E 1988 Antibiotic treatment: Aerosol therapy. Chest 94 (suppl): 156S–163S

Hodson M E 1990 Personal communication

Hodson M E, Penketh A R L, Batten J C 1981 Aerosol carbenicillin and gentamicin treatment of *Pseudomonas aeruginosa* infection in patients with cystic fibrosis. Lancet ii: 1137–1139

Hofmyer J, Webber B A, Hodson M E 1986 Evaluation of positive expiratory pressure as an adjunct to chest physiotherapy in the treatment of cystic fibrosis. Thorax 41: 951–954

Hoiby N 1988 *Haemophilus influenzae, Staphylococcus aureus, Pseudomonas cepacia* and *Pseudomonas aeruginosa* in patients with cystic fibrosis. Chest 94: 975–1015

Hoiby N, Pedersen S S 1989 Estimated risk of cross-infection with *Pseudomonas aeruginosa* in Danish cystic fibrosis patients. Acta Paediatrica Scandinavica 78: 395–404

Holselaw D S, Grand R J, Shwachmann H 1970 Massive haemoptysis in cystic fibrosis. Journal of Pediatrics 76: 829

Isles A, Maclusky I, Corey M et al 1984 *Pseudomonas cepacia* infection in cystic fibrosis: An emerging problem. Journal of Pediatrics 104: 206–210

Jones K, Higgenbottam T, Wallwork J 1988 Successful heart–lung transplantation for cystic fibrosis. Chest 93: 644–645

Kelly N M, Fitzgerland M X, Tempany E et al 1982 Does *Pseudomonas* cross infection occur between cystic fibrosis patients? Lancet ii: 688–690

Kerem B-S, Rommens J M, Buchanan J A et al 1989 Identification of the cystic fibrosis gene: Genetic analysis. Science 245: 1073–1080

Knowles M R, Carson J L, Collier A M et al 1981 Measurement of nasal transepithelial elective potential difference in normal human subjects in vivo. American Review of Respiratory Disease 124: 484–496

Knowles M R, Church N J, Waltner W E et al 1990 A pilot study of aerosolised amiloride for the treatment of lung disease in cystic fibrosis. New England Journal of Medicine 322: 1189–1194

Kohler D, App E, Schmitz-Schumann M et al 1986 Inhalation of amiloride improves the mucociliary and the cough clearances in patients with cystic fibrosis. European Journal of Respiratory Diseases 69 (suppl 146): 319–326

Kuzenko J A 1988 Home treatment of pulmonary infections in cystic fibrosis. Chest 94: 1625–1655

Levy L D, Durie P R, Rencharz P B 1985 Effects of long-term nutritional rehabilitation on body composition and clinical status in malnourished children and adolescents with cystic fibrosis. Journal of Pediatrics 107: 225–250

Lewin L O, Byard P J, Davis P B 1990 Effects of *Pseudomonas cepacia* colonization on survival and pulmonary function in cystic fibrosis patients. Journal of Clinical Epidemiology 43: 125–131

Littlewood J M 1986 An overview of the management of cystic fibrosis. Journal of the Royal Society of Medicine 79 (suppl 12): 55–63

McIntosh I, Strain L, Brock D J H 1988 Prenatal diagnosis of cystic fibrosis where single affected child has died: Guthrie spots and microvillar enzyme sampling. Lancet ii: 1085

McIntosh I, Raeburn J A, Curtis A et al 1989 First trimester prenatal diagnosis of CF by direct gene probing. Lancet ii: 972

Nagel R A, Westaby D, Javaid A et al 1989 Liver disease and common bile duct abnormalities in adults with cystic fibrosis. Lancet ii: 1422–1425

Neijens H J 1989 Strategies and perspectives in treatment of respiratory infections. Acta Paediatrica Scandinavica (suppl) 363: 66–73

Palmer J, Dilloon-Baker C, Tecklin J S et al 1983 Pregnancy in patients with cystic fibrosis. Annals of Internal Medicine 99: 596–600

Pedersen S S, Jensen T, Hoiby N et al 1987 Management of *Pseudomonas aeruginosa* lung infection in Danish cystic fibrosis patients. Acta Paediatrica Scandinavica 78: 395–404

Penketh A R L, Wise A, Mearns M B et al 1987 Cystic fibrosis in adolescent and adults. Thorax 42: 526–532

Pryor J A, Webber B A, Hodson M E et al 1979 Evaluation of the forced expiration technique as an adjunct to postural drainage in treatment of cystic fibrosis. British Medical Journal 2: 417–418

Pryor J A, Webber B A, Hodson M E 1990 Effects of chest physiotherapy on oxygen saturation in patients with cystic fibrosis. Thorax 45: 77

Regelmann E W, Elliot G R, Warwick W J et al 1990 Reduction of sputum *Pseudomonas aeruginosa* density by antibiotics improves lung function in cystic fibrosis more than do bronchodilators and chest physiotherapy alone. American Review of Respiratory Disease 141: 914–921

Ringe D, Petski G A 1990 A transport problem? Nature 346: 312–313

Roberts G, Stanfield M, Black A et al 1988 Screening for cystic fibrosis: A four year regional experience. Archives of Disease in Childhood 63: 1438–1443

Robinson P J, Olinsky A, Smith A L et al 1989 High compared with standard dose lipase pancreatic supplements. Archives of Disease in Childhood 64: 143–145

Ryley H C, Deam S M, Williams J et al 1988 Neonatal screening for cystic fibrosis in Wales and the West Midlands: I. Evaluation of immunoreactive trypsin test. Journal of Clinical Pathology 41: 726–729

Saiki R V, Gelfand D H, Stoffel S et al 1988 Primer-directed enzymatic amplification of DNA with a thermostable DNA polymerase. Science 239: 487–491

Salh W, Bilton D, Dodd M et al 1989 Effect of exercise and physiotherapy in aiding sputum expectoration in adults with cystic fibrosis. Thorax 44: 1006–1008

Sato K, Sato F 1984 Defective beta adrenergic response of cystic fibrosis sweat glands in vivo and in vitro. Journal of Clinical Investigation 73: 1763–1771

Schwartz M, Super M, Schmidtke J et al 1988 Prenatal diagnosis of cystic fibrosis using linked DNA probes. Prenatal Diagnosis 8: 619–624

Scott J, Higenbottam T, Hutter J et al 1988 Heart lung transplantation for cystic fibrosis. Lancet ii: 192–194

Shepherd R W, Holt T L, Thomas B J et al 1986 Nutritional rehabilitation in cystic fibrosis: Controlled studies of effects on nutritional growth retardation, body protein turnover and course of pulmonary disease. Journal of Pediatrics 109: 788–794

Shepherd S L, Hovell M F, Harwood I R et al 1990 A comparative study of the psychological assets of adults with cystic fibrosis and their healthy peers. Chest 97: 1310–1316

Sinaasappel M 1989 Hepatobiliary pathology in patients with cystic fibrosis. Acta Paediatrica Scandinavica (suppl) 363: 45–51

Sitrin M D, Lieberman F, Jansen W E et al 1987 Vitamin E deficiency and neurologic disease in adults with cystic fibrosis. Annals of Internal Medicine 107: 51–54

Smith M H, Efthimiou J, Hodson M E et al 1984 Mycobacterial isolations in young adults with cystic fibrosis. Thorax 39: 369–375

Speert D P, Campbell M E 1987 Hospital epidemiology of *Pseudomonas aeruginosa* from patients with cystic fibrosis. Journal of Hospital Infection 9: 11–21

Speert D P, Campbell M E, Farmer S W et al 1989 Use of a pilin gene probe to study molecular epidemiology of *Pseudomonas aeruginosa*. Journal of Clinical Microbiology 2589–2593

Standvik B 1989 Relation between essential fatty acid metabolism and gastrointestinal symptoms in cystic fibrosis. Acta Paediatrica Scandinavica (suppl) 363: 58–65

Stead R J, Skypala I, Hodson M E 1987 Enteric coated microspheres of pancreatin in the treatment of cystic fibrosis: Comparison with a standard enteric coated preparation. Thorax 42: 533–537

Stutts M J, Knowles M R, Gatzy J T 1986 Oxygen consumption and oubain binding sites in cystic fibrosis nasal epithelium. Pediatric Research 20: 1316–1320

Super M, Ivinson A, Schwartz M et al 1987 Clinical experience of prenatal diagnosis of cystic fibrosis by use of linked DNA probes. Lancet ii: 782–784

Sutton P P, Parker R A, Webber B A et al 1983 Assessment of the forced expiration technique, postural drainage and directed coughing in chest physiotherapy. European Journal of Respiratory Diseases 64: 62–68

Sweezy N B, Fellows K E 1990 Bronchial artery embolisation for severe haemoptysis in cystic fibrosis. Chest 97: 1322–1326

Tablan O C, Chorba T L, Schidlow D V et al 1985 *Pseudomonas cepacia* colonization in patients with cystic fibrosis, risk factors and clinical outcome. Journal of Pediatrics 107: 382–387

Thomassen M J, Demko C A, Klinger J D et al 1985 *Pseudomonas cepacia* colonization among patients with cystic fibrosis: A new opportunist. American Review of Respiratory Disease 131: 791–796

Thomassen M J, Demko C A, Doershuk C F et al 1986 *Pseudomonas cepacia*: Decrease in colonization in patients with cystic fibrosis. American Review of Respiratory Disease 134: 669–671

Van Bever H P, Gigase P L, de Clerck L S et al 1988 Immune complexes and *Pseudomonas aeruginosa* antibiotics in cystic fibrosis. Archives of Disease in Childhood 63: 1222–1228

Vernon S A, Neugebauer M A Z, Brimlow G et al 1989 Conjunctival xerosis in cystic fibrosis. Journal of the Royal Society of Medicine 82: 46–47

Wang E L, Prober C G, Manson B et al 1984 Association of respiratory viral infections with pulmonary deterioration in cystic fibrosis. New England Journal of Medicine 311: 1653–1658

Watson E et al 1990 Genetic counselling for cystic fibrosis based upon mutation/haplotype analysis. Lancet ii: 190–191

Webber B A, Hofmeyr B A, Morgan M D L et al 1986 Effects of postural drainage incorporating the forced expiration technique on pulmonary function in cystic fibrosis. British Journal of Diseases of the Chest 80: 353–359

Wilken B, Chalmers G 1985 Reduced morbidity in patients with cystic fibrosis detected by neonatal screening. Lancet ii: 1319–1321

Wilken B, Brown A R D, Urwin R et al 1983 Cystic fibrosis screening by dried blood spots trypsin assay: Results in 75 000 newborn infants. Journal of Pediatrics 102: 383–387

Williams C, Williamson R 1988 Same-day first-trimester antenatal diagnosis for cystic fibrosis by gene amplification. Lancet ii: 102–103

Williams C, Weber L, Williamson R et al 1988 Guthrie spots for DNA-based carrier testing in cystic fibrosis. Lancet ii: 693

Wolz C E, Kiosz G, Ogle J W et al 1989 *Pseudomonas aeruginosa* cross-colonization and persistence in patients with cystic fibrosis: use of a DNA probe. Epidemiology of Infection 102: 205–214

Yacoub M H, Bonner N R 1990 Recent developments in lung and heart–lung transplantation. In: Morris P, Tilne N L (eds) Transplantation reviews, vol 3. Saunders, Philadelphia, pp 1–29

Zentler-Munro R L, Fine D R, Batten J C et al 1985 Effects of cimetidine on enzyme inactivation, bile acid precipitation and lipid solubilization in pancreatic steatorrhoea due to cystic fibrosis. Gut 26: 892–901

Zimakoff J, Hoiby N, Rosendal K et al 1983 Epidemiology of *Pseudomonas aeruginosa* infection and the role of contamination of the environment in a cystic fibrosis clinic. Journal of Hospital Infection. 4: 31–40

13

Occupational lung disease

A. J. Newman Taylor

The nature of the respiratory diseases caused by occupation is changing. Increasingly strict control of conditions at work has greatly reduced occupational exposure to mineral dusts and subsequently to the incidence of silicosis, coal-worker's pneumoconiosis and asbestosis. Although the conditions of the past continue to be the cause of new cases of these diseases, their numbers are falling and the risk of their developing in those now entering employment in the UK is small. Respiratory diseases caused by current conditions at work, such as asthma, chronic air flow limitation and lung cancer are less specifically related to occupation, their causes are widely distributed in industry and therefore they are often difficult to appreciate.

Estimation of the contribution of occupational causes to the burden of respiratory illness in the community is difficult. The number of cases compensated by the Department of Social Security is likely to be a considerable underestimate: not all occupational lung disease is compensatable and not all eligible cases apply for compensation. Since January 1989 respiratory and occupational physicians have voluntarily reported cases of newly diagnosed work related respiratory illness to SWORD (Surveillance of Work-Related and Occupational Respiratory Disease). During the first year, 1989, 2101 cases were notified, of which the most frequent diagnoses were asthma (26%), mesothelioma (16%), pneumoconiosis (15%), benign pleural disease (11%) and allergic alveolitis (6%). Asbestos exposure accounted for the majority of cases of pneumoconiosis (58%), lung cancer (65%) and mesothelioma (87%). Of 554 cases of occupational asthma, 282 (51%) were attributed to agents on the then prescribed list. Incidence rates calculated using denominators from the Labour Force Survey showed considerable differences between occupational groups, particularly for asthma and asbestos-related diseases. The incidence of occupational asthma in the general working population was estimated to be 22 per million, but in excess of 100 per million in several occupational groups which included spray painters, chemical process workers, bakers, laboratory technicians and solderers. Similarly, the incidence of asbestos-related diseases in the general working population was 22 per million but in excess of 100 per million among electricians and power plant operators and in building and construction, which included lagging, and in excess of 1000 per million in boiler operators and shipyard and dock workers (Meredith et al 1991). Occupational lung disease caused by a wide variety of agents in many different occupations clearly continues to make an important contribution to respiratory ill health.

In this review topics of current interest and continuing importance as well as those illuminated by the results of recent investigations have been selected. These fall into three major groups: (1) the respiratory effects of inorganic dusts (see Table 13.1); (2) the effects of metals; and (3) the allergic lung diseases.

RESPIRATORY EFFECTS OF INHALED INORGANIC DUSTS

Coal dust

Respirable coal dust retained in sufficient concentration in the lungs of coal-miners causes 'dust macules' which, superimposed, are visible on the chest radiograph as small rounded opacities scattered throughout both lungs ('simple' pneumoconiosis). The profusion of simple pneumoconiosis is related to the concentration of coal dust retained in the lungs. In some cases 'simple' pneumoconiosis becomes complicated by the development of large opacities — 'progressive massive fibrosis' (PMF). Whereas simple pneumoconiosis does not increase in profusion after avoidance of exposure, and does not appear to cause impairment of lung function or shorten life, PMF can progress (and may develop) after avoidance of exposure and is

Table 13.1 Respiratory effects of inorganic dusts

Inorganic dust	Respiratory effect
Coal	Simple pneumoconiosis Complicated by: Progressive massive fibrosis Mucus hypersecretion, emphysema and reduced FEV_1

Silica	Simple silicosis
	Complicated by:
	    Conglomerate silicosis
	    Pulmonary TB
	    Lung Cancer

Asbestos	Benign pleural disease:
	    Pleural plaques
	    Pleural effusions
	    Pleural thickening
	
	Asbestosis (interstitial fibrosis)
	Complicated by:
	    Lung cancer
	    Malignant mesothelioma

associated with both impairment of lung function and shortening of life (Cochrane 1976). The risk of developing PMF increases with increasing profusion of simple pneumoconiosis (Cochrane 1962).

Two different pathological patterns of PMF can be distinguished. In one the lesions are formed by conglomeration of smaller whorled nodules of collagen. These are very similar to the characteristic nodules of silicosis and seem likely to be a response to the silica present in coal dust. In the other, the lesions are large amorphous pigmented masses which contain fibronectin and little collagen and are caused by coal dust with little or no silica (Seaton 1989). Several hypotheses have been advanced to account for the development of these pigmented lesions, including an atypical response to tuberculosis or an autoimmune reaction. More recently Seal et al (1986) have suggested that the lesions may be caused by dust-laden activated macrophages which re-enter the lungs, after rupturing through the capsule of lymph nodes where they had accumulated following migration from the lungs.

The ability of coal dust to cause both simple and complicated pneumoconiosis is no longer questioned, although until Gough's observation of pneumoconiosis occurring in coal-trimmers exposed to quartz-free coal (Gough 1940) coal-worker's pneumoconiosis was generally believed to be wholly caused by the silica present in coal dust. More recently interest has focused on whether inhaled coal dust also causes disabling air flow limitation. This involves two separate but related questions: (1) does inhaled coal dust cause chronic bronchitis, emphysema or chronic air flow limitation; if so, (2) is this of sufficient severity to cause clinically important respiratory disability?

The first question has been examined in two ways: firstly, to determine whether there is an excess of respiratory symptoms, or functional and pathological abnormalities in coal-miners as compared to the population from which they came, and secondly, to examine for evidence of a gradient of effect in relation to exposure. For both questions the potential confounding effects of age and cigarette smoking need to be accounted for and the potential biases from self-selection into and out of the study populations need to be recognized. The results of several studies have now shown that coal dust inhaled during a working lifetime causes mucus hypersecretion (chronic bronchitis), reduced forced expiratory volume in 1 second (FEV_1) and emphysema. Cockroft et al (1982) found an excess of centri-acinar emphysema in the lungs of 39 coal-workers as compared with 48 non-coal-workers, after age and smoking history had been taken into account. The prevalence of emphysema in the miners' lungs was related to the amount of coal dust present in the lungs. To overcome the potential bias inherent in studying the lungs of miners, who would be more likely than non-miners with respiratory disease to have post-mortem examinations. The post-mortems were undertaken in men in South Wales who had died of an unrelated condition, ischaemic heart disease. Love & Miller (1982) found that the loss of FEV_1 measured in three consecutive cross-sectional surveys of 1677 coal-miners over 11 years was related to age, height and smoking, and to the measured cumulative respirable mine dust exposure. Cochrane (1982) criticized this study because the 1677 miners studied represented less than 30% of the original study population of 6191. In a subsequent study (Marine et al 1988) of 3380 of the 3995 coal-miners eligible for inclusion there was an association in both smokers and non-smokers between cumulative mine dust exposure and chronic bronchitis and the rate of decline in FEV_1.

Marine et al (1988) also examined the related question of whether the increased loss of FEV_1 in coal-miners caused clinically important disability. They estimated the proportions of their study population, both smokers and non-smokers, who would at age 47 years have an FEV_1 of less than 65% of predicted in three exposure groups — zero, intermediate and high. Their results, which showed a similar gradient of effect on FEV_1 in relation to cumulative dust exposure in smokers and non-smokers, suggested an additive effect of smoking with dust exposure. The estimated proportion whose FEV_1 at age 47 years was less than 65% was as shown in Table 13.2. The relative risk of a reduced FEV_1 in the high dust exposure group was similar in non-smokers (2.4) and smokers (2.8).

Table 13.2 Cumulative dust exposure

	Zero	Intermediate (on average between 3.1 and 3.7 mg/m for 35 years)	High (on average between 6.1 and 7.2 mg/m for 35 years)
Non-smokers	3.2%	5.5%	7.7%
Smokers	5%	8.5%	14.2%

Silica

The inhalation of respirable quartz causes nodular fibrosis of the lungs (silicosis), which produces small rounded opacities on the chest radiograph. Silicosis may be complicated by pulmonary tuberculosis and the fibrotic nodules may conglomerate to form the large lesions of PMF. Exposure to silica occurs in many different occupations, which include quarrying, mining, tunnelling, pottery work, stone masonry (using sandstone) and sandblasting, and continues to occur. Silicosis now often develops unexpectedly and may, at least initially, be unrecognized. The rate of progression of silicosis is dependent upon the intensity of silica exposure. Accelerated silicosis with rapid progression to PMF, silico-tuberculosis and, when exposure is particularly intense, silico-proteinosis, has been reported in sandstone tunnellers and in sandblasters, most recently in the Gulf of Mexico (Ziskind et al 1977). The hazards of sandblasting were cogently expressed in a notorious workshop notice: 'Join the Navy and see the world. Become a sandblaster and see the next.'

Current interest in silica is centred on its possible carcinogenicity. There is a clear excess of lung cancer deaths among compensated cases of silicosis, although in the most convincing study (Rivard et al 1989) the threefold excess of lung cancer was confined to smokers. An increased incidence of lung cancer has, however, not been consistently observed in populations occupationally exposed to silica dust. Hessel et al (1990) found no evidence for an association between silica exposure and lung cancer in a post-mortem case-referent study, and McDonald et al (1978) found no increase in lung cancer deaths in a cohort study of miners sufficiently exposed to silica dust to have suffered a marked excess of deaths from pneumoconiosis and silico-tuberculosis.

Asbestos

Asbestos is the name given to fibrous silicates of commercial value. They comprise two major groups: the wavy serpentine chrysotile (white) asbestos, and the straight amphiboles which include crocidolite (blue), amosite (brown) and tremolite asbestos. The biological effects of inhaled asbestos fibres have been widely reported and reviewed; probably no other cause of occupational disease has received so much attention. There is general agreement that occupational asbestos exposure can cause:

1. Benign pleural disease — pleural plaques, pleural effusions and pleural thickening which may cause respiratory impairment by compression of the underlying lungs
2. Interstitial fibrosis of the lungs (asbestosis) which causes impairment of lung function and shortens life
3. Lung cancer
4. Malignant mesothelioma.

Several studies have shown that the incidence of lung cancer increases with increasing asbestos exposure (McDonald et al 1986) and that asbestos and smoking interact to increase the risk of lung cancer (Berry et al 1985). The question of whether the increased risk of lung cancer is a complication of asbestosis or is an independent risk of asbestos exposure continues to be debated. A considerable excess of lung cancer definitely occurs among cases of asbestosis. In a study of compensated cases of asbestosis, Berry (1981) found that 39% died of lung cancer, a risk 9.1 greater than expected. Few studies have tried to separate the risk to those exposed to asbestos from those with asbestosis. Of those which have, Farebrother et al (1983) found no excess of asbestos exposure among cases of lung cancer as compared with their referents, and Hughes & Weill (1991) found the excess of lung cancer cases in a cohort of asbestos cement workers to be confined to men with pneumoconiosis (asbestosis). It would not be surprising if the increased risk of lung cancer was a complication of asbestosis, as the risk of lung cancer is markedly increased in cryptogenic fibrosing alveolities, a disease clinically, radiographically and pathologically very similar to asbestosis. In patients with cryptogenic fibrosing alveolitis, Turner-Warwick et al (1980) found a 14-fold increase in male and a 7-fold increase in female smokers dying of lung cancer as compared to the rate 'expected' for smokers of their age.

Mesothelioma is now the most feared consequence of asbestos exposure. It may follow exposure to asbestos for only a few months and is invariably fatal, causing death on average between one to two years from diagnosis. To date no form of treatment has been reported which improves survival. The initial description by Wagner et al (1960) drew attention to its association with crocidolite and to the risk of environmental (both vicinity and domestic) as well as occupational exposure. Subsequent studies have confirmed that amphiboles (crocidolite, amosite and tremolite) are associated with a markedly greater risk of mesothelioma than chrysotile, and mesothelioma in chrysotile workers may in fact be caused by tremolite which contaminates chrysotile deposits (McDonald et al 1989). Tremolite also contaminates vermiculite and talc deposits and is probably the cause of mesothelioma among miners of these minerals (McDonald et al 1986, Kleinfeld et al 1967). The carcinogenicity of amphiboles for mesothelial tissues seems primarily related to their physical characteristics and specifically to the durability and dimensions of the fibres retained in the lungs, long thin fibres (length greater than 8 μm, diameter less than 0.25 μm) being most carcinogenic. Amphiboles are extremely durable in biological tissue, and at equivalent inhaled doses some ten times more amphibole than chrysotile is retained in the lungs (Wagner et al 1974), probably because the wavy chrysotile fibres penetrates the lung less well and because they are more rapidly cleared than amphiboles. This selective retention of amphiboles has been observed in chrysotile miners; although the proportion of tremolite in asbestos dust in the chrysotile mines in Thetford, Quebec is only about 1%, some 80% of the fibres recovered at post-mortem from the lungs of these miners is tremolite (Sebastien et al 1989).

Consistent with the 'long thin' fibre hypothesis, malignant mesothelioma is endemic in some remote villages in Cappadocia where the population is environmentally exposed to a fibrous zeolite, erionite, one of a family of silicate minerals entirely different from either serpentine or amphibole asbestos. In one village, Karain, mesothelioma accounted for 44% of 55 deaths; in another, Tuzkoy, for 40% of 67 deaths (Baris et al 1979). These observations have caused concern regarding similar risks from man-made mineral fibres (MMMFs) of similar dimensions. The results of two large studies — one in Europe and the other in the USA (Doll 1987) — provided no evidence of an increased risk of mesothelioma. This is probably because MMMFs are less durable in the lungs than amphibole fibres; whereas asbestos breaks longitudinally into increasingly thin fibrils, MMMFs tend to break laterally into shorter fragments. However, workers who produced fibrous wool from rock or slag experienced a 30% increase in lung cancer 20 or more years after initial exposure. It remains unclear whether this excess is attributable to MMMFs or to other exposures experienced during their production, such as arsenic which contaminated the slag (Enterline 1990).

Industrial exposures to asbestos experienced during the first half of this century by those who subsequently developed asbestosis, lung cancer and mesothelioma were uncontrolled and often in excess of 100 fibres/ml. Increasingly strict and legally enforceable control limits have been introduced, and exposure to asbestos is now undertaken in the workplace under controlled conditions of less than 1 fibre/ml. Considerably lower fibre concentrations are present in the general environment and in buildings where asbestos products have been used. Whether such environmental exposure constitutes a risk to health has become an important social and practical issue. Current occupational exposure limits are intended to eliminate the risk of asbestosis and thereby also the risk of lung cancer. Similar confidence cannot be expressed about mesothelioma because of more limited knowledge regarding its exposure–response relationship. The risk of mesothelioma from occupational exposure is related to both intensity and duration of exposure (Newhouse et al 1985) and to fibre type (e.g. amphiboles). However, the description of vicinity, domestic and neighbourhood cases implies a risk at relatively low levels of exposure.

The incidence of mesothelioma during this century in countries where asbestos has been used, and is now present in the environment, could provide some insight into the importance of environmental asbestos exposure. Biologically significant exposure to asbestos in the general environment would be expected to increase the incidence of mesothelioma in both males and females from early adult life onward, and the progressive increase in asbestos use during the first half of the century should be reflected in increasing mesothelioma deaths in both sexes from about the middle of the century. Mesothelioma mortality rates in the USA, Canada and the UK are remarkably similar: until the early 1950s, annual mortality from mesothelioma was 1–2 per million in both men and women; subsequently there has been a consistent increase in mortality in males but not females from middle life (Jones & Thomas 1986), consistent with important occupational but not environmental asbestos exposure starting some 30–40 years previously.

THE RESPIRATORY EFFECTS OF INHALED METALS

Metals and their salts can cause a remarkable array of respiratory disorders (Table 13.3). Tin, barium and iron, inhaled as dust or fume, when retained in the lungs in sufficient concentration cause widespread nodular opacities

Table 13.3 Metals and the lung

Respiratory effect	Metal
Dust retention causing nodules on chest X-ray	Barium Tin Iron
Mixed dust fibrosis	Iron with silica
Lung cancer	Hexavalent chromium salts Nickel subsulphide Arsenic Haematite miners[a] Tin miners[a]
Giant cell interstitial pneumonitis and interstitial fibrosis ('hard metal disease')	Cobalt
Emphysema	Cadmium
Asthma	Complex platinum salts
Acute pulmonary oedema	Cadmium Beryllium Mercury Lead

[a] Probably due to ionizing radiation from radon daughters.

on the chest radiograph. Because they are not fibrogenic they do not appear to impair lung function or shorten life. Iron attenuates the fibrogenicity of inhaled silica so that haematite (iron ore) miners and iron foundry workers, who are exposed to both, develop a mixed dust fibrosis with a stellate rather than a nodular pattern of fibrosis. Occupational exposure to several metals has been associated with an excess of lung cancer: nickel subsulphide is the probable cause of nasal and lung cancers in nickel refinery workers, and hexavalent chromium salts of lung cancer in chromate production workers. The excess of lung cancer among haematite and tin miners is probably caused by ionizing radiation from radon daughters present in the mines.

Interstitial fibrosis of the lungs caused by exposure to hard metal has been recognized for many years, but only recently has its cause been identified and the characteristic nature of the pathological response in the lungs described. Davison et al (1983) reported three cases of so-called 'hard metal disease' which showed giant cell transformation, both of type 2 epithelial cells and of alveolar macrophages. This suggested that giant cell interstitial pneumonia (GIP) might be a characteristic pathological reaction to a constituent of hard metal, either tungsten carbide or cobalt. Subsequently, Demedts et al (1984) reported similar giant cell transformation in the lungs of diamond polishers with interstitial fibrosis. Cobalt is used as a binding agent for both polishing diamonds and hard metal, suggesting that it rather than tungsten carbide might be the cause of GIP and hard metal disease. Subsequent reports have now confirmed the association between hard metal and GIP. Davison et al (1983) also identified tungsten by electron microprobe analysis within giant cell macrophages recovered by bronchoalveolar lavage (BAL). This now allows the diagnosis of hard metal disease to be made from a lavage specimen.

Inhalation of cadmium fumes has been reported to cause acute pulmonary oedema, and inhaled or ingested cadmium can cause chronic renal tubular disease. The question of whether inhaled cadmium causes air flow limitation and emphysema, originally suggested in the 1950s, has until recently remained unclear. Parkes concluded in 1982 that there was little or no evidence to suggest that cadmium caused emphysema. However, Armstrong & Kazantzis (1983) reported an excess mortality from 'bronchitis' in those with 'ever high' exposure to cadmium, a category which included producers of copper–cadmium alloy who were exposed to cadmium fume. In a subsequent study of cadmium alloy producers, Davison et al (1988) reported a significant excess of radiographic and functional abnormalities consistent with emphysema. These were not accounted for by tobacco smoking or α_1-antitrypsin deficiency and showed a clear relationship with cumulative cadmium exposure and cadmium body burden, estimated by neutron activation analysis of cadmium in liver. Gas transfer coefficient (KCO) showed a linear decrease with increasing cumulative cadmium exposure with no evidence of a threshold. The results of these two studies taken together strongly suggest that cadmium exposure, at least in the concentrations experienced in the recent past, causes emphysema and, because of its effects on respiratory function, shortens life.

ALLERGIC REACTIONS TO AGENTS INHALED AT WORK

Allergic reactions of the lungs caused by agents inhaled at work cause two patterns of tissue response: asthma (and associated airway hyperresponsiveness), probably the expression of an eosinophilic bronchitis of the airways; and granulomatous inflammation of the peripheral gas-exchanging parts of the lungs caused by organic dusts — extrinsic allergic alveolitis (hypersensitivity pneumonitis) — and beryllium — beryllium disease.

In this group of diseases particularly, early case recognition and identification of the specific cause with avoidance of further exposure can prevent the progression to irreversible disease.

Occupational asthma

Occupational asthma is asthma initiated by an agent inhaled at work; the specific agent 'switches on' asthma and airway hyperresponsiveness. This occurs either as the result of direct damage to the airway epithelium by a reactive chemical inhaled in toxic concentrations — reactive airways dysfunction syndrome (RADS) (Brookes et al 1985) — or as the outcome of an acquired specific hypersensitivity response. In general, asthma caused by an inhaled toxic chemical such as chlorine follows an identifiable incident which is also the cause of respiratory symptoms in other exposed individuals. The effects are usually transient, resolving in weeks or months. In contrast, asthma induced by a specific hypersensitivity response is usually initiated by exposure concentrations which are not toxic and which do not cause reactions in the majority of others similarly exposed. Asthma, often of increasing severity, occurs while exposure to its cause at work continues; in many cases, particularly when caused by low-molecular-weight chemicals, asthma persists indefinitely despite subsequent avoidance of exposure. Some of the more important causes of occupational asthma are listed in Table 13.4

Incidence of occupational asthma

Asthma was the most frequent diagnosis (26%) in the 2101 cases reported to the SWORD scheme (Meredith et al 1991). Estimated incidence rates using denominators calculated from the Labour Force Survey showed considerable differences between occupational groups and between geographical regions. The high-risk occupations with their incidence are shown in Table 13.5 (after Meredith et al 1991). These groups experienced between 5 and 30 times the risk of occupational asthma in the general population (22 per million per annum). The regional variations were only partly explained by the regional distribution of high-risk occupations and were considered also to be due to differences in ascertainment and reporting. Meredith et al (1991) suggest that the true incidence of occupational asthma might be three times higher than that reported.

Table 13.4 Some causes of occupational asthma

	Proteins	Low-molecular-weight chemicals
Animal	Excreta of: rats, mice, etc.; locusts, grain mites	
Vegetable	Grain/flour Castor bean Green coffee bean Ispaghula	Plicatic acid (western red cedar) Colophony (pinewood resin)
Microbial	Harvest moulds *Bacillus subtilis* enzymes	Antibiotics, e.g. penicillins, cephalosporins
'Minerals'		Acid anhydrides Isocyanates Complex platinum salts Polyamines Reactive dyes

Table 13.5   Incidence of occupational asthma in high-risk occupations

Occupational group	Cases	Population	Rate/million/per year
Welders/solderers/electronic assemblers	35	220 068	159
Laboratory technicians and assistants	26	127 478	204
Metal-making and treating	14	56 270	249
Plastics-making and processing	27	66 005	409
Bakers	29	70 839	409
Chemical processors	31	73 189	424
Coach and spray painters	35	54 737	639
Other painters	21	201 225	104

Occupational asthma as a hypersensitivity response

Occupational asthma fulfils the criteria for a specific acquired hypersensitivity response:

1.   It occurs in a proportion, usually a minority, of those exposed to the specific agent. The risk of developing asthma in laboratory animal workers and isocyanate workers, for instance, is between 5% and 10%.

2.   Asthma only develops after an initial symptom-free period of exposure. This is usually several weeks or months, but can be years. The majority of cases of occupational asthma in laboratory animal workers, platinum refinery and isocyanate workers occur within the first 2 years of exposure. Subsequently the risk of developing asthma seems considerably reduced.

3.   Asthmatic reactions (both reduction in airway calibre and increase in non-specific airway responsiveness) are provoked by inhalation of the specific agent in atmospheric concentrations which were previously tolerable and which do not provoke airway responses in others similarly exposed. In toluene diisocyanate (TDI)-sensitive individuals, asthma may be provoked by atmospheric concentrations of 0.001 parts per million (p.p.m.) (about one five-hundredth of the concentration irritant to mucosal surfaces, 0.05 p.p.m.).

These characteristics have stimulated a search for evidence of a specific immunological response (in particular evidence of specific immunoglobulin E (IgE) to the agents responsible for occupational asthma. The presence of specific IgE antibody is usually inferred from the ability of a water-soluble extract of the responsible allergen or a hapten protein conjugate to provoke an immediate 'wheal and flare' reaction in the skin. Alternatively, specific IgE antibody can be directly identified in the serum by the radioallergosorbent test (RAST). Specific IgE has been demonstrated by one or other of these methods in patients with occupational asthma caused by proteins of animal, vegetable or microbial origin. These include secreta and excreta of laboratory animals, both small mammals (Newman Taylor et al 1977) and locusts (Tee et al 1988), wheat and rye flour (Bjorksten et al 1977) and the proteolytic enzyme alcalase derived from *Bacillus subtilis* (Pepys et al 1973). Specific IgE has also been identified in the serum of those with asthma caused by low-molecular-weight chemicals, phthalic (PA) (Maccia et al 1973), tetrachlorophthalic (TCPA) (Howe et al 1983) and trimellitic (TMA) (Zeiss et al 1977) anhydrides and several reactive dyes (Luczynska & Topping 1986). The determinants of allergenicity of low-molecular-weight organic chemicals was investigated by comparing the properties of two β-lactams: clavulanic acid, which is non-allergic, and a carbapenam MM22383, which is allergenic in experimental animals and can cause occupational asthma with specific IgE production in man (Edwards et al 1988). The characteristics relevant to the allergenicity of MM22383 were: (1) reactivity with body proteins (recognized originally by Landsteiner); (2) homogeneity with respect to the chemical hapten; and (3) stability of the conjugate formed.

The demonstration of a specific immunological response to an inhaled allergen is not itself sufficient evidence for an immunological mechanism of disease. Supportive evidence of a causal relationship is that, in exposed populations, the specific immunological response, such as specific IgE antibody, is associated with the tissue response (asthma), and does not simply reflect exposure to the causal allergen. This has been investigated in relatively few situations, but a clear relationship between specific IgE antibody and asthma has been demonstrated in populations exposed to laboratory animals (Venables et al 1988), to locusts (Tee et al 1988) and to the acid anhydride TCPA (Howe et al 1983).

For several of the low-molecular-weight chemicals which cause asthma, including isocyanates and colophony, either no evidence of a specific immunological response has been found, or if found no consistent relationship demonstrated between the immunological response and asthma. This may reflect the difficulties of working with highly reactive chemicals in in vitro systems, or the failure to prepare the relevant in vivo chemical hapten for the in vitro test. Reactants of the isocyanate water reaction, for instance, may be formed in the water-saturated respiratory tree and these, rather than the parent isocyanate, may bind to tissue proteins and be the immunogen.

Failure to find consistent evidence of a relationship between a specific immunological response and asthma caused by these agents has led to the suggestion that asthma may be caused by a pharmacological rather than an immunological mechanism. TDI inhibits the in vitro stimulation of lymphocyte adenyl cyclase by isoprenaline in a dose-related fashion (Davies et al 1977), possibly by covalent binding of the isocyanate group to the membrane receptor, and could hypothetically cause asthma by β-adrenoceptor inhibition in those with pre-existing airway hyperresponsiveness. This does not, however, explain the well-documented latent interval between initial exposure to TDI and the development of asthma, or the observation that in sensitized individuals inhalation of TDI induces an increase in non-specific airway responsiveness in those without pre-test airway hyperresponsiveness (Durham et al 1987). Furthermore, TDI fails to inhibit isoprenaline-induced tracheal smooth muscle relaxation (Mackay & Brooks 1983).

Outcome of occupational asthma

Respiratory symptoms and airway hyperresponsiveness continue for several years after avoidance of exposure in many cases of occupationally induced asthma. Malo et al (1988) studied 31 snowcrab workers up to 5 years from last exposure with occupational asthma, diagnosed by specific inhalation tests. All denied exposure to crabmeat by inhalation or ingestion during this period. All had continuing respiratory symptoms and 26 had measurable bronchial hyperresponsiveness. The FEV_1, FEV_1/FVC and PC20 improved during the initial period of follow-up, but the FEV_1 and FEV_1/FVC plateaued after one year and the PC20 after 2 years. Venables et al (1987) followed up 6 cases of TCPA-induced asthma 4 years after avoidance of exposure, and found that 5 had continuing respiratory symptoms consistent with airway hyperresponsiveness, and all 5 in whom it was assessed had measurable bronchial hyperresponsiveness. The rate of decline of specific IgE against a TCPA–human serum albumin conjugate after avoidance of exposure was exponential and parallel in all 6 subjects, with a half-life of one year. The half-life of specific IgE injected into normal persons is about 2.5 days, suggesting continuing specific IgE production in the absence of further antigenic exposure in these cases.

The continuing symptoms and airway hyperresponsiveness in these cases seem likely to be manifestations of chronic airway inflammation. Paggiaro et al (1990) investigated 10 patients with TDI-induced asthma who had continuing respiratory symptoms and airway hyperresponsiveness between 4 and 40 months from their last exposure. Bronchial mucosal biopsies obtained from 8 of the 10 showed basement membrane thickening and infiltration of the submucosa by eosinophils, lymphocytes and neutrophils. Four of the 5 patients in whom airway responsiveness had persisted unchanged had an increased eosinophil count in BAL fluid, whereas this was the case in only one of the 5 whose airway hyperresponsiveness had improved.

The only important determinant of continuing asthma so far identified is the duration of exposure to the initiating cause after the onset of respiratory symptoms. Chan Yeung (1987) found that 60% of 136 cases of occupational asthma caused by western red cedar (*Thuja plicata*) continued to have episodes of asthma at review on average 4 years from last contact with wood dust. The mean interval from onset of symptoms to diagnosis was 2¹/₂ years longer in those with continuing asthma than in those whose symptoms resolved.

Smoking, respiratory irritants and occupational asthma

Cigarette smoking has been associated with an increased rate of specific IgE antibody production and asthma in populations exposed in the workplace to airborne proteins and some low-molecular-weight chemicals. There is an increased risk of four to five fold of developing specific IgE (detected as an immediate 'weal and flare' skin test response or in serum by RAST) in smokers as compared with non-smokers in workers exposed to green coffee bean and ispaghula (Zetterstrom et al 1981), to the acid anhydride TCPA (Venables et al 1985) and in platinum refinery workers (Venables et al 1989). All seven cases of occupational asthma in the TCPA-exposed workforce were smokers (Howe et al 1983). The platinum refinery workers who smoked had a twofold increase in risk of developing respiratory symptoms — a level of risk similar to that observed in smokers processing snowcrabs (Cartier et al 1984). This 'adjuvant' effect of smoking in enhancing IgE production and asthma is probably local and non-specific.

Several studies in animals have found that inhaled respiratory irritants as well as inhaled tobacco smoke potentiate sensitization. Experimental smoking increases sensitization of rats who develop IgE to ovalbumin when inhaled but not when injected subcutaneously (Zetterstrom et al 1985). Concurrent inhalation of ozone enhanced sensitization (both IgE and airway responses) in cynomolgus monkeys to complex platinum salts (Biagini et al 1986), and concurrent inhalation of sulphur dioxide increased in a dose-dependent fashion the rate of sensitization of guinea-pigs who inhaled nebulized ovalbumin (Riedel et al 1988). Taken together these observations suggest that the risk of allergy and asthma caused by agents inhaled at work probably during the initial months of exposure to novel antigen is increased almost certainly by inhalation of tobacco smoke and also possibly by inhalation of other respiratory irritants such as ozone and sulphur dioxide which may be encountered at work.

Occupational lung diseases with granulomatous responses

Extrinsic allergic alveolitis

Extrinsic allergic alveolitis (hypersensitivity pneumonitis) is a T-cell-dependent granulomatous inflammatory condition response, caused by a variety of inhaled organic dusts, which predominantly involves the peripheral gas-exchanging parts of the lungs.

The list of causes of the disease is long, and continues to grow; some of the more important are listed in Table 13.6. In general these fall into two

Table 13.6 Some causes of extrinsic allergic alveolitis

Disease	Antigen source	Antigen
Farmer's lung	Mouldy hay, etc.	*Micropolyspora faeni*
Pigeon-financer's lung	Avian excreta and bloom	Avian serum proteins
Budgerigar-fancier's lung		
Bagassosis	Mouldy bagasse	*Thermoactinomyces sacchari*
Malt-worker's lung	Mouldy maltings	*Aspergillus clavatus*
Mushroom-worker's lung	Spores generated during mushroom spawning	Thermophilic actinomycetes
Maple bark stripper's lung	Removing bark from stored maple, sycamore etc	*Cryptostroma corticale*
'Ventilation pneumonitis'	Contaminated air-conditioning systems	Thermophilic actinomycetes

groups: (1) microbial spores which mould vegetable matter such as hay and barley, mushroom compost, bagasse and wood bark; (2) foreign animal proteins, such as pigeon and budgerigar serum proteins and bovine and porcine pituitary extract.

The colourful names given to many of these diseases reflect the varied occupational circumstances in which exposure to the particular organic dust occurs. It is important to appreciate that the different organic dusts provoke the same tissue response in the lungs.

Modern work practices have considerably reduced the risk of exposure to many of the classical spore-related causes of extrinsic allergic alveolitis. Malt-worker's lung is now confined to maltings where the traditional 'open floor' method is still used; the introduction of mechanical spawning has reduced the risk of the developing mushroom-worker's lung; bagassosis may be prevented by drying raw bagasse and spraying it with propionic acid to prevent moulding.

Farmer's lung and bird-fancier's lung, however, remain important causes of extrinsic allergic alveolitis. Changed conditions of work also create new hazards; air-conditioning systems with reservoirs of heated water allow circumstances in which thermophilic actinomycetes can grow and cause the inelegantly named 'ventilation pneumonitis'.

Beryllium disease

Beryllium inhaled acutely in high concentration usually causes acute pulmonary oedema. Beryllium and its salts may also cause chronic beryllium disease, which is in many important respects no different from sarcoidosis. Beryllium has been widely used and chronic beryllium disease has been reported in many occupations, which include those where exposure occurs to beryllium fume in beryllium–copper alloy manufacture and to beryllium oxide dust contaminating beryllium phosphors in the manufacture of fluorescent strip-lighting. The use of beryllium in industry in the UK is now subject to strict control and new cases of beryllium disease are uncommon, but beryllium disease remains a tantalizing model for sarcoidosis.

Extrinsic allergic alveolitis and beryllium disease as hypersensitivity granulomatous diseases

Inhaled organic dusts and beryllium salts stimulate a granulomatous inflammatory response in the lungs and, in the case of beryllium salts, in other organs of the body as well. Granulomas are focal accumulations of macrophages, and epithelioid and giant cells are derived from them. Local recruitment and activation of macrophages at disease sites is probably the outcome of a specific T-lymphocyte response to inhaled antigen and the formation of granulomas a reflection of antigen persistence in the lungs. Understanding of the immunopathogenesis has increased greatly since the advent of fibreoptic bronchoscopy and BAL. This technique has allowed the study of the cells, in particular lymphocytes, participating in these reactions.

Diseases characterized by widespread granuloma formation in the lungs, which include pulmonary tuberculosis and sarcoidosis as well as extrinsic allergic alveolitis and beryllium disease, have an increase in the proportion of lymphocytes among the cells recovered at BAL (Haslam 1984). About 90% of the cells recovered from normal individuals are macrophages, the remainder being small numbers of lymphocytes and neutrophils. In sarcoidosis and beryllium disease the proportion of lymphocytes is increased to about 50% of the total cell count and in extrinsic allergic alveolitis to 60–70% or more. In sarcoidosis and beryllium disease, the ratio of helper to suppressor (CD4 : CD8) T-lymphocytes is increased from a normal value of between 1.5 and 2:1 to 5:1 (Hunninghake & Crystal 1981). In extrinsic allergic alveolitis, suppressor (CD8) T-cells can form some 40% of the total lymphocytes recovered and the helper to suppressor ratio can be less than 1 (Leatherman et al 1984).

The specificity of T-lymphocytes recovered from blood at BAL has been investigated in patients with both extrinsic allergic alveolitis and beryllium disease. Schuyler et al (1978) reported that pigeon serum stimulated transformation of lymphocytes recovered from BAL, but not blood, from a pigeon fancier 5 days before and 10 weeks after the inhalation test with pigeon serum. In contrast, one week after the inhalation test, pigeon serum stimulated transformation of blood but not BAL lymphocytes. Specific T-lymphocytes responsive to pigeon serum seemed to be present in lungs but not blood yet following antigen exposure specific lymphocytes were found in blood but not BAL. Santini et al (1989) developed T-cell lines and clones obtained from peripheral blood and BAL from eight patients with beryllium disease. They found that the in vitro T-cell response to beryllium was confined to CD4 T-lymphocytes, was MHC Class 2 restricted and dependent upon functional IL2 receptors — characteristics consistent with beryllium disease being the outcome of a specific response to beryllium.

An increase in lymphocytes with helper to suppressor ratios similar to those found in farmers with allergic alveolitis has also been found in the cells recovered from BAL in asymptomatic farmers (Solal et al 1982). Thus, although the evidence would now suggest that the granulomatous inflammation of extrinsic allergic alveolitis is T-cell dependent (rather than, as was previously suggested, due to immune complex deposition in the lungs), asymptomatic farmers seem no different from those with disease with respect to the number, responsiveness and phenotype of T-lymphocytes recovered from BAL. Two different observations may help explain this paradox. It is possible that those who develop disease have a defect in antigen-specific suppressor T-lymphocyte function which allows inhaled allergen to provoke a T-lymphocyte-dependent inflammatory response. The translation of the specific immunological response into granulomatous inflammation is inhibited in the asymptomatic farmers by antigen-specific suppressor T-lymphocytes. The concept of allergic alveolitis as an inflammatory expression of impaired immunoregulation is supported by studies of the response in mice to granuloma-provoking stimuli such as BCG. 'High' responder strains develop antigen-specific suppressor T-lymphocytes able to reduce T-cell-dependent granulomatous inflammation. 'Low' responder strains, on the other hand, do not develop these suppressor T-lymphocytes and so develop granulomatous disease (Allen et al 1981). These antigen-specific suppressor T-cells are sensitive to cyclophosphamide, which can transiently convert 'high' into 'low' responders (Moore et al 1979). Thus a disease-free BCG-primed 'high' responder mouse develops granulomatous inflammation following cyclophosphamide therapy.

In addition to the increase in T-lymphocytes in BAL, patients with extrinsic allergic alveolitis have an increase in the number of mast cells (Haslam et al 1987). It has been suggested that the initiation of a delayed hypersensitivity response depends upon the release of vasoactive mediators from mast cells activated by antigen-specific T-cell-derived factors. It is possible, although as yet unproven, that an important difference between those with disease and those without is the ability to release cytokines from sensitized T-cells which are able to recruit mast cells and stimulate them to release vasoactive mediators initiating the local inflammatory response.

REFERENCES

Allen E M, Sternick J L, Schrier D J, Moore V L 1981 BCG induced chronic pulmonary inflammation and splenomegaly in mice: Suppression of PHA-induced proliferation, delayed hypersensitivity to sheep erythrocytes and chronic pulmonary inflammation by soluble factors from adherent spleen cells. Cellular Immunology 58: 61
Armstrong B G, Kazantzis G 1983 The mortality of cadmium workers. Lancet i: 1425–1427
Baris Y I, Artivinli M, Sakin A A 1979 Environmental mesothelioma in Turkey. Annals of the New York Academy of Sciences 330: 423
Berry G 1981 Mortality of workers certified by pneumoconiosis medical panels as having asbestosis. British Journal of Industrial Medicine 38: 130–137
Berry G, Newhouse M L, Antonis P 1985 Combined effect of asbestos and smoking on mortality from lung cancer and mesothelioma in factory workers. British Journal of Industrial Medicine 42: 12–18

Biagini R E, Moorman W J, Lewis T R, Bernstein I L 1986 Ozone enhancement of platinum asthma in a primate model. American Review of Respiratory Disease 134: 719–725

Bjorksten F, Backman A, Jarvinen A J, Savilahti E K, Syvanen P, Karkkainen T 1977 Immunoglobulin E specific to wheat and rye flour. Clinical Allergy 7: 473–483

Brookes S M, Weiss M A, Bernstein I L 1985 Reactive airways dysfunction syndrome (RADS) persistent asthma syndrome after high level irritant exposures. Chest 88: 376–384

Cartier A, Malo J-L, Forest F et al 1984 Occupational asthma in snow crab processing workers. Journal of Allergy and Clinical Immunology 74: 261–269

Cochrane A L 1962 The attack rate of progressive massive fibrosis. British Journal of Industrial Medicine 19: 52–64

Cochrane A L 1976 An epidemiologist's view of the relationship between simple pneumoconiosis and morbidity and mortality. Proceedings of the Royal Society of Medicine 69: 12–14

Cochrane A L 1983 (Letter). Thorax 877–878

Cockroft A, Seal R M E, Wagner J C, Lyons J P, Ryder R, Anderson N 1982 Post-mortem study of emphysema in coal workers and non-coal workers. Lancet i: 600–603

Davies R J, Butcher B T, O'Neil C E, Salvaggio J E 1977 The in vitro effect of toluene di-isocyanate on lymphocyte cyclic adenosine monophosphate production by isoproterenol, prostaglandin and histamine. Journal of Allergy and Clinical Immunology 60: 223–229

Davison A G, Haslam P L, Corrin B et al 1983 Interstitial lung disease and asthma in hard metal workers: Bronchoalveolar lavage, ultrastructural, and analytical findings and results of bronchial provocation tests. Thorax 38: 119–128

Davison A G, Fayers P M, Newman Taylor A J et al 1988 Cadmium fume inhalation. Lancet i: 663–667

Demedts M, Gheysens B, Nagels J et al 1984 Cobalt lung in diamond polishers. American Review of Respiratory Disease 130: 130–135

Doll R 1987 Symposium on MMF, Copenhagen, October 1986: Overview and conclusions. Annals of Occupational Hygiene 31: 805–819

Durham S R, Graneek B J, Hawkins R, Newman Taylor A J 1987 The temporal relationship between increases in airway responsiveness to histamine and late asthmatic responses induced by occupational agents. Journal of Allergy and Clinical Immunology 79: 398–406

Edwards R G, Dewdney J M, Dobrzanski R J, Lee D 1988 Immunogenicity and allergenicity studies on two beta-lactam structures, a clavam, clavulanic acid and a carbapenem: Structure–activity relationships. International Activities of Allergy and Applied Immunology 85: 184–189

Enterline P E 1990 Role of manmade mineral fibres in the causation of cancer. British Journal of Industrial Medicine 47: 145–146

Farebrother M J B, Heller R F, O'Brien I M, Azzopardi A, Telfer T P, Young M 1983 Occupation and lung cancer in a naval dockyard area. Thorax 38: 225(P)

Gough J 1940 Pneumoconiosis of coal trimmers. Journal of Pathology and Bacteriology 51: 277–285

Haslam P L 1984 Bronchoalveolar lavage. Seminars in Respiratory Medicine 6: 55–70

Haslam P L, Dewar A, Butchers P, Primett Z S, Newman Taylor A, Turner-Warwick M 1987 Mast cells, atypical lymphocytes and neutrophils in bronchoalveolar lavage in extrinsic allergic alveolitis. American Review of Respiratory Disease 135: 35–47

Hessel P A, Sluis-Cremer G K, Huizdo E 1990 Silica exposure, silicosis and lung cancer: A necropsy study. British Journal of Industrial Medicine 47: 4–9

Howe W, Venables K, Topping M et al (eds) 1983 Tetrachlorophthalic acid anhydride asthma: Evidence for specific IgE. Journal of Allergy and Clinical Immunology 71: 5–11

Hughes J, Weill H 1991 Asbestosis as a precursor of asbestos related lung cancer: Results of a prospective mortality study. British Journal of Industrial Medicine 48: 229–233

Hunninghake G W, Crystal R G 1981 Pulmonary sarcoidosis: A disorder mediated by excess helper T lymphocyte activity at sites of disease activity. New England Journal of Medicine 305: 429–434

Jones R, Thomas P 1986 Incidence of mesothelioma in Britain. Lancet i: 1275 and ii: 167

Kleinfeld M, Messite J, Koogman O, Zaki M H 1967 Mortality among talc miners and millers in New York State. Archives of Environmental Health 14: 663–667

Leatherman J W, Michael A F, Schwartz B A, Hordal J R 1984 Lung T cells in hypersensitivity pneumonitis. Annals of Internal Medicine 100: 390–392

Love R G, Miller B G 1982 Longitudinal study of lung function in coalminers. Thorax 37: 193–197

Luczynska C M, Topping M D 1986 Specific IgE antibodies to reactive dye-albumin conjugates. Journal of Immunological Methods

Maccia C A, Bernstein I L, Emmett E A, Brooks S M 1976 In vitro demonstration of specific IgE in phthalic anhydride sensitivity. American Review of Respiratory Disease 113: 701–704

MacKay R T, Brooks S M 1983 Effect of toluene di-isocyanate in beta adrenergic receptor function. American Review of Respiratory Disease 128: 50–53

Malo J L, Cartier A, Ghezzo J, Lafrance M, McCante M, Lehrer S B 1988 Patterns of improvement in spirometry, bronchial hyperresponsiveness and specific IgE antibody levels after cessation of exposure in occupational asthma caused by snow crab processing. American Review of Respiratory Disease 138: 807–812

Marine W M, Gurr D, Jacobsen M 1988 Clinically important respiratory effects of dust exposure and smoking in British coal miners. American Review of Respiratory Disease 137: 106–112

McDonald J C 1980 Asbestos and lung cancer: Has the case been proven. Chest 78: 374–376

McDonald J C, Gibbs G W, Liddell F D K, McDonald A D 1978 Mortality after long exposure to cummingtonite-grunerite. American Review of Respiratory Disease 118: 271–277

McDonald J C, McDonald A D, Armstrong B, Sebastien P 1986 Cohort study of vermiculite miners exposed to tremolite. British Journal of Industrial Medicine 436: 444

McDonald J C, Armstrong B, Case B et al 1989 Mesothelioma and asbestos fiber type: Evidence from lung tissue analysis. Cancer 63: 1544–1547

Meredith S K, Taylor V M, McDonald J C 1991 Occupational respiratory disease in the United Kingdom. British Journal of Industrial Medicine (in press)

Moore V L, Pederson G M, Mondloch V J, Schrier D J, Allen E M 1979 BCG induced chronic pulmonary inflammation in mice controlled by a cyclophosphamide-sensitive cell. Journal of the Reticuloendothelial Society 25: 50

Newhouse M L, Berry G, Wagner J C 1985 Mortality of factory workers in East London 1933–1980. British Journal of Industrial Medicine 42: 4–11

Newman Taylor A J, Longbottom J L, Pepys J 1977 Respiratory allergy to urine proteins of rats and mice. Lancet ii: 847–849

Paggiaro P, Bacci E, Paoletto P et al 1990 Bronchoalveolar lavage and morphology of the airways after cessation of exposure in asthmatic subjects sensitised to toluene diisocyanate. Chest 98: 536–542

Pepys J, Wells E D, D'Souza M, Greenburg M 1973 Clinical and immunological responses to enzymes of *Bacillus subtilus* in factory workers and consumers. Clinical Allergy 3: 143–160

Riedel F, Kramer M, Scheinbenbogen C, Rieger C H L 1988 Effects of SO_2 exposure on allergic sensitisation in the guinea pig. Journal of Allergy and Clinical Immunology 82: 527–534

Rward C I, Armstrong B, Petitclerc M, Cloutier L-G, Theriault G 1989 Lung Cancer mortality and silicosis in Quebec 1938–1985. Lancet i: 1504–1506

Santini C, Winestock K, Kirby M, Pinkston P, Crystal R G 1989 Maintenance of alveolitis in patients with chronic beryllium disease by beryllium specific helper T cells. New England Journal of Medicine 320: 1103–1109

Schuyler M R, Thypen T P, Salvaggio J E 1978 Local pulmonary immunity in pigeon breeders' disease. Annals of Internal Medicine 88: 355–357

Seal R M E, Cockroft A, Kung I, Wagner J C 1986 Central lymph node changes and progressive massive fibrosis in coalworkers. Thorax 41: 531–537

Sebastien P, McDonald J C, McDonald A D, Case B, Harley R A 1989 Respiratory cancer in chrysotile textile and mining industries: Exposure inferences from lung analysis. British Journal of Industrial Medicine 46: 180–187

Solal Celigny P, Laviolette M, Herbert J, Cormier Y 1982 Immune reactions in the lungs of asymptomatic dairy farmers. American Review of Respiratory Disease 126: 964–967

Tee R D, Gordon D J, Hawkins E R et al 1988 Occupational allergy to locusts: An investigation of the sources of the allergen. Journal of Allergy and Clinical Immunology 81: 517–525

Turner-Warwick M, Lebowitz M, Burrows B, Johnson A 1980 Cryptogenic fibrosing alveolitis and lung cancer. Thorax 35: 496-499

Venables K M, Topping M D, Nunn A J, Howe W, Newman Taylor A J 1987 Immunologic and functional consequences of chemical (tetrachlorophthalic anhydride) induced asthma after 4 years of avoidance of exposure. Journal of Allergy and Clinical Immunology 80: 212–218

Venables K M, Tee R D, Hawkins E R et al 1988 Laboratory animal allergy in a pharmaceutical company. British Journal of Industrial Medicine 45: 660–666

Venables K M, Dally M B, Nunn A J et al 1989 Smoking and occupational allergy in workers in a platinum refinery. British Medical Journal 299: 939–942

Wagner J C, Sleggs C A, Marchand P 1960 Diffuse pleural mesothelioma and asbestos exposure in the North Western Cape Province. British Journal of Industrial Medicine 17: 260–271

Wagner J C, Berry G, Skidmore J W, Timbreel U 1974 The effects of the inhalation of asbestos in rats. British Journal of Cancer 29: 252–269

Zeiss C R, Patterson R, Pruzansky J J, Miller M M, Rosenberg M, Levitz D 1977 Trimellitic anhydride induced airway syndromes. Journal of Allergy and Clinical Immunology 60: 96–103

Zetterstrom O, Osterman K, Machado L, Johansson S G O 1981 Another smoking hazard: Raised serum IgE concentrations and increased risk of occupational allergy. British Medical Journal 283: 1215–1217

Zetterstrom O, Nordvall S L, Bjorksten B, Ahlstedt S, Stelander M 1985 Increased IgE antibody responses in rats exposed to tobacco smoke. Journal of Allergy and Clinical Immunology 75: 594

Ziskind M, Jones R M, Weill H 1977 In: Murray J F (ed) Silicosis in lung disease: State of the art. American Lung Association, New York

MINI SYMPOSIUM:
Lung transplantation

14

Patient selection and preoperative work-up

P. A. Corris

By 1980 progress in organ transplantation had established kidney, liver and heart transplantation as successful treatments for selected patients with irreversible failure of these organs (Egan et al 1989). Progress with lung transplantation, however, lagged behind and Veith in 1983 noted that there had been 'no unmitigated long-term successes' among 38 reported attempts. Reasons for this early dismal experience can be explained not only by technical problems unique to lung transplantation (Dubois et al 1984) but also by problems due to poor recipient selection. Many early recipients were acutely ill, dependent upon ventilatory support, infected systemically and had multi-organ failure (Veith 1988). The successful establishment of lung transplantation as a viable therapeutic option during the 1980s started with heart–lung transplantation in 1982 (Reitz et al 1982), followed by single lung transplantation in 1983 (Toronto Lung Transplant Group 1986) and double lung transplantation in 1986 (Cooper et al 1988). Success reflected improvements in surgical technique, the introduction of cyclosporin (Borel et al 1986) and a more rigorous selection of recipients. All transplant centres now have intensive preoperative assessment programmes which apply stringent selection criteria to patients referred for consideration of lung transplantation. Such an approach is necessary to maintain success and to ensure that the best use is made of donor lungs, which remain a scarce resource due to the current marked shortfall compared to the number of potential recipients. This chapter discusses the general and specific criteria for selecting recipients, and describes the preoperative work-up of such individuals.

INDICATIONS AND GENERAL SELECTION CRITERIA FOR LUNG TRANSPLANTATION

The major indications for lung transplantation are pulmonary vascular disease, including primary pulmonary hypertension and Eisenmenger's syndrome and irreversible primary pulmonary disease (see Table 14.1). The large number of patients with pulmonary fibrosis in our series reflects our interest in single lung transplantation for this condition. The patients with emphysema are generally homozygous for α_1-antitrypsin deficiency.

251

252 RECENT ADVANCES IN RESPIRATORY MEDICINE

Table 14.1 Diagnosis of patients accepted for assessment for lung transplantation at Freeman Hospital, Newcastle

	Number	Mean age
Pulmonary fibrosis	46	40
Emphysema	31	44
Cystic fibrosis	21	23
Bronchiectasis	17	40
Pulmonary vascular disease	18	28
Miscellaneous	7	34

With the potential exception of alveolar cell carcinoma, patients with primary lung cancer are not suitable for consideration. Similarly patients with adult respiratory distress syndrome do not conform to requirements and are currently not considered (Dark & Corris 1989). The shortfall in suitable donor organs leads to an upper age limit of 50 years for transplantation of heart and lungs or both lungs alone, and an upper age limit of 60 years for transplantation of a single lung. The higher age limit for single lung reflects the increased availability of suitable single lungs and the less rigorous postoperative course such patients follow compared to those following heart–lung transplantation.

Transplantation is usually considered for a patient when estimated life expectancy is less than 18 months. As the majority of lung diseases lack features which permit accurate prediction of survival, estimates are based on the current lung function, the rate of decline over previous years and the date of onset of cor pulmonale. In contrast, the mixed venous oxygen saturation may be used as a predictor of survival in primary pulmonary hypertension as only 17% remain alive at 3 years from diagnosis if the saturation is less than 63% (Dinh Xuan et al 1990, Fuster et al 1984). The aim is to place a patient on the active waiting list when a balance has been achieved between a significant degree of functional deterioration and the increased probability of surviving transplantation when less ill. The degree of impairment of lung function in patients with primary lung disease accepted for transplantation varies. Lung function for patients with different lung diseases who have been accepted for transplantation in Newcastle are shown in Table 14.2.

In patients with cystic fibrosis or bronchiectasis, an increased number of hospital admissions for infective exacerbations or progressive weight loss is a further guide to deterioration which may predate an accelerated loss of lung function. The early unsuccessful transplant recipients were all bed-bound and the majority of transplant centres now require that recipients are capable of self-care and able to participate in gentle exercise rehabilitation to maintain muscle bulk and physical fitness.

Table 14.2 Lung function in patients accepted for transplantation in Newcastle (results for group expressed as mean)

		FEV$_1$	VC	TLCO[a]
		% predicted		
Pulmonary fibrosis	$n=38$	38	35	30
Emphysema	$n=25$	22	48	29
Cystic fibrosis	$n=16$	20	33	39
Bronchiectasis	$n=15$	23	39	47

[a]FEV$_1$, forced expiratory volume in 1 second; VC, vital capacity; TLCO, diffusing capacity

Many patients reaching the end-stage of chronic pulmonary disease suffer from cachexia and malnutrition (Hunter et al 1981). All recipients lose weight in the first week following transplantation and severe preoperative nutritional deficiency leads to an inability to withstand the rigours of the postoperative period, increased susceptibility to infection and poor wound healing. Obesity, on the other hand, increases surgical risk, predisposing to atelectasis and impairing postoperative mobility, which is essential following lung transplantation. Ideally recipients should be within 15 kg of ideal body weight. There is an increased mortality in adult patients whose body weight is less than 40 kg. As experience with adult lung transplantation has grown, this form of treatment has been offered with success to children with terminal respiratory failure and hence recipient selection has expanded now to include children.

SPECIFIC EXCLUSION CRITERIA FOR LUNG TRANSPLANTATION

Presence of systemic disease or other major organ dysfunction

The presence of uncontrolled systemic disease in addition to respiratory failure precludes consideration. Good renal and hepatic function are essential particularly in view of cyclosporin toxicity (Bennett & Pulliam 1983). A creatinine clearance of over 50 ml/min is required and only minor abnormalities of liver function are acceptable. This is of importance in patients with α_1-antitrypsin deficiency or cystic fibrosis who may have abnormalities of hepatic function as a result of their disease. Portal hypertension precludes consideration of transplantation of heart and lungs alone or lungs alone. In systemic diseases such as collagen vascular disease, when transplantation is being considered for the pulmonary disease the non-pulmonary features may preclude transplantation. Examples include lack of mobility due to destructive rheumatoid arthritis or evidence of nephritis complicating systemic lupus erythematosus. Type I diabetes mellitus, if well controlled, no longer rules out transplantation.

Infection

Localized sepsis preoperatively may lead to severe systemic infection postoperatively because of the need for immunosuppressive therapy. Extrapulmonary sepsis therefore mitigates against successful transplantation. Patients with recurrent or persistent pulmonary infection are not suitable for single lung transplants. Patients with cystic fibrosis or bronchiectasis require double lung or heart lung transplantation. Chronic bacterial sinusitis is very common in cystic fibrosis patients, yet current experience suggests that although there is potential for contamination of the lower respiratory tract complications appear no more common than in other patients (Scott et al 1988). Sinusitis alone does not therefore constitute a contraindication. Oral hygiene is important and all patients should have any dental sepsis eradicated preoperatively.

The presence of an aspergilloma is a contraindication to any form of lung transplant. Removal of the lung containing an aspergilloma is likely to result in seeding of the pleural space with *Aspergillus*, leading to fungal empyema. Removal of the contralateral lung for a single lung transplant leaves the aspergilloma in situ and subsequent immunosuppression will inevitably lead to disseminated *Aspergillus* infection.

Previous surgery

In contrast to single lung transplantation, heart–lung transplantation requires cardiopulmonary bypass with associated anticoagulation. There is a risk of life-threatening haemorrhage when the native lungs are removed if there are pleural scars or adhesions (Griffith et al 1987). There is clearly a gradation of risk from scarring left by previous open lung biopsy via a limited thoracotomy to previous total pleurectomy, and the latter is a general contraindication for heart–lung transplantation. This has important consequences for the management of pneumothorax in potential future recipients, in particular cystic fibrosis patients. If pleurodesis is required, surgeons should be advised to perform a limited anterior pleurodesis. The use of the antifibrinolytic aprotinin (Trasylol) during transplant surgery may reduce bleeding in such circumstances (Bidstrup et al 1989), and the recent development of bilateral lung transplantation via a transverse anterior incision allows the surgeon better access to the pleural space.

Systemic corticosteroids

Animal studies have shown that previous deaths resulting from tracheal or bronchial dehiscence were linked in part to preoperative use of systemic corticosteroids, which presumably interfered with healing (Goldberg et al 1983). Although early lung transplant programmes insisted on patients being weaned from corticosteroids, this proved very difficult to achieve in practice, particularly in patients with fibrotic lung disease. In view of this, in Newcastle we are prepared to accept patients for transplantation on up to 15 mg of prednisolone daily, providing there is no evidence of steroid-induced thinning of skin, osteoporosis or myopathy.

Cardiac disease

Patients under consideration for single lung transplantation or double lung transplantation ideally should have sufficient preservation of right ventricular function to sustain the recipient during single lung anaesthesia, obviating the need for cardiopulmonary bypass. It is imperative that ventricular function is preserved sufficiently to allow improvement after surgery. There are no studies which help to determine the level of right ventricular function which will predict outcome with regard to these points. The Toronto group have successfully performed a single lung transplant in a patient with a right ventricular ejection fraction of only 12%, although the mean right ventricular ejection fractions in a series of patients reported by this group were 31% and 38% for their single and double lung transplant candidates, respectively (Morrison et al 1990). Cardiac catheterization both before and up to 18 months following single lung transplantation for pulmonary fibrosis has shown that pulmonary vascular resistance, pulmonary artery pressure and right ventricular performance return to normal even when they are markedly abnormal preoperatively (Doig et al 1990). The presence of cor pulmonale is no longer a contraindication for single lung transplantation.

Psychosocial factors

There is no procedure in medicine which provides more stress for recipient and family than lung transplantation. The process begins from the time of initial referral and lasts until postoperative rehabilitation is complete. Any potential recipient must be well motivated, be able to cope and have demonstrated a willingness to comply. A supportive family or circle of close friends is essential. Underlying psychiatric illness, abuse of drugs or alcohol constitute contraindications. It is an absolute requirement for potential recipients to want a lung transplant.

FORMAL IN-PATIENT ASSESSMENT

Once a referral has been received, the preliminary data are reviewed by the transplant team and a decision is made whether or not to admit the patient to hospital for a full assessment. Initial screening data of value to transplant units are the height and weight, serial lung function tests, 6-minute walking distance, arterial blood gases, chest radiograph, creatinine clearance and liver function tests. A formal admission for assessment takes 5 days and enables specific investigations to be carried out and also sufficient time for members of the transplant team to discuss all aspects of transplantation with the patient and family. During these discussions members of the transplant team make a psychological assessment of the potential recipient, individuals with a high degree of confidence and self-motivation being best suited. The main investigations which are performed during the in-hospital evaluation are as follows:

1. Respiratory evaluation
   (a) Pulmonary function tests
   (b) Arterial blood gases breathing air
   (c) Quantitative ventilation–perfusion radionuclide scan
   (d) Symptom-limited progressive exercise test on bicycle ergometer (usually inspiring 50% oxygen)
   (e) Six-minute walk test with oximetry to measure desaturation
   (f) Computed tomographic scan of thorax
2. Cardiac evaluation
   (a) ECG
   (b) Two-dimensional echocardiogram with Doppler estimate of pulmonary artery pressure
   (c) Gaited nuclear angiogram
   (d) Cardiac catheterization with coronary angiography (for patients under assessment for single lung transplantation)
3. Microbiology
   (a) Cytomegalovirus, human immunodeficiency virus, hepatitis B, *Toxoplasma* serology and *Aspergillus* precipitins
   (b) Sputum for culture, including *Aspergillus*
   (c) Nose and throat swabs and Mid Stream Specimen of Urine for Culture (MSSU)
4. Haematology and biochemistry
   (a) Full blood count
   (b) ABO blood grouping
   (c) Lymphocyte cross-match
   (d) Clotting studies
   (e) Full biochemical profile, including creatinine clearance
5. Nutritional assessment
   (a) Creatinine height ratio
   (b) Albumin and total protein

CONCLUSION

The uniformly unsuccessful outcome of lung transplantation up to the early 1980s has been dramatically improved over the last decade (Hutter et al 1988), with a one-year actuarial survival of up to 74% (Scott et al 1988, Smyth et al 1989) now being reported. The improvement in success reflects more careful choice of suitable recipients as well as advances in surgical technique and immunosuppressive therapy. Careful selection is important not only to afford recipients the best chance of surviving the operation and living longer but also to allow an enhanced quality of life. Furthermore the shortfall in suitable donor organs also demands that this rare resource is given to those who are most likely to benefit.

REFERENCES

Bennett W M, Pulliam J P 1983 Cyclosporin nephrotoxicity. Annals of Internal Medicine 99: 851–854
Bidstrup B P, Royston D, Sapsford R N, Taylor K M 1989 Reduction in blood loss and blood use after cardiopulmonary bypass with high dose Aprotinin (Trasylol). Journal of Thoracic and Cardiovascular Surgery 97: 364–372
Borel J F, Feurer C, Gubler H B, Stahelin H 1976 Biological effects of cyclosprin A: A new antilymphocyte agent. Agents and Actions 6: 465–475
Cooper J D, Patterson G A, Grossman R, Maurer J 1988 Double lung transplant for advanced chronic obstructive lung disease. American Review of Respiratory Disease 139: 303–307
Dark J, Corris P A 1989 The current state of lung transplantation. Thorax 44: 689–692
Dinh Xuan A T, Higgenbottam T W, Scott J P, Wallwork J 1990 Primary pulmonary hypertension: Diagnosis, medical and surgical treatment. Respiratory Medicine 84: 189–197
Doig J C, Richens D, Corris P A et al 1990 Resolution of pulmonary hypertension after single lung transplantation. British Heart Journal 64: 72
Dubois P, Choiniere L, Cooper J D 1984 Bronchial omentopexy in canine lung allotransplantation. Annals of Thoracic Surgery 38: 211–214
Egan T, Kaiser L R, Cooper J D 1989 Lung transplantation. Current Problems in Surgery 26: 673–751
Fuster V, Steele P M, Edwards E D, Gersh B J, McGoon M D, Frye R L 1984 Primary pulmonary hypertension, national history and the importance of thrombosis. Circulation 70: 580–587
Goldberg M, Lima O, Morgan E et al 1983 A comparison between cyclosporin A and methylprednisolone plus azothiaprine on bronchial healing following canine lung allotransplantation. Journal of Thoracic and Cardiovascular Surgery 85: 821–826
Griffith B P, Hardisty R L, Trento A et al 1987 Heart lung transplantation: Lessons learned and future hopes. Annals of Thoracic Surgery 43: 6–16
Hunter A M B, Carey M A, Larsh H W, 1981 The nutritional status of patients with chronic obstructive pulmonary disease. American Review of Respiratory Disease 124: 376–381
Hutter J A, Despins P, Higgenbottam T et al 1988 Heart lung transplantation: Better use of resources. American Journal of Medicine 85: 4–11
Morrison D L, Maurer J R, Grossman P F 1990 Preoperative assessment for lung transplantation. Clinics in Chest Medicine 2: 207–215
Reitz B A, Wallwork J L, Hunt J A et al 1982 Heart lung transplantation: Successful therapy for patients with pulmonary vascular disease. New England Journal of Medicine 306: 557–564
Scott J, Higgenbottam T, Hutter J et al 1988 Heart lung transplantation for cystic fibrosis. Lancet ii: 192–194
Smyth R L, Higgenbottam T W, Scott J P, Wallwork J 1989 Transplantation of the lungs. Respiratory Medicine 83: 459–465
Toronto Lung Transplant Group 1986 Unilateral transplant for pulmonary fibrosis. New England Journal of Medicine 314: 1140–1145
Veith F J 1988 Lung transplantation in perspective. New England Journal of Medicine 314: 1186–1187
Veith F J, Kamhol S L, MollenKopf F P, Montefusco C M 1983 Lung Transplantation 35: 271–278

15

Technical aspects

J. H. Dark

Although it is more than 25 years since the first lung transplant, clinical success was only achieved in 1981 (Reitz et al 1981). That initial report was of a combined heart and lung transplant (HLT), but over the past decade two separate approaches have developed.

The en-bloc heart and lung transplant was first applied to patients with pulmonary vascular disease (either primary pulmonary hypertension or various forms of Eisenmenger's syndrome). Indications were subsequently widened to include various pulmonary conditions (Penketh et al 1987). Although survival rates were relatively good at some centres, many patients received a new heart unnecessarily, and it was then recognized that even replacement of both lungs was not required.

The alternative approach has been to transplant only lung tissue — if possible, just one lung. Success with single lung transplantation (SLT) for restrictive lung disease was first achieved by the Toronto group in 1983 (Cooper et al 1986). The technique was subsequently applied to obstructive lung disease, predominantly emphysema (Trulock et al 1989), and even to pulmonary hypertension (Fremes et al 1990). The philosophy of preserving the recipient's own heart lay behind the development of the double lung transplant (DLT) (Patterson et al 1988) and subsequently the 'bilateral' or 'sequential single' lung transplant for patients with septic lung disease.

The shortage of donor organs, particularly of heart–lung blocs, and particularly in North America, has accelerated the use of these more 'economical' lung transplants. The heart of the donor can always be used for a cardiac recipient in all of these procedures. Opinions still differ, but there is now some agreement about the indications for and the technical approaches to each particular procedure. There seems little doubt that in the future only a minority of pulmonary transplants will be of both heart and lungs.

THE SINGLE LUNG TRANSPLANT

General considerations: the importance of the other lung

At present, indications for the SLT fall into three groups: restrictive lung disease (predominantly fibrosing alveolitis), obstructive lung disease (principally emphysema) and pulmonary hypertension. The procedure is well established for the first two, but at a much more preliminary stage for pulmonary vascular disease. In all three, the outcome is significantly affected by the behaviour of the remaining, native, lung.

Specific considerations

Restrictive lung disease

It was realized at an early stage that pulmonary fibrosis is the ideal indication for the SLT. The transplanted lung is both preferentially ventilated, because it is more compliant, and perfused, because it has a lower pulmonary vascular resistance. Thus the native lung makes a very small contribution to gas exchange. However, all its defence mechanisms (e.g. ciliary function) are left intact, so it does not pose a septic threat to the transplant. Evidence of infection in the lung to be left behind is a relative contraindication to SLT. A particular problem in fibrosing alveolitis is *Aspergillus* infection. The combination of 'honeycombed' lungs, with cavities, and the steroid-induced immunosuppression used in treating these patients, may lead to the development of an aspergilloma. We would regard this as an absolute contraindication to lung transplant. Even if localized in the lung to be removed, the cavity would almost certainly be breached during surgery, and the resultant fungal contamination of the pleural space would prove unmanageable in the post-transplant immunosuppressed patient.

Obstructive lung disease

Historical reports of SLT in emphysema (Stevens et al 1970) suggested that the native lung would expand and compress the transplant lung. It is now known that this does not happen, although the native lung may continue to be ventilated, and pulmonary function, as assessed by spirometry, may be disappointing (Mal et al 1989). There will be mediastinal shift and elevation of the hemidiaphragm on the side of the transplant, because the donor lung will never fill the pleural cavity vacated by the overexpanded emphysematous lung.

Infection in the native lung is a particular problem in these patients, many of whom describe occasional production of purulent sputum. It is difficult to control in the immunosuppressed patient after transplant, and requires aggressive management, even amounting to contralateral pneumonectomy.

Air leaks, from either native or transplant lung, can also be a major postoperative problem in these patients. The size discrepancy between the transplanted lung and the hemithorax prevents sealing of parenchymal leaks, and pneumothoraces may persist for many days. The native lung, especially if it contains large bullae, may overexpand during anaesthesia, and go on to cause mediastinal shift that requires management as for a tension pneumothorax. The fragile surface may continue to leak post-transplant, and even necessitate pleurodesis on the native side.

Pulmonary vascular disease

This is at present a controversial indication for SLT. Although there are a number of unsolved problems and clinical experience is small, it will undoubtedly be an area of great activity in the future.

Success depends upon the premise that pulmonary artery pressure will become normal when faced with a normal vascular bed, even in a single lung. This is a reasonable assumption — pulmonary pressure is virtually normal after pneumonectomy if the remaining lung is normal; pulmonary pressure becomes normal after SLT for fibrosing alveolitis, when most of the blood is passing through one lung (Doig et al 1990).

For patients with pulmonary hypertension and a structurally normal heart, i.e. those with primary pulmonary hypertension or thromboembolic pulmonary hypertension, a question remains over the reversibility of their right ventricular failure. Clinical anecdote and some animal studies both suggest considerable scope for recovery, and it is clear that the limits of right ventricular dysfunction have not yet been explored.

The final group for whom SLT is being proposed are patients with Eisenmenger's syndrome due to an easily correctable cardiac defect. SLT and concomitant division of a patient ductus arteriosus has already been described (Fremes et al 1990). Patients with straightforward atrial or ventricular septal defects are suitable, as are the occasional individuals with worsening pulmonary hypertension after closure of an intracardiac shunt at a late age.

Surgical considerations

The need for cardiopulmonary bypass

Most patients with fibrosing alveolitis (Conacher et al 1990) and probably most with emphysema do not require cardiopulmonary bypass, although it should be available at short notice for all single lung transplants (and the femoral vessels should be accessible for cannulation). Intensive monitoring is essential, and despite aggressive ventilation of the remaining lung many patients are unstable, with an inexorable rise of arterial carbon dioxide tension ($PaCO_2$) prior to reperfusion of the transplanted lung. Recipients who are hypercapnic before surgery are those most likely to require supportive bypass during the period of one lung anaesthesia.

Choice of side

In general, we would avoid the side of previous surgery, and obviously aim to remove any unilateral focus of infection. If bypass is not required it is a little easier to transplant the left lung — the patient is likely to be more stable maintained on the slightly larger right lung, and the atrial anastomosis is easier on the left. On the other hand, cannulation for bypass is a good deal easier on the right. Preoperative isotope perfusion scanning will often help to predict the appropriate (i.e. the 'worst') lung to remove.

Correction of an intracardiac shunt is most easily performed through a median sternotomy, followed by implantation of the right lung on bypass.

The airway anastomosis

Bronchial dehiscence was an apparently insuperable problem before the modern era of lung transplantation. A major contribution by the Toronto group was to introduce the wrapping of the bronchial anastomosis in a pedicle of greater omentum (Lima et al 1982) to ensure anastomotic revascularization. Rigid avoidance of steroids both before and after surgery was also thought to be essential (Cooper et al 1986, Pearson 1989). With increased experience in bronchial anastomosis, it is no longer essential to use the omentum, which means that previous abdominal surgery is no longer a contraindication to single lung transplant. A further result of increased experience is that pre- and postoperative steroids are permissible at low dosages (e.g. 10–15 mg/day).

Contraindications to single lung transplant

In addition to the general requirements discussed in Chapter 14, a number of specific contraindications to SLT are shown in Table 15.1.

HEART AND LUNG TRANSPLANTATION

Almost any form of end-stage lung disease, with or without cardiac dysfunction, can be treated by the combined heart–lung transplant. When originally introduced, for the treatment of patients with pulmonary hypertension, it was the only successful lung transplant operation (Reitz et al 1981). In contrast to previous attempts (Veith et al 1983), anastomotic

Table 15.1 Contraindications to single lung transplantation

Pleurectomy on intended side

Absence of femoral pulses

Oral prednisolone > 15 mg/day or severe Cushingoid appearance

Coronary artery disease (> 2 vessels)

healing was consistently good. Inclusion of the heart with the lungs gave a systemic blood supply to the donor trachea via coronary to bronchial collaterals (Jamieson et al 1984). This technical advance coincided with the introduction of cyclosporin A, and with it the prospect of avoiding high-dose corticosteroids in the early postoperative period.

Mortality was initially high; in the first period of the Stanford series, only 65% of patients left hospital (McCarthy et al 1990). The technique was slow to expand. By 1988, only 200 procedures had been performed throughout the world, and over half of these had been in the UK.

Surgical considerations

The combined heart–lung transplant is a major procedure for both patient and operator. During extraction of the organs the phrenic nerves are at risk, as is the recurrent laryngeal nerve underneath the aortic arch. Vocal cord palsy is not infrequent, and should be managed by early injection of the vocal cord affected.

A major problem is bleeding; in early series as many as 30% of patients needed re-thoracotomy to deal with excessive blood loss. Adhesions between the chest wall and the lung, the result of previous surgery or lung sepsis, can be relatively difficult to control through a median sternotomy. Previous pleurectomy or decortication, extensive chest wall to pulmonary collaterals (as can occur in pulmonary atresia after any thoracotomy) and a grossly thickened pleura on plain X-ray are all contraindications to HLT (Griffith et al 1987).

Haemostasis in the posterior mediastinum must be perfect. Any bleeding points are completely inaccessible after the new organs are implanted. On the other hand, overzealous use of diathermy in the area in front of the oesophagus can result in vagal damage; gastric outlet obstruction and recurrent aspiration have both been described (Reid et al 1990).

There are various strategies to deal with particularly troublesome bleeding. If the adhesions are limited to one side, they can be divided at a separate thoracotomy before heparinization. Alternatively, there is some evidence that the antifibrinolytic drug aprotinin can reduce bleeding in this situation.

As has been mentioned, inclusion of the heart in the transplanted bloc usually ensures reliable tracheal healing. It was also hoped that monitoring of rejection of the transplanted bloc would be possible by the well-established technique of endomyocardial biopsy. This hope has not been realized, and isolated pulmonary rejection was recognized as early as 1985 (MacGregor et al 1985). Indeed, as the lung is almost invariably rejected first, routine cardiac biopsy has largely been abandoned after HLT. Despite this preferential rejection of the lung, chronic cardiac rejection, as manifest by accelerated coronary disease, also undoubtedly occurs.

As a true perspective of the importance (or otherwise) of the heart in the HLT was gained, and as it was realized that many HLT recipients with

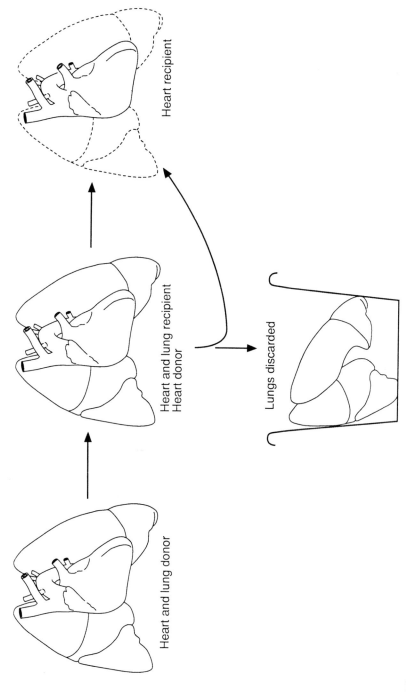

Fig. 15.1   The 'Domino' concept in heart-lung transplantation.

respiratory disease had good cardiac function, attempts were made to rationalize the procedure so as to avoid wasting valuable donor hearts. In North America, where the pressure on donor hearts was greatest, the double lung and subsequently the bilateral lung transplant were developed (see below). In the UK the favoured approach, until very recently, has been the 'Domino' concept.

The 'Domino' heart–lung transplant

The use of the heart of an HLT recipient was probably first performed by Yacoub et al (1990) (Fig. 15.1). The main technical difference is the need for separate caval anastomoses (as opposed to a single right atrial anastomosis in the standard operation) so as to preserve the whole of the right atrium for the cardiac recipient. The small increase in technical difficulty should not affect the operative risk for the HLT recipient.

Hearts made available by this technique possess a number of advantages. They are removed from stable, anaesthetized patients, often young, who will have had extensive preoperative cardiac investigations. If the cardiac transplant is performed at the same institution ischaemic time will be short and there will be cost savings on donor organ transport. Many HLT recipients who are 'domino donors' will have mild to moderate pulmonary hypertension and their hearts will function well in recipients with elevated pulmonary vascular resistance. Finally, since both recipient and donor are identified before the operation, some forms of simple immunological matching may be carried out.

There remain some unanswered questions: the ethics of investigating a patient, perhaps even by cardiac catheterization, and then increasing the difficulty of his operation, all for the benefit of another, merit debate. The usability of hearts with signs of right ventricular failure is unresolved.

DOUBLE AND 'BILATERAL' LUNG TRANSPLANTS

The en-bloc double lung transplant (DLT) was developed by the Toronto group once it was realized that cardiac biopsy was not a particular advantage to the patient after HLT, and that many 'respiratory' patients had adequate cardiac function (Fig. 15.2). Ischaemia of the airway, because of the absence of the coronary to bronchial collaterals important in the HLT, was the potential major disadvantage, but this was thought to be outweighed by the preservation of the patient's own innervated heart, and by some simplification of the operation. The basic operation had tracheal, left atrial and pulmonary arterial anastomoses (Dark et al 1986). Although satisfactory airway healing was demonstrated in the laboratory (Patterson et al 1986), tracheal dehiscence was to be a major clinical problem (Patterson et al 1990). In addition, the operation was if anything more complex than the HLT, and the extensive mediastinal dissection frequently led to denervation of the

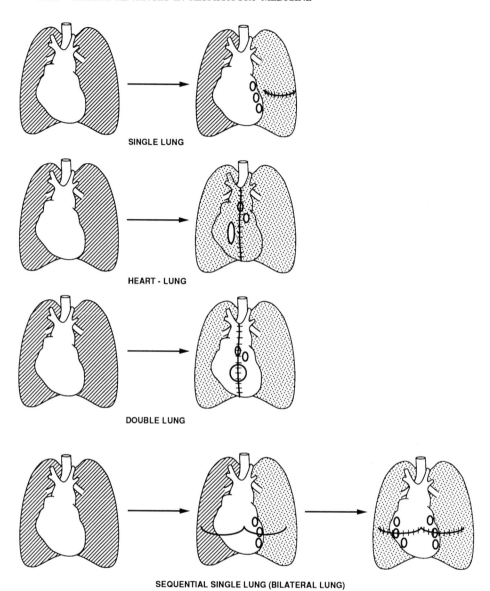

Fig. 15.2 Currently available pulmonary transplant operations. Heart–lung and double lung transplants are carried out through a median sternotomy. There is relatively poor access to the pleural spaces and the central position of the anastomoses requires extensive mediastinal dissection. The bilateral lung transplant with its hilar anastomoses leaves the mediastinum undisturbed. There is excellent access to all parts of the chest through the transverse thoracotomy.

recipient's heart (Schafers et al 1988). Bleeding was at least as great a problem as after HLT, and by 1989 the procedure as originally described had been largely abandoned.

Bilateral lung transplantation

Noirclerc et al (1990) provided a solution to the problem of airway healing by performing two separate bronchial anastomoses. As was shown in the SLT, the bronchus is better vascularized close to the lung parenchyma. The concept has been further developed by Pasque et al (1990) with the bilateral or sequential single lung transplant. As its name implies, two separated lungs are implanted with separate hilar anastomoses (each of bronchus, pulmonary artery and left atrial cuff). The heart and mediastinum are left largely undisturbed. The incision is a transverse bilateral thoracotomy, dividing the sternum horizontally. This gives superb exposure to any pleural adhesions. Bypass is often unnecessary and the lack of mediastinal dissection further reduces the chance of troublesome bleeding. The heart, of course, remains innervated.

On the other hand, the incision is undoubtedly much more painful than the standard median sternotomy and this is a major postoperative problem. With six anastomoses rather than three, it takes longer than an HLT, and there is an extended ischaemic time for the second lung. Experience is still very limited, but the bilateral lung transplant shows great promise. It is likely to become the treatment of choice for patients with adequate cardiac function who have bilateral lung sepsis, i.e. cystic fibrosis or bronchiectasis.

CONCLUSION: MATCHING THE PATIENT TO THE PROCEDURE

The SLT is simple, economical of donor organs, and is the least traumatic for the patient. Bilateral sepsis will remain the principal contraindication, but the SLT will become the most commonly performed pulmonary transplant. Combined HLT will probably be superseded by the bilateral approach for patients with infected lungs, principally the large group of young adults with cystic fibrosis.

There will remain a need for HLT for patients with uncorrectable congenital heart disease, and suitable organ blocs should still be made available for such patients. The current indications for the various procedures are set out in Table 15.2.

Table 15.2   Current indications for the various pulmonary transplants

Single lung transplant	Restrictive lung disease Emphysema Pulmonary hypertension (probably)
Bilateral lung transplant	Septic lung disease Cystic fibrosis, bronchiectasis Plus any of the above with recurrent infection
Heart–lung transplant	Uncorrectable congenital heart disease with pulmonary hypertension Any of the above with irreversible cardiac disease

REFERENCES

Conacher I D, Dark J H, Hilton C J, Corris P A 1990 Isolated lung transplantation for pulmonary fibrosis. Anaesthesia 45: 971–975

Cooper J D, Ginsberg R J, Goldsberg M, Toronto Lung Transplant Group 1986 Unilateral lung transplantation for pulmonary fibrosis. New England Journal of Medicine 314: 1140–1145

Dark J H, Patterson G A, Al Jilaihawi A W et al 1986 Experimental en-bloc double lung transplantation. Annals of Thoracic Surgery 42: 394–398

Doig C, Dark J H, Corris P A, Bexton R S 1990 Resolution of pulmonary hypertension after single lung transplantation. British Heart Journal 64: 72P

Fremes S E, Patterson G A, Williams W G et al 1990 Single lung transplantation and closure of patent ductus arteriovenous for Eisenmenger's syndrome. Journal of Thoracic and Cardiovascular Surgery 100: 1–5

Griffith B P, Hardisty R L, Trento A et al 1987 Heart lung transplantation: Lessons learned and future hopes. Annals of Thoracic Surgery 43: 6–16

Jamieson S, Bladwin J C, Stinson E et al 1984 Clinical heart–lung transplantation. Transplantation 37: 81–85

Lima O, Goldberg M, Peters W J et al 1982 Bronchial omentopexy in canine lung transplantation. Journal of Thoracic and Cardiovascular Surgery 83: 418–421

Mal H, Pariente R, Andreassin B 1989 Unilateral lung transplantation in severe panacinar emphysema. American Review of Respiratory Disease 139 (4, part 2): A268

McCarthy P M, Starnes V A, Theodore J et al 1990 Improved survival after heart lung transplantation. Journal of Thoracic and Cardiovascular Surgery 99: 54–60

McGregor C G A, Baldwin J C, Jamieson S W et al 1985 Isolated pulmonary rejection after combined heart lung transplantation. Journal of Thoracic and Cardiovascular Surgery 90: 623–626

Noirclerc M, Chazalette J P, Metras D, Camboulives J, Vaillant A, Dumon J F, Carcassomme M 1989 Lestransplantations bi-pulmonaire: rapport de la premiére observation français et commentaires des cinq suivantes. Annales chirugeri 43: 597–600

Pasque M K, Cooper J D, Kaiser L R et al 1990 Improved technique for bilateral lung transplantation: Rationale and initial clinical experience. Annals of Thoracic Surgery 49: 785–791

Patterson G A, Cooper J D, Dark J H et al 1988 Experimental and clinical double lung transplantation. Journal of Thoracic and Cardiovascular Surgery 95: 70–74

Patterson G A, Todd T R, Cooper J D et al 1990 Airway complications after double lung transplantation. Journal of Thoracic and Cardiovascular Surgery 99: 14–21

Pearson F G 1989 Lung transplantation. Archives of Surgery 124: 535–538

Penketh A, Higgenbotham T, Hakin M, Wallwork J 1987 Heart and lung transplantation in patients with end stage lung disease. British Medical Journal 295: 311–314

Reid K R, McKenzie F N, Menkis A H et al 1990 Importance of chronic aspiration in recipients of heart–lung transplants. Lancet 336: 206–208

Reitz B A, Wallwork J, Hunt S A et al 1981 Heart lung transplantation: Successful therapy for patients with pulmonary vascular disease. New England Journal of Medicine 306: 557–564

Schafers H J, Frost A E, Waxman M B et al 1988 Cardiac denervation following double lung transplantation. American Review of Respiratory Disease 137: 245 (Abstract)

Scott J, Higenbotham T, Hutter J et al 1988 Heart lung transplantation for cystic fibrosis. Lancet ii: 192–194

Stevens P M, Johnson P C, Bell R L, Beall A C et al 1970 Regional ventilation and perfusion after lung transplantation in patients with emphysema. New England Journal of Medicine 282: 245–249

Trulock E P, Egan T M, Kouchoukos N T et al 1989 Single lung transplantation for severe chronic obstructive lung disease. Chest 96: 738–742

Veith F J, Kanholz S L, Hallenkopf F P, Montefusco C M 1983 Lung transplantation. Transplantation 35: 271–278

Yacoub M H, Bonner N R, Khaghani A et al 1990 Heart lung transplantation for cystic fibrosis and subsequent domino heart transplantation. Journal of Heart Transplantation 9: 459–467

16

The donor for heart–lung transplantation

D. J. Aravot   J. Wallwork

Combined heart–lung transplantation (HLT) has become established for selected patients with end-stage pulmonary or cardiopulmonary disease (Aravot et al 1990, Hakim et al 1988). The success and expansion of a heart–lung transplant programme depends on an adequate supply of suitable organs (Haverich et al 1990), which in turn relies on successful procurement. Only a small proportion of organ donors are suitable for heart–lung donation. This is due to the delicate structure of the lung, making it more susceptible to trauma, neurogenic pulmonary oedema associated with brain death and the risk of infection from prolonged assisted ventilation. Initially, the lack of a satisfactory method for lung preservation necessitated moving the donor to the hospital of the recipient, with the attendant ethical and emotional problems further reducing donor availability (Haverich et al 1985).

It was not until methods of cardiopulmonary preservation were developed (Hardesty & Griffith 1985, Harjula et al 1988, Wallwork et al 1987), allowing successful distant organ procurement, that the supply of donor organs began to improve.

At Papworth Hospital we have developed a simple and inexpensive preservation technique that has enabled reliable distant procurement of organs for HLT with excellent postoperative graft function (Hakim et al 1988, Wallwork et al 1987).

Almost a hundred heart–lung transplants have been performed at Papworth during the last 6 years (Aravot et al 1990). In this chapter we describe our experience with donor selection and management, retrieval and preservation of organs and postimplantation graft function.

DONOR SELECTION

Selection criteria for donors for HLT are more strict than those for heart transplant alone. It has been estimated that less than 20% of potential heart donors are suitable for HLT (Jamieson et al 1984b). Most victims of road traffic accidents are unsuitable for lung donation. Deterioration of lung function may occur in potential donors who are brain dead as a result of accumulation of secretions, atelectasis, aspiration of gastric contents or pulmonary oedema. Pulmonary oedema can occasionally be neurogenic in origin, but it is more frequently the result of overinfusion of fluid, particularly crystalloid (Gosh et al 1990). Lung infections are common after prolonged periods of ventilation and 65% of the donors have tracheal aspirates that are culture positive for bacteria (Harjula et al 1987). Contusion of the heart and lungs is also a cause of impaired organ function in donors who have sustained trauma even in the absence of overt thoracic injury.

Finally, a close size match between donor and recipient is required.

To ensure satisfactory graft function, a potential donor should meet the following criteria:

Age: Less than 40 years for male and 45 years for female to reduce the risk of ischaemic heart disease.

Past medical history: The donor should be a non-smoker with no history of lung or heart disease.

Cardiac function: A brief period of cardiac arrest at the time of injury or during resuscitation is not a contraindication, providing a stable circulation is restored. This should, however, be without high-dose inotropic support, which impairs the performance of the heart after transplantation (English et al 1984).

Pulmonary function: Adequate gas exchange is essential. The arterial oxygen tension (PaO_2) should be greater than 100 mmHg (13 kPa) on 30% oxygen, and greater than 300 mmHg (40 kPa) on 100% oxygen. Lung compliance should exceed 0.1 litres/cmH_2O at a tidal volume of 10 ml/kg. Peak inspiratory pressure should not rise above 30 mmHg. The chest X-ray should be clear of major pulmonary collapse or post-traumatic opacifications.

Infective potential: Mechanical ventilation of more than a week in brain-dead subjects will usually preclude use of the lungs because of increased infection risk. Despite a normal chest X-ray most donors will have bacterial or fungal colonization. Specimens should be taken for Gram stain and cultures. Purulent sputum with positive Gram stain is a relative contraindication to donation. Because of the morbidity and mortality from donor-transmitted cytomegalovirus (CMV) infection, we have developed a rapid latex agglutination test to screen out CMV-positive donors who would infect CMV-negative recipients (Gray et al 1987).

MATCHING DONOR AND RECIPIENT

Donor and recipient are matched for ABO blood group. A direct cross-match is not performed unless testing of the recipient's blood against a random pool of lymphocytes shows cytolytic antibodies.

A close size match of thoracic cavities is mandatory for HLT. Transplanting a donor heart–lung block which is bigger than the recipient thoracic cavity can result in atelectasis and cardiac tamponade. Use of small donor organs can cause repeated pneumothoraces and empyema. The ideal is to select donor lungs that are smaller than the recipient's chest cavity by up to 10% (Bethune & Wheeldon 1990).

The size of the donor and recipient are matched according to the total lung capacity of the recipient measured at the time of assessment, and predicted values for the donor based largely on the height of the donor, together with comparison of chest X-rays.

PREOPERATIVE MANAGEMENT OF DONOR

Left-sided arterial and right-sided central venous lines should be inserted. The right subclavian artery and brachiocephalic vein are divided early in the donor operation so monitoring and access from right-sided arterial and left-sided venous cannulae is lost.

Hypotension is usually the result of vasodilatation and hypovolaemia, and rarely requires the use of inotropes. Donors may be on a dopamine infusion at doses necessary for support of renal function, the need for higher doses being avoided by judicious titration of fluids against central venous pressure. The preferred fluid replacement is with colloid and this should be either 20% human albumin or blood.

Prevention of deterioration in lung function can be achieved by regular physiotherapy with tracheal suction, the avoidance of overinfusion of crystalloid, and rigorous early treatment of pulmonary oedema. Pulmonary oedema, whether neurogenic or the result of fluid overload, can usually be treated with diuretics combined, if necessary, with positive end-expiratory pressure.

THE DONOR OPERATION

Attention to detail in the procurement procedure is vital if satisfactory organ function is to be achieved. In the case of the multi-organ donor (Odorm 1990), the kidneys and liver are mobilized first, but are not removed until the heart and lungs have been excised. This is accomplished through a median sternotomy. The thymic tissue is removed, both pleurae are opened and the lungs are mobilized completely, including division of both pulmonary ligaments. The pericardium is opened in the mid-line and the right side of the pericardium is excised back to the pulmonary veins. Division of the left brachiocephalic artery improves access to the trachea. The pulmonary trunk is mobilized from the ascending aorta. The superior and inferior venae cavae are mobilized and the azygos vein is ligated and divided. After systemic heparin (3 mg/kg) is administered, a small cannula (5 mm external diameter) is inserted into the pulmonary artery and a prostacyclin infusion (10–20 mg/kg per minute) is commenced. The infusion rate is titrated to a maximum to avoid significant hypotension and tachycardia. The trachea is encircled with a tape as high as possible without dissection of peritracheal tissue in the immediate supracarinal region. After ligation and division of the superior vena cava and just before the heart is arrested, the left side of the pericardium is excised back to the pulmonary veins. The inferior vena cava and the aorta are then cross-clamped and the heart arrested with St Thomas' Hospital cardioplegic solution (10 ml/kg), which is infused into the aortic root at 4°C. The inferior vena cava is then divided and the left side of the heart is decompressed by excision of the tip of the left atrial appendage. On completion of the cardioplegic infusion, the pulmonary artery is perfused with the cold flushing solution at 4°C (400 ml donor blood, 700 ml Ringer's solution, 200 ml salt-poor albumin, 100 ml 20% mannitol, 63 ml citrate–phosphate–dextrose and 10 000 units heparin). When the pulmonary artery flush (Fig. 16.1) is completed the aorta is

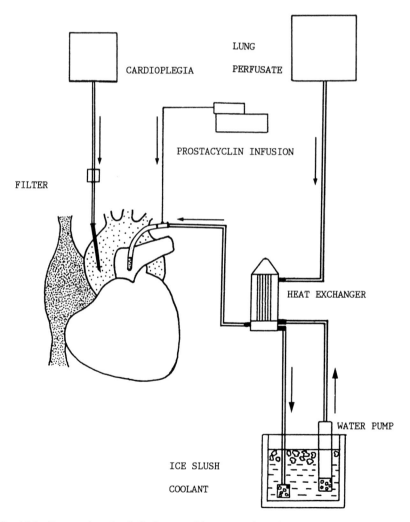

Fig. 16.1 Preservation circuit for heart and lung transplantation.

transected as far distally as possible. Extreme care is taken in dissecting the trachea with the surrounding tissues to preserve the collaterals that supply the bifurcation and the distal part of the trachea. Before the trachea is clamped and divided, the lungs are held partially inflated with room air above their functional residual capacity. This has been shown experimentally to enable lungs to tolerate longer periods of ischaemia (Veith et al 1971). Dissection in the posterior mediastinum then proceeds from above downwards, with initial separation of the posterior wall of the trachea from the oesophagus. The two pulmonary arteries are than dissected out, and the posterior pericardium is incised transversely to liberate both hilar regions. The trachea is then stapled below the clamp, and the organs are transported in an insulated box maintained at 4°C by using eutectic mixture (Wheeldon et al 1988).

METHODS OF HEART–LUNG PRESERVATION

Following the long-term survival of a patient who underwent combined HLT in 1981, the question arose as to how to preserve the integrity of the delicate structures of the lung to allow distant procurement. Following numerous animal experiments four main modalities of preservation are currently in clinical use.

Hypothermic flush perfusion with blood

As previously described, this is the method which we developed and now use (Bethune & Wheeldon 1990, Gosh et al 1990, Hakim et al 1988, Wallwork et al 1987). The donor is pretreated with prostacyclin, which is infused into the main pulmonary artery immediately prior to flush perfusion. The objective is to obtain maximal vasodilation of the pulmonary vasculature in order to achieve uniform distribution of the preservation solution. The rate of the infusion is titrated against the systemic blood pressure, which is not allowed to drop more than 20 mmHg. Prostacyclin also has a cytoprotective effect, inhibiting complement activation and platelet aggregation, thus preventing endothelial damage. Following the administration of prostacyclin the lungs are perfused by cold donor blood with the addition of anticoagulants, buffer and protein solution (Bethune & Wheeldon 1990, Hakim et al 1988). The high osmolarity of the flushing solution due to the addition of mannitol and albumin helps reduce interstitial oedema. Mannitol may also inhibit further complement activation. The presence of blood in the flushing solution increases buffering capacity and provides oxygen (Singh et al 1982). The flushing solution is infused into the pulmonary artery by gravity and the left atrium is vented through the auricle. This prevents any significant rise in pressure within the pulmonary vascular bed, which has been shown to lead to an increase in lung water (Gaan et al 1967). This approach is simple and yields excellent early lung function following ischaemic periods of up to 4 hours (Gray et al 1987, Wallwork et al 1987), thus enabling use of donors from all over Britain and Western Europe (Fig. 16.2).

Hypothermic flush perfusion with crystalloid solution

The modified Euro-Collins solution, which is a buffered solution with increased osmolarity compared to serum, is preferred by some centres (Haverich et al 1990, Locke et al 1988, Wahlers et al 1986). It is administered at a flow rate of 60 ml/kg body weight over 4 minutes. While the infusion is taking place, the heart and lungs are irrigated externally with cold (4°C) saline. Pretreatment with prostacyclin is also used. In terms of technical and instrument requirements, this approach is as simple to perform as our own. The next two methods to be described are more complex.

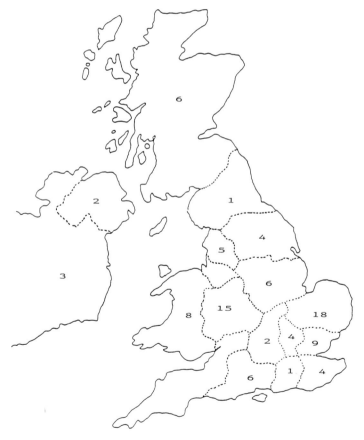

Fig. 16.2 The number of heart and lung donors harvested from the various health regions and transported for transplant at Cambridge ($n = 94$).

Cooling by means of extracorporeal circulation

This method was described in 1984 (Ladowski et al 1984) and is used by the Harefield group (Banner et al 1987), who have now performed more than 300 HLTs using this method. Cardiopulmonary bypass is used to cool the donor to 10°C with topical cooling of the lungs, prior to excision of the heart–lung block. The major disadvantage of this technique is the need to transport a heart–lung machine to the donor centre and the need for a perfusionist in the procurement team. Experiments in dogs (Wahlers et al 1986) have shown a reduced post-transplant capacity for oxygen exchange by lungs preserved by this method when compared to lungs preserved by flush perfusion with Euro-Collins solution.

Autoperfusion heart–lung preparation

Following extensive animal investigations (Ladowski et al 1985, Longmore et al 1969, Robincsek et al 1985), this method was used clinically by the Pittsburg group (Hardesty & Griffith 1987). The disadvantages of this technique were, firstly, hypostatic pulmonary oedema and functional impairment (Taft et al 1976), and secondly, increased risk of introducing infection during ventilation of the lungs during transplantation. For these reasons this method has been abandoned.

Though these last two methods appear to have yielded acceptable preservation in clinical use, they are rather cumbersome. Our method is simple, inexpensive and allows the lungs to be capable of providing immediate and almost normal oxygenation after implantation.

RESULTS

HLT has now been performed in 94 patients at Papworth Hospital. Sixty-four patients are alive between one and 73 months after surgery (Aravot et al 1990). Actuarial probability of survival was calculated at 77% at one year and 63% at 2 years (Fig. 16.3). A major cause of early death in our series was CMV infection due to mismatch between donor and recipient. This is now uncommon due to the rapid CMV screening test.

All but five surviving patients now enjoy an unrestricted lifestyle and most have returned to their previous occupation. One patient is undergoing advanced combat training in the army and another gained a gold medal in swimming at the World Transplant Games. Immediate function of the graft was satisfactory in all cases. Eighty per cent of patients were extubated within 8 hours post-transplant and were able to maintain a normal PaO_2, breathing air, within a week after surgery. Eighty-five per cent of recipients had a normal forced expiratory volume in 1 second (FEV_1) and forced vital capacity (FVC) at 6 months. The cardiac graft function was initially poor in 3 cases, one was probably due to subendocardial infarction prior to

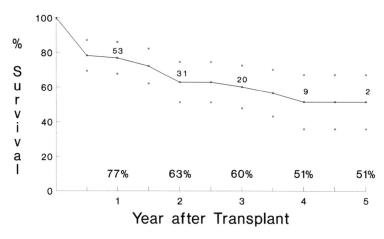

Fig. 16.3   Heart and lung transplant: actuarial survival at Papworth Hospital (n = 94).

excision from the donor, and in the others, to poor donor selection. In the Sixth Report of the International Registry (Heck et al 1989) actuarial survival based on 501 HLT was 60% at one year and 57% at 2 years. The Stanford group recently reported a survival of 70% at one year, and a one-year survival of 52% was reported by the Pittsburgh group (Griffith et al 1987).

CONCLUSION

Successful HLT programmes depend entirely on an adequate supply of suitable organs. Selection criteria for donors for HLT are more rigorous than for other organs in view of the greater tendency for the lung to become damaged and so unsuitable for transplant (Jamieson et al 1984a). Meticulous technique during the procurement operation is critical in this regard. A further problem has been organ preservation before engraftment to the recipient. This has now been largely circumvented as a result of the development of improved techniques of organ preservation, including our own technique of hypothermic flush perfusion, which is simple, inexpensive and yields excellent results.

ACKNOWLEDGEMENT

We wish to thank our colleagues P. Mullins, J. P. Scott, C. Dennis, L. Doolan, S. Kendall and D. Wheeldon for their help in preparing this chapter.

REFERENCES

Aravot D J, Scott J P, Mullins P et al 1990 Recent advances in heart–lung transplantation. In: Sokolic J, Soltic Z, Biocina B (eds) Organ Transplantation II. Medicenska Akademija Havatsche, Zagreb, pp 73–83

Banner N R, Fitzgerald M, Khaghani A et al 1987 Cardiac transplantation at Harefield Hospital. In: Terasaki P (ed) Clinical transplants 1987. UCLA Tissue Typing Laboratories, pp 17–26

Bethune D, Wheeldon D R 1990 Anesthetic management. In: Cooper DKC, Novitzky D (eds) The transplantation and replacement of thoracic organs. Kluwer, London, pp 283–287

English T A H, Spratt P, Wallwork J et al 1984 Selection and procurement of hearts for transplantation. British Medical Journal 288: 1889–1891

Gaan K A, Taylor A E, Owens L J, Guyton A C 1967 Pulmonary capillary pressure and filtration coefficient in the isolated perfused lung. American Journal of Physiology 213: 910–914

Gosh S, Bethune D W, Hardy I et al 1990 Management of donors for heart and heart–lung transplantation. Anaesthesia 45: 672–675

Gray J J, Alvey B, Smith D J, Wreghitt T G 1987 Evaluation of a commercial latex agglutination test for detecting antibodies to cytomegalovirus in organ donors and transplant recipients. Journal of Virological Methods 16: 13–20

Griffith B P, Hardesty R L, Trento A 1987 Heart–lung transplantation: Lessons learned and future hopes. Annals of Thoracic Surgery 43: 6–16

Hakim M, Higenbottam T, Bethune D et al 1988 Selection and procurement of combined heart and lung grafts for transplantation. Journal of Thoracic and Cardiovascular Surgery 95: 474–479

Hardesty R L, Griffith B P 1985 Procurement for combined heart–lung transplantation. Journal of Thoracic and Cardiovascular Surgery 89: 795–799

Hardesty R L, Griffith B P 1987 Autoperfusion of the heart and lungs for preservation during distant procurement. Journal of Thoracic and Cardiovascular Surgery 93: 11–17

Harjula A, Baldwin J C, Staines V A et al 1987 Proper donor selection for heart–lung transplantation. Journal of Thoracic and Cardiovascular Surgery 94: 874–880

Harjula A, Baldwin J C, Shumway N E 1988 Donor deep hypothermia or donor pre-treatment with prostaglandin E, and single pulmonary flush for heart–lung graft preservation: An experimental primate study. Annals of Thoracic Surgery 46: 553–555

Haverich A, Scott W C, Jamieson S W 1985 Twenty years of lung preservation: A review. Heart Transplantation 4: 234–240

Haverich A, Novitzky D, Cooper DKC 1990 Selection of the donor: Excision and storage of donor organs. In: Cooper D K C, Novitky D (eds) The transplantation and replacement of thoracic organs. Kluwer, London pp 273–282

Heck C F, Shumway S J, Kaye M P 1989 The Registry of the International Society for Heart Transplantation: Sixth Official Report 1989. Journal of Heart Transplantation 8: 271–276

Jamieson S W, Stinson E B, Oyer P E et al 1984a Operative techniques for heart–lung transplantation. Journal of Thoracic and Cardiovascular Surgery 87: 930–935

Jamieson S W, Baldwin J, Stinson E B et al 1984b Clinical heart–lung transplantation. Transplantation 37: 81–85

Ladowski J S, Hardesty R L, Griffith B P 1984 Protection of the heart–lung allograft during procurement: Cooling of the lungs with extracorporeal circulation or pulmonary artery flush. Heart Transplantation 3: 351–358

Ladowski J S, Kapelauski D P, Teodoric M D et al 1985 Use of autoperfusion for distant procurement of heart lung allografts. Journal of Heart Transplantation 4: 330–333

Locke T J, Hooper T L, Flecknell P A, McGregor C G A 1988 Preservation of the lung. Journal of Thoracic and Cardiovascular Surgery 96: 789–795

Longmore D B, Cooper D K C, Hall R W et al 1969 Transplantation of the heart and both lungs. II. Experimental cardiopulmonary transplantation. Thorax 24: 391–399

Odom N J 1990 Organ donation I. Management of the multi-organ donor. British Medical Journal 300: 1571–1573

Robincsek F, Masters T N, Duncan G D et al 1985 An autoperfused heart–lung preparation: Metabolism and function. Journal of Heart Transplantation 4: 334–339

Singh A K, Farivgia R, Teplitz C, Karlson K E 1982 Electrolytes versus blood cardioplegia: Randomized clinical and myocardial ultrastructural study. Annals of Thoracic Surgery 33: 218–227

Taft P M, Collins G M, Grotke G T, Halosz N A 1976 Warm ischaemic injury of the lung. Journal of Thoracic and Cardiovascular Surgery 72: 784–789

Veith F J, Sinha S B P, Graves J S et al 1971 Ischaemic tolerance of the lung: The effect of ventilation and inflation. Journal of Thoracic and Cardiovascular Surgery 61: 804–819

Wahlers T, Haverich A, Filguth H G et al 1986 Flush perfusion using Euro-Collins solution vs cooling by means of extracorporeal circulation in heart–lung preservation. Journal of Heart Transplantation 5: 89–98

Wallwork J, Jones K, Cavarocchi N et al 1987 Distant procurement of organs for clinical heart–lung transplantation using single flush technique. Transplantation 44: 654–658

Wheeldon D R, Wallwork J, Bethune D W, English T A H 1988 Storage and transport of heart and heart–lung donor organs with inflatable cushions and eutectoid cooling. Journal of Heart Transplantation 7: 265–272

17

Postoperative complications and follow-up

C. Dennis   T. W. Higenbottam

Until the 1980s, heart–lung transplantation (HLT) was experimentally and clinically unsuccessful. Failure was due to poor initial graft function, severe lung rejection, overwhelming infection, or dehiscence of the tracheal anastomosis. The introduction of cyclosporin, by allowing a reduction in perioperative corticosteroid therapy, may have improved healing of the airway anastomosis. Following the success of experimental studies in primates, the first clinically successful HLT in man was performed at Stanford in 1981 (Reitz et al 1982).

Surgical techniques have advanced rapidly, with concomitant reduction in postoperative mortality rates. In the last decade further advances have included the development of a highly effective and simple pulmonary artery flush technique for lung preservation (Jones et al 1986, Wallwork et al 1987; see also Chapter 16) and the early, precise histological diagnosis of rejection by transbronchial biopsies (Higenbottam et al 1987). These advances have led to impressive improvements in the postoperative mortality rates for HLT. In the best centres these are below 10% and the one-year survival from operation can be as high as 78% (Hutter et al 1989a). The principal causes of mortality remain, however, acute rejection and subsequent chronic rejection of the lungs, together with opportunistic pulmonary infections.

IMMUNOSUPPRESSION AND POSTOPERATIVE MANAGEMENT

Most patients are extubated less than 36 hours after surgery and then begin an active programme of mobilization. Fluid intake is restricted in the early postoperative period and a diuresis encouraged, to avoid accumulation of fluid in the lungs. Antibiotics are given prophylactically for 48 hours (flucloxacillin and a third-generation cephalosporin) and subsequently according to known sensitivity of pathogens. At present patients receive azathioprine, rabbit antihuman thymocyte globulin and methylprednisolone during the immediate postoperative period. Cyclosporin is gradually introduced in the early postoperative period and combined with azathioprine to provide maintenance immunosuppression (Table 17.1). Rejection episodes

Table 17.1 Immunosuppressive regime for HLT. Antithymocyte globulin (ATG) is given in the first three postoperative days according to lymphocyte levels

Perioperative	Maintenance
Cyclosporin 4–6 mg/kg	Cyclosporin 6–10 mg/kg per day
Azathioprine 2 mg/kg	Azathioprine adjusted to keep white blood cells > 5000/mm³
Methylprednisolone 1 g + 125 mg × 3	
Rabbit ATG for 3 days	

are treated with 3 days of i.v. methylprednisolone (1 g) followed by oral therapy (1 mg/kg), which is subsequently tapered by 5 mg/day.

ASSESSMENT OF GRAFT FUNCTION

In the first few postoperative days analysis of arterial blood gases and examination of the chest radiograph are used to monitor graft function. Thereafter chest radiographs are performed daily for approximately one week and lung function is monitored by daily spirometry and regular measurement of lung volumes and diffusing capacity.

CLINICAL DIAGNOSIS OF PULMONARY COMPLICATIONS

The principal problem in the management of HLT patients is that clinically it is impossible to separate opportunistic infection of the lungs from lung rejection. Both complications can present with respiratory symptoms of dyspnoea and chest tightness, together with cough. The physical signs are comparable on auscultation of the chest. There may be evidence of both crackles and wheezes (Higenbottam et al 1988). The chest radiograph is also unhelpful in this situation; bilateral pulmonary shadows are often seen in both infection and rejection. Additionally the chest radiograph may be entirely normal in patients experiencing acute rejection. This is particularly true after the first month following transplantation. After this time up to 70% of patients with acute rejection may have a clear chest radiograph (Millet et al 1989).

PULMONARY FUNCTION MONITORING

During most episodes of acute rejection and infection the dynamic lung volumes (forced expiratory volume in 1 second (FEV_1) and forced vital capacity (FVC)) diminish significantly. This change in function recovers with treatment. It is possible to measure these lung volumes, FEV_1 and FVC on each day with a pocket battery-operated spirometer. Changes as small as a 5% reduction on two consecutive days are sufficient to require the patient to attend for assessment and possible biopsy (Otulana et al 1990). Hence, unlike other solid organ transplants, the HLT patient can be monitored very closely and easily in terms of the physiological function of the graft. These patients can also undergo repeated biopsies of the lung if necessary.

DIAGNOSIS OF REJECTION

The diagnosis is considered on the basis of clinical symptoms and signs, chest radiograph changes and results of pulmonary function tests. Patients with breathlessness and fever, crackles or wheezes on auscultation have transbronchial lung biopsies. Further indications for biopsy are shadows on chest radiograph or a reduction in FEV_1 and FVC. The use of alligator forceps (Higenbottam et al 1987) enables specimens to be taken with sufficient tissue for histological assessment of vascular, parenchymal and mucosal change. Up to four biopsies are taken from any region where there is a radiographic abnormality, but more usually three biopsies are taken from each lobe even when the radiograph is normal.

The principal morphological changes found in acute rejection are circumscribed perivascular infiltrates. The infiltrate may extend into alveolar septa at later stages of rejection and indeed may cause alveolar infiltration. The presence of perivascular lymphocytic infiltrates is clearly distinguishable from the changes seen in opportunistic infection of the lung. With infection, perivascular oedema without densely cellular circumscribed adventitial infiltrations occurs. Intra-alveolar exudates are common, together with the pathognomonic features of the organism causing the infection. In our prospective study of 95 occasions when transbronchial biopsies were performed, in just under half was rejection found alone. Seventeen per cent were entirely normal and 8% showed infection alone. In just under one-quarter of the biopsies, both infection and rejection were found. Indeed, on three occasions two infections in addition to rejection were found. This illustrates the importance of systemically sampling each of the lobes in turn, as in one case infection was found in one lobe whilst rejection was found in another (Igboaka et al 1989).

OPPORTUNISTIC LUNG INFECTION

Sputum bacteriology and viral serological studies are performed regularly. Bronchial lavage is combined with transbronchial biopsy. Cytomegalovirus (CMV) infection is diagnosed by viral culture or by histological demonstration of viral inclusion bodies in the lung tissue. *Pneumocystis carinii* pneumonia is diagnosed by the demonstration of foamy exudate containing cysts on silver staining of tissue obtained by transbronchial biopsy. Herpes simplex virus (HSV) pneumonia may also occur and is usually diagnosed histologically. Both previous CMV infection and augmented immunosuppression are associated with the development of HSV pneumonia. Likewise, invasive aspergillosis of the lung has essentially developed in patients who have had pre-existing CMV infection. Close monitoring and repeated biopsy of patients has made it possible to reduce the number of fatalities due to infection. In our first 80 patients only 13 deaths were attributable to fatal infections. Three of these were due to bacterial pneumonia associated with donor lung infection and only one was due to *Aspergillus*.

CMV pneumonia has caused the death of four patients. Three of these were where donor and recipient were not matched for CMV. This meant that organs from a donor who was CMV positive were used in a recipient who was CMV negative. In our first 17 patients this occurred on 7 occasions and 6 of these developed primary CMV infection. Five infections occurred in the lung and one in the gastrointestinal tract (Hutter et al 1989b). Although effective treatment is now available for CMV pneumonia in the form of i.v. ganciclovir (Collaborative DHPG treatment study group 1986), it is our current policy to match all donors and recipients for CMV, so that no recipient who is CMV negative will receive organs from a donor who is serologically positive for CMV.

Following the institution of this policy there have been only two instances of primary CMV pneumonia, one of which was related to the use of CMV-infected blood. In addition there have been 11 cases of reactivation of CMV. All of these patients had sustained at least one episode of rejection requiring augmentation of immunosuppression prior to the development of the infection. We infer from this that an increase in immunosuppression is a major contributing cause to the reactivation of CMV (Hutter et al 1989b).

HSV pneumonia has occurred in seven of our patients. All seven patients had positive serology for HSV prior to transplantation or had developed mucocutaneous lesions prior to the development of pneumonia. As a result of these observations, patients who are HSV positive prior to transplantation now receive acyclovir for a period of 3 months following surgery. Furthermore, patients receiving augmentation of immunosuppression with corticosteroids for episodes of acute rejection are given prophylactic treatment with trimethoprim/sulphamethoxazole for *Pneumocystis carinii*. Selected patients who have sustained an episode of CMV infection are considered for prophylactic therapy with econazole for *Aspergillus*.

OBLITERATIVE BRONCHIOLITIS

This process can be defined as irreversible severe air flow obstruction as measured by lung function tests (FEV_1) where decline in lung function has not been prevented by recurrent use of augmented immunosuppression (Burke et al 1986; Fig. 17.1). The pathology of the condition is one of obliteration of the bronchioli which are left as fibrous bands extending out to the pleura, with associated dilatation and bronchiectasis of the proximal airways (Higenbottam et al 1987). This unusual pattern of distribution of fibrosis and dilatation indicates that the major impact of the disease process falls on the airways. The transplanted lung relies upon the pulmonary artery for intrapulmonary airway blood flow, which follows a retrograde course up the bronchial arteries (Sadeglu et al 1982). This is likely to be compromised during acute rejection since the rejection process principally affects blood vessels (venules and arteries) not only of the lung but also of the airways (Hutter et al 1989c).

Transbronchial biopsy specimens have revealed obliteration of the airways, but in addition submucosal fibrosis is seen in association with vascular sclerosis (Higenbottam et al 1987). Whilst these changes are found in obliterative bronchiolitis they are by no means diagnostic of the condition, which requires, as we have defined, irreversible air flow obstruction to be present clinically. Our observations clearly suggest that the development of obliterative bronchiolitis is closely related to the incidence and severity of rejection which occurs during the first 6–12 months following transplantation.

The strategy to overcome the problem has involved close monitoring of patients with lung function measurements via home spirometry and repeated transbronchial biopsy to establish the presence of rejection, its severity on histological grounds and to monitor the response to augmented immunosuppression. As a result, the incidence of obliterative bronchiolitis in our long-term survivors is currently 18%. This represents a considerable reduction from the initial figures of early experience, in which between 20% and 50% of patients developed this complication.

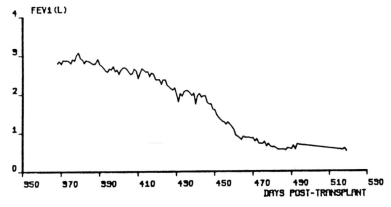

Fig. 17.1 A plot of home FEV_1 recording in a 35-year old male heart–lung transplant recipient who developed obliterative bronchiolitis diagnosed at open lung biopsy 15 months post-transplantation. A single lung transplantation had to be carried out at 20 months to arrest deteriorating lung function.

UNCOMMON PROBLEMS

Lymphoproliferative disorders

An association between immunosuppression and lymphoproliferative disorders is well recognized. The most common form appears to affect the B-cell lineage, resulting in B-cell non-Hodgkin's lymphomas. These are usually associated with the Epstein–Barr virus. The abnormal lymphatic tissue has been found within the lung parenchyma itself, in the mediastinal nodes and finally in peripheral lymph organs (tonsil). The condition usually responds firstly to a reduction in the level of immunosuppression and secondly to administration of acyclovir.

Graft-versus-host phenomena

The transplanted heart–lung block contains a significant amount of donor lymphoid tissue. This is situated within the pulmonary lymphatics themselves and also in the bronchial associated lymphoid tissue and the transplanted hilar nodes. In the early postoperative period observations have been made which suggest that a form of graft-versus-host disease can occur in HLT. This consists of skin rash, acute colitis, liver dysfunction and pancytopenia, usually in association with sepsis. We have observed chimerism (presence of donor lymphocytes in blood and bronchoalveolar lavage fluid) in association with the syndrome. This acute form may be particularly severe and prove to be fatal but usually responds to increased immunosuppression.

CONCLUSION

Heart–lung transplantation now offers an effective therapy for patients with end-stage pulmonary and pulmonary vascular disease. Opportunistic infection and graft rejection remain the major problems in the postoperative management of the transplant recipient. It is impossible to differentiate between infection and rejection on clinical grounds alone, and the use of the pocket spirometer to detect small asymptomatic falls in lung function, coupled with early transbronchial lung biopsy, have allowed rapid and sensitive diagnosis of rejection together with the ability to differentiate it from opportunistic infection. The incidence of opportunistic infection is closely related to the incidence of rejection and the repeated use of augmented immunosuppression treatment. Prophylactic therapy for the major opportunistic organisms may have a role in reducing morbidity and mortality due to such infections. Obliterative bronchiolitis remains the major long-term problem facing heart–lung transplantation and is associated with frequent episodes of acute lung rejection.

ACKNOWLEDGEMENT

We wish to thank our colleagues D. J. Aravot and J. Wallwork for their help in preparing this chapter.

REFERENCES

Burke C M, Theodor J, Baldwin J C 1986 Twenty-eight cases of human heart–lung transplantation. Lancet i: 517

Collaborative DHPG treatment study group 1986 Treatment of serious cytomegalovirus infections with 9-(1, 3-dihydroxy-2-proproxymethyl) guanine in patients with AIDS and other immuno deficiencies. New England Journal of Medicine 314: 801–805

Higenbottam T, Stewart S, Penketh A, Wallwork J 1987 The diagnosis of lung rejection and opportunistic infection by transbronchial biopsy. Transplantation Proceedings 19: 3777–3778

Higenbottam T, Stewart S, Penketh A, Wallwork J 1988 Transbronchial lung biopsy for diagnosis of rejection in heart–lung transplant patients. Transplantation 46: 532–539

Hutter J A, Scott J P, Despins P, Stewart S, Higenbottam T, Wallwork J 1989a Heart–lung transplantation at Papworth Hospital. European Journal of Cardiothoracic Surgery 3: 300–304

Hutter J, Stewart S, Higenbottam T, Scott J P, Wallwork J 1989b The importance of cytomegalovirus in heart–lung recipients. Chest 95: 627–631

Hutter J, Stewart S, Higenbottam T, Scott J, Wallwork J 1989c The characteristic histological changes associated with rejection in heart–lung recipients. Transplantation Proceedings 21: 435–436

Igboaka G U A, Higenbottam T W, Scott J P, Smyth R L, Wallwork J 1989 The distribution of lung rejection and infection in heart–lung transplantation. American Review of Respiratory Disease 139: A242

Jones D K, Cavarocchi N, Hakim M 1986 A single flush technique for successful distant organ procurement in heart–lung transplantation. Journal of Heart Transplantation 4: 614

Millet B, Higenbottam T, Flower C, Stewart S, Wallwork J 1989 The radiographic appearances of infection and acute rejection of the lung after heart–lung transplantation. American Review of Respiratory Disease 140: 62–67

Otulana B A, Higenbottam T, Ferrari L, Scott J, Igboaka G, Wallwork J 1990 The use of home spirometry in detecting acute lung rejection and infection following heart–lung transplantation. Chest 97: 353–357

Reitz B A, Wallwork J, Hunt S et al 1982 Heart–lung transplantation: Successful therapy for patients with pulmonary vascular disease. New England Journal of Medicine 306: 557–564

Sadeglu A M, Guthaner D F, Wexler L 1982 Healing and revascularization of the tracheal anastomosis following heart–lung transplantation. Surgical Forum 33: 236–238

Wallwork J, Jones D K, Cavarocchi N et al 1987 Distant procurement of organs for heart–lung transplantation using a single flush technique. Transplantation 44: 654–658

Index